A
WOMAN'S COMPLETE
GUIDE TO NATURAL HEALTH

ALSO BY ELLEN BROWN AND LYNNE WALKER

Nature's Pharmacy
Nature's Pharmacy for Kids (with Lendon Smith, M.D.)
Menopause and Estrogen: Natural Alternatives to Hormone Replacement Therapy
(formerly *Breezing Through the Change*)
The Informed Consumer's Pharmacy

ALSO BY ELLEN BROWN

Healing Joint Pain Naturally
The Key to Ultimate Health (with Richard Hansen, D.M.D.)
Forbidden Medicine
With the Grain: Eat More, Weigh Less, Live Longer

A WOMAN'S COMPLETE
GUIDE TO NATURAL HEALTH

LYNNE PAIGE WALKER, D.Pharm., D.Hom., L.Al.,

and ELLEN HODGSON BROWN

Avery
a member of
Penguin Group (USA) Inc.
New York

Most Avery books are available at special quantity discounts for bulk purchase for sales promotions, premiums, fund-raising, and educational needs. Special books or book excerpts also can be created to fit specific needs. For details, write Penguin Group (USA) Inc. Special Markets, 375 Hudson Street, New York, NY 10014.

a member of
Penguin Group (USA) Inc.
375 Hudson Street
New York, NY 10014
www.penguin.com

Published simultaneously in Canada

Library of Congress Cataloging-in-Publication Data

Walker, Lynne Paige.
A woman's complete guide to natural health / Lynne Paige Walker and Ellen Hodgson Brown.
    p.   cm.
Includes bibliographical references and index.
ISBN 1-58333-155-7
    1. Naturopathy.   2. Women—Diseases—Alternative treatment.   3. Women—Health and hygiene.
I. Brown, Ellen Hodgson.   II. Title.

RZ440.W297   2003   2002033041
615.5'35'082—dc21

Printed in the United States of America
10 9 8 7 6 5 4 3 2 1

Book design by Mauna Eichner

ACKNOWLEDGMENTS

The authors wish to acknowledge the many patients, friends, and relatives who have shared their beneficial results when they switched to a natural, body-supporting approach to their own and their children's ailments.

Special thanks to our agent and friend, Bob Silverstein of Quicksilver Books, for his invaluable aid and advice with this and other projects over the years, and to Ed Claflin and Ernie Tremblay for their editorial help.

CONTENTS

PART ONE

WOMEN'S HEALTH: KEEPING YOUR BALANCE IN A DEMANDING WORLD

PART TWO

AN A-TO-Z GUIDE TO COMMON WOMEN'S AILMENTS AND THEIR BEST TREATMENTS

INTRODUCTION

Women today are leading lives that are, in many ways, more stressful than our grandmothers' lives were. We make 130 million more annual doctor visits than men do—a fact largely attributable to our female hormones, which can keep us on a physical and emotional roller coaster. We have not only more but also different kinds of health complaints—complaints our mothers did not teach us how to deal with. To regain and maintain our health, we need more than a doctor's prescription. We need to understand what is going on in our bodies.

The conventional approach to disease is to chart symptoms and suppress them with drugs. Physicians are taught to diagnose the patient's disease from a list of symptoms, and then prescribe the appropriate drug for that disease. The problem with this approach is that symptoms are the body's response to imbalance and represent its efforts to cure itself. Coughing, sneezing, and diarrhea are obvious eliminatory processes; fever "cooks out" germs; high blood pressure is the body's attempt to keep the rate at which blood moves through the body constant when the arteries have become narrowed and constricted by toxins and cholesterol buildup. Stopping these processes thwarts what the body itself is trying to do. Putting the system right requires supporting rather than suppressing the body's natural functions.

From our perspective, the underlying imbalances in a range of women's diseases are precipitated by stress, an overloaded liver, and a lifetime of accumulated dietary and lifestyle abuses. Hormone levels can be thrown into imbalance not only by mental stress (from overwork, moving too fast or pushing too hard, worry, and negative emotions) but also by physical stressors, including toxic chemical overload, pesticides, overeating or eating the wrong kinds of food, and physical injury. Adrenal burnout from these stressors can cause irritability and an inability to sleep. Thyroid burnout can cause weight gain, tiredness, hair loss, and other symptoms.

Taking supplemental nutrients, hormones, and herbal and homeopathic remedies can help, but simply substituting specific herbs or nutrients for drugs won't necessarily cure the problem. Natural remedies need an uncongested lymphatic system and a well-functioning liver in order to work. The lymphatics move toxins through the body; the liver is responsible for detoxifying whatever is ingested or inhaled. Taking handfuls of nutritional supplements can actually increase the stress on an overloaded liver.

Correcting the problem at its source requires locating and relieving stresses, correcting the diet, and detoxifying the body of toxic chemical and heavy metal buildup. Liver cleansing and other detoxifying measures can help get the organs into operational shape so they can make productive use of natural remedies.

There is another important difference between "quick fix" drug treatments and the natural approach. While drugs may make you feel better in the short term but worse in the long term, homeopathic and other natural remedies may make you feel worse before you feel better. Years of taking antibiotics and other drugs suppress the immune system and the elimination of pathogenic and drug residues. These toxins then settle throughout the body. Homeopathic remedies and detox therapies "stir up" these toxins, and you reexperience them as they are moved out. However, the long-term result is greater health and well-being.

Part One of this book provides an overview of women's bodies, their hormones, and a variety of natural approaches designed to keep them in balance. Part Two catalogs more than 140 women's complaints and offers the safest and most effective treatment approaches. The text is illustrated throughout with actual case histories. Drawing from a number of treatment options—drugs, herbs, nutritional supplements, homeopathic remedies, Chinese patent medicines, flower essences, and essential oils—this book provides a broad and diverse approach to the treatment of women's illnesses, allowing you to choose the best, most appropriate, and safest therapies for your condition.

Dr. Lynne Walker is trained in both the conventional and alternative approaches to disease. Her first doctorate was in pharmacy; but after working for a number of years as a hospital pharmacist, she became aware of the limitations of pharmaceuticals. She went on to acquire doctorates in Chinese medicine and homeopathy. Her experience includes ten years as a hospital pharmacist; five years as pharmacist at the largest and busiest homeopathic pharmacy in the country, Capitol Drugs; fourteen years in private practice as a homeopath and acupuncturist; and ten years as proprietor of herb companies in Idaho, New York, and California. She currently lectures on speaking tours and is the proprietor of Vivid, a vibrational hypothecary in Malibu, California. As a result of this varied experience, she has seen the effects and side effects of drugs and the benefits of a broad range of natural remedies in virtually all of the ailments discussed in the following pages. She has coauthored four other books with Ellen Brown, including the best-selling *Nature's Pharmacy*.

Ellen Brown's expertise is in research and writing. She practiced for ten years as an attorney in Los Angeles before switching her focus to medical research. She has written nine books and numerous articles in the field of alternative health care.

Most of the products discussed in this book are readily available in health food stores, but if you have trouble finding them, they can be ordered from the website www.alternative pharmacy.com or by calling (800) 578-4104.

PART ONE

WOMEN'S HEALTH: KEEPING YOUR BALANCE IN A DEMANDING WORLD

WHAT MAKES WOMEN DIFFERENT: UNDERSTANDING HORMONES

There is no better time to be a woman. We have more choices and more opportunities than ever before. Birth control has freed us from the baby-a-year cycle that bound so many of our grandmothers. We have equality with men, at least potentially, not only at the polls but also in the workplace. While we're equal, we retain our differences: our female bodies have their own special health needs.

These needs stem largely from the fact that we are designed to bear children. We have ovaries, mammary glands, and moist internal areas with openings for the implantation of a fetus. Regulating this system are the female hormones, powerful substances that can wreak physical and emotional havoc when they go out of balance. The hormones and neurotransmitters regulating body functions—estrogen, progesterone, thyroid hormone, cortisol, adrenaline, melatonin, serotonin, norepinephrine, testosterone, and so on—are all interrelated. When one is thrown off, the others are too. When stress depletes the adrenals, the reproductive hormones also get depleted, since they are all drawing from the same well. The hormone edifice is a delicate one requiring special understanding and care.

THE HORMONE CASCADE

The steroid glands produce about thirty known hormones from the cholesterol distributed throughout the body. These hormones are of five types, as follows:

1. *Estrogens* (estrone, estradiol, and estriol) are primarily produced by the ovarian follicles. They maintain female secondary characteristics, such as a higher-pitched voice and breasts that are more developed than those of men.

2. *Androgens* (testosterone and androsterone) are typical products of the testes in males, but are produced in much smaller amounts by the ovaries and adrenal glands in women. These hormones maintain male secondary characteristics in men, and in women help to regulate sex drive, muscle mass, assertiveness, and mood.

3. *Gestagens* (for example, progesterone) are released by the ovaries' corpus luteum, the "yellow body" that remains after an egg is released. Gestagens support and maintain pregnancy.

4. *Glucocorticoids* (for example, cortisol and its precursor, cortisone) are products of the adrenal cortex. They transform proteins into glucose, causing blood sugar to rise. Cortisol is the adrenal hormone responsible for the "fight-or-flight" response.

5. *Mineralocorticoids* (for example, aldosterone) maintain mineral and water balance in the body.

The two major hormones produced by the ovaries are estrogen and progesterone. Estrogen builds up the endometrium (the lining of the uterus) in preparation for supporting a developing fetus. It does this by building endometrial cells into a thickened tissue. Progesterone is released after the ovary drops an egg into the fallopian tube, about two weeks into the monthly cycle. It prepares the lining of the uterus to nurture a fertilized egg. If the egg isn't fertilized, progesterone breaks down the thickened endometrial lining into layers for shedding.

Estrogen and progesterone have opposite metabolic effects and act to balance each other in the body, so we call progesterone estrogen's "antagonist." Estrogen causes salt and fluid retention, lowers blood sugar, and promotes blood clotting. Progesterone has the opposite effect in each case. Estrogen stimulates the manufacture of cells and the growth of tumors, while progesterone arrests their growth. Estrogen increases the risk of blockages in your arteries, fibroid tumors in your uterus, high blood pressure, fibrocystic breasts, and cancer of the breast and endometrium, while progesterone reduces these risks by holding estrogen in check.[1]

When progesterone is depleted, estrogen gets the upper hand. And progesterone can easily get depleted because it is used to make other hormones. When you are under stress, for example, your progesterone is converted to the stress hormone cortisol. The result is a hormone deficiency in your reproductive system. This deficiency is particularly troublesome during menopause, when hormone production is already rapidly declining. That may be why stress has been shown in laboratory studies to increase the frequency of hot flashes.[2]

Progesterone also enhances the action of the thyroid, which regulates energy levels, while estrogen impairs it.[3] Women taking estrogen supplements often complain of chronic fatigue or lack of energy, symptoms of an underactive thyroid. When thyroid tests are found to be normal, the symptoms are attributed to old age; however, if natural progesterone is given to these women, their symptoms often disappear.[4]

THE STRESS RESPONSE

Stress is a major culprit in unbalancing the hormone system. In moments of stress, animals (including humans) suspend nonessential functions like digestion and prepare either to fight or run away. This happens when adrenaline is secreted from the interior of the adrenal glands, which sit on top of the kidneys. Noradrenaline, secreted by the same glands, serves to increase blood pressure during emergencies. Other hormones are secreted by the adrenal cortex, a separate gland of the adrenals. Adrenaline, cortisol, and other steroids are "uppers," which cause cells to age and degenerate.

In preparation for fight or flight, the liver releases sugar into the blood. The liver, stomach, and intestinal wall also give up protein for energy. Calcium is drawn from the bones to support the muscles and nerves. Vitamin C, the B-complex vitamins, magnesium, sodium, potassium, and zinc wind up in short supply. Environmental chemicals add to this burden, depleting free-radical scavengers, including vitamin A, vitamin E, selenium, cysteine, and methionine. Unless these key nutrients are replaced by sufficient nutritional supplementation, the result is inflammation and degenerative disease.

The fight-or-flight response was a critical survival mechanism for our primitive ancestors, but it spells trouble for modern men and women. Modern humans under stress usually flee or attack only in their minds. We carry anger, fear, and anxiety around with us, often for years at a time, generating low but continuous levels of stress chemicals that impair the functioning of our bodies. Suppressed fear becomes worry; suppressed anger becomes irritability. Keeping fear or anger suppressed costs us even more energy, leaving us feeling tense and rigid. Psychic rigidity and tension—for example, fear of letting go, an inability to express emotion, and other subconscious tensions—cause a corresponding physical tension and endocrine imbalance. The rush of adrenaline, which is meant to propel the body around, merely gnaws at the organs and joints and degenerates them.

Cortisol has other functions besides activating the body for fight or flight. It helps to regulate blood sugar; the movement of carbohydrates, proteins, and fats in and out of the cells; inflammation; and muscle function. Chronically elevated levels of cortisol from chronic stress result in weight gain, blood sugar imbalances, thinning skin, muscle wasting, memory loss, high blood pressure, dizziness, hot flashes, and excessive facial hair and other masculinizing tendencies. Symptoms of overtaxed adrenals include chronic fatigue, irritability, inability to concentrate, frustration, insomnia, addictions to either sweet or salty foods, allergies, nervousness, depression, premenstrual syndrome (PMS), sensitivity to cold, diabetes, headaches, and chronic low blood pressure.[5]

Compounding the problem is the stress caused by the variety of roles women are expected to play in today's world. A woman is supposed to bear and raise children, hold down a job, clean the house, cook, and still have energy for sex and to dote on her man. Held-in resentments add to the havoc in her body. Small things can set her off—her husband looks at another woman or makes a comment that pushes her adrenaline buttons. She manages to cope until some last straw—an added physical or emotional trauma such as a death in the family, financial crisis, or auto injury—drives her over the edge. Add to this the stress caused by normal monthly fluctuations in her hormone levels and the result is often physical disease.

ADRENAL STRESS AND MENOPAUSE

Stress can always cause problems, but it can really wreak havoc at menopause, when hormone levels are already in decline. Nature seems to have intended menopause to be a gradual process, wherein the ovaries gradually reduce hormone output. The complex of glands to which the ovaries belong are all under the control of the pituitary, which sends signals to the adrenals to increase their hormone output as ovarian function falls off and hormone levels drop. What was lost from the ovaries is then partly replaced by these glands.

At least, that's how it's supposed to work. Chinese doctors say that the menstrual flow should stop without symptoms between the ages of 49 and 56 (the later the better, since menstruation is considered an internal cleansing process). Studies show that Japanese women rarely experience hot flashes and other menopausal complaints.[6] Mayan women, too, have virtually no menopausal symptoms.[7] Women in certain non-Western countries also manage to escape the degenerative diseases that plague older American women: osteoporosis, heart disease, and cancer.[8] How do they do it, and why can't we?

The blame, again, has been put on adrenal exhaustion, caused by stress, low blood sugar, and poor nutrition. Menopause is a time when the abuses of a lifetime of bad eating habits, insufficient exercise, exposure to environmental toxins, and psychological stress finally take their toll. Pharmaceutical hormone replacement therapy, the conventional answer, not only won't correct these problems but also adds a possible 120 side effects of its own.[9] Reversing the underlying problem requires rebuilding the reserves of the adrenals, which entails dietary and lifestyle changes and natural therapies that help balance hormone levels and reduce stress.

PREMENSTRUAL SYNDROME: WHEN HORMONES START TO FAIL

The same adrenal stress that causes more severe menopausal symptoms among Western women helps explain the greater prevalence of premenstrual syndrome (PMS) today than when our mothers were young. Premenstrual syndrome is a complex of symptoms that can include headaches, abdominal bloating, breast swelling, fluid retention, and mood swings, beginning about seven to ten days before a woman starts her period. The condition normally begins sometime during a woman's thirties, when hormone production begins to slow down. PMS is now thought to plague from 25 to 90 percent of all women, depending on how it is defined.

As with menopause, PMS symptoms result from a hormone imbalance, and they are compounded by stress. During the normal menstrual cycle, immediately after ovulation, levels of both estrogen and progesterone rise, and they continue to rise until menstruation. The progesterone acts as an estrogen antagonist, keeping estrogen levels from going too high. But progesterone stores can be depleted by stress—physical, emotional, dietary, or environmental—and stress causes progesterone to be converted to cortisol. Without enough progesterone, estrogen levels get too high. Excess estrogen can then produce the symptoms associated with PMS, including salt and fluid retention, low blood sugar, blood clotting, breast tenderness, thyroid problems, and weight gain. These physical imbalances then produce the mood swings and other psychological effects that are associated with PMS.

Typically, a woman with PMS also has congestion in her liver, the organ assigned the task of breaking down hormones and other metabolic waste products as well as any other toxins that find their way into her body. Environmental stressors, such as the formaldehyde in new carpets and fabrics and the chemicals in food additives and drugs, add to the load on the liver. In the days preceding menstruation, this burden is made even worse by an onslaught of hormones.

When the liver becomes overloaded, a woman may feel angry, irritable, sluggish, and depressed. She may yell at the kids; she may yell at the supermarket checker. She may feel "on edge" and ready to explode, but she doesn't know why she is behaving this way. In fact, it's because her liver is seriously overworked.

DIGESTIVE STRESSORS

The liver's burden is increased if the foodstuffs reaching it are insufficiently digested. Many health problems begin with poor assimilation and elimination of foods. Inadequate digestion, in turn, can result from an insufficient volume of digestive enzymes. Enzymes are destroyed by poisonous pesticides and chemicals, genetic engineering, food irradiation, hydrogenated oils, microwaves, radiation, fluoridation, heavy metals, and mercury amalgam dental fillings. Enzyme deficiencies can lead to food intolerances and allergies, a compromised immune system, chronic infections, fluid retention, chronic constipation, hypoglycemia, moodiness, depression, irritability, anxiety, impaired bone metabolism and osteoporosis, blood clots, diabetes, high cholesterol, high blood pressure, and varicose veins.

Besides insufficient digestive enzymes, digestive ills can be caused by an overgrowth of *Candida albicans,* a ubiquitous yeast that can wreak havoc on the immune system. Thought to affect as many as one in three American women, this toxic yeast overgrowth, known as candidiasis, is caused by eating excess sugar and by using antibiotics, birth control pills, cortisone, and estrogen therapy. Not only can excess sugar consumption cause candidiasis, but *Candida* can cause a craving for sugar. Because this yeast wants sugar, you will too. Parasite infection can make the condition worse by suppressing the immune system, encouraging *Candida* overgrowth. Symptoms of candidiasis include depression, anxiety attacks, mood swings, lack of concentration, drowsiness, poor memory, headaches, insomnia, fatigue, bloating, constipation, bladder infections, menstrual cramps, vaginal itching, muscle and joint swelling, pain, hypothyroidism, and skin problems.[10]

2

HORMONE REPLACEMENT THERAPY: PROS, CONS, AND ALTERNATIVES

The pharmaceutical industry's response to the loss of female hormones at menopause is supplemental hormones. They either extract the hormones from animals or make them in the laboratory. But pharmaceutical hormone replacement therapy (HRT) is an imperfect solution. Drugs cannot duplicate the body's own hormones—not because it cannot be done, but because substances found naturally in plants or animals cannot be patented. As a result, natural substances cannot generate sufficient profits to underwrite the FDA-approval process, which now costs in excess of $100 million for a single drug or device. (Contrary to popular belief, the FDA does not pay for this process. Drug companies pay for it, although the government sometimes subsidizes the development of new medications.)

The result is that more expensive, less natural products with more potential for side effects wind up obtaining FDA approval. Meanwhile, cheaper and more effective natural products that duplicate the body's own hormones go unheralded and unnoticed.

THE HORMONE THERAPY CRAZE

The first and still the leading pharmaceutical estrogen was Ayerst's Premarin, introduced in 1942. Premarin is an estrogen extract synthesized from the urine of pregnant mares, from which it took its name. When it first came on the market, Premarin seemed to be a wonder drug for many women. It eliminated their hot flashes and revived their lost interest in sex. Moreover, estrogen replacement therapy was linked to a reduction in the risk of heart disease and osteoporosis. Premarin soon rose to the top of the drug charts. It continued to be popular for menopausal complaints until 1975, when an epidemic of uterine cancer was traced to its use.[1] Later studies showed that pharmaceutical estrogen increased the risk of endometrial cancer (cancer of the lining of the uterus) by 400 to 800 percent.[2] What was worse, the increased risk did not stop when a woman stopped taking the drug but continued for many years afterward.[3]

This alarming result was soon explained as a problem of imbalance. Estrogen was being supplied without its antagonist, progesterone. In a normal menstrual cycle, estrogen is released in the first part of the cycle to build up the lining of the endometrium. Without the progesterone normally released midway through the cycle, the uterine lining continues to build up, producing the uncontrolled proliferation of cells known as cancer. To correct for this imbalance, progesterone was added to the hormone replacement formula.

The prevailing trend in the United States since the mid-1970s has been toward an estrogen/progesterone mixture called hormone replacement therapy (HRT). Prempro is a popular estrogen/progestin (synthetic progesterone) product consisting of Premarin and Provera (the progestin component) combined. By the 1990s, Premarin— either alone or as Prempro—had become the number-one selling drug on the U.S. market. In 2002, it generated more than $2 billion in sales for Wyeth.[4]

Then, in July 2002, another bombshell study hit. Prempro, which was being used by more than 6 million women in the United States, was found to *increase* the risk of heart disease, breast cancer, and stroke. The Women's Health Initiative had lasted more than five years and was supposed to continue until 2005; but the study was abruptly halted in late May 2002, after researchers determined that the risks of taking Prempro outweighed the benefits. The study involved 16,000 women who still had their uteruses. Compared to a placebo group, the estrogen-plus-progestin group had a 41 percent increase in strokes, 29 percent increase in heart attacks, a doubling of the rate of venous thromboembolism (blood clots), a 22 percent increase in total cardiovascular disease, and a 26 percent increase in breast cancer. Just a few days later, the National Cancer Institute made public a study linking the use of estrogen-only replacement therapy to an increased risk of ovarian cancer in women without uteruses (but with one or more ovaries). Women who took estrogen for at least ten years were twice as likely to develop ovarian cancer, and those who took it for twenty years or more were three times as likely to develop ovarian cancer compared to those who did not take the hormone. Both studies were published in *The Journal of the American Medical Association* (*JAMA*) on July 17, 2002.[5]

These studies had an impact like the adverse findings of 1975. Guidelines were hastily issued recommending that combined postmenopausal hormones for primary prevention of coronary artery disease not be begun, and not be continued if already begun. Law firms began advertising for women who might have lawsuits against Wyeth, for side effects incurred from the drug (stroke, blood clots, or thromboembolic disease). Physicians were at a loss what to recommend to their patients, and women took an increased interest in finding alternatives.

PROBLEMS WITH SYNTHETIC PROGESTERONE

While it is the estrogen fraction of Prempro that is most suspected of stimulating malignancy, the progestin fraction is blamed for the most unpleasant side affects. Although allowed to go under the name of progesterone, the progestin compounds used in HRT are actually synthetic products. Pure progesterone was isolated from animals and its chemical structure was determined in 1934; however, this crystalline progesterone could not be taken in pill form because it was converted by the liver and excreted too rapidly to be absorbed into the bloodstream. It had to be injected, a process that was cumbersome, expensive, and ran the risk of leaving toxins at the injection site. So interest in it waned, as the drug industry succeeded in developing patentable synthetic forms of steroid hormones—progestins, estrogens, and glucocorticoids.

Provera (the "pro" of Prempro) is the most popular brand of progestin used in pharmaceutical HRT. It is generally used for the last one or two weeks of each twenty-five-day course of estrogen to protect against uterine cancer. Many women report, however, that the progestin phase of their HRT is particularly difficult. It makes them feel heavy, bloated, and depressed. Long-term dangers aside, women are often deterred from taking HRT simply because they don't feel well on the drugs. At one clinic, two-thirds of the women who started on hormone replacement therapy wound up abandoning the pursuit. Most women, it seems, don't stay on HRT more than nine months.[6] Side effects result because pharmaceutical hormones are only imperfect copies of our own. Hormones act in the body like keys in a lock. The slightest variation in the key can prevent it from performing its intended functions and result in adverse reactions.

No synthetic progesterone has ever been able to duplicate the hormonal activities of the native hormone. Provera and other chemically altered forms of progesterone cannot, like natural progesterone, be converted in the body to other hormones as needed. The result is a host of side effects, including bloating, water retention, nausea, insomnia, jaundice, mental depression, fever, masculinization, weight changes, breast tenderness, abdominal cramping, anxiety, irritability, and allergic reactions. Fluid retention can exacerbate asthma, migraines, epilepsy, and heart and kidney problems.[7] Some progestin compounds are as much as 2,000 times more potent than the progesterone found in the body. Some are made strictly from chemicals. Others are made from the male hormone testosterone. These react like male hormones and can result in masculine characteristics.

Eighty-five percent of women taking progestins continue to have monthly bleeding (along with 25 percent of women on estrogen alone). The other negative side effects come just before this bleeding, or in the "premenstrual" phase. They are similar to the symptoms of PMS except that they are drug-induced. Some of these side effects can be avoided by switching brands of progestins, since different brands are more or less androgenic; all of them have side effects, however. The androgenic types (Norlutin and Norlutate) can cause acne and greasy skin and hair. The estrogenic types (Provera and Amen) can cause depression and anxiety.[8]

While the estrogen in Premarin is more natural than synthetic progesterone, it too can have side effects, since the mares' urine from which it is derived contains equilin and other estrogens not normally found in humans. Because they don't have the same molecular structure as human estrogens (estrone, estradiol, and estriol), they cannot be used by human estrogen receptors.[9] Potential adverse reactions to Premarin listed in the *Physician's Desk Reference* or *PDR* (the standard medical reference on drugs) include PMS-like symptoms; breast tenderness, enlargement, and secretion; nausea, vomiting, abdominal cramps, and bloating; skin and eye sensitivities; headaches, dizziness, and depression; weight gain and water retention; bleeding between periods or missed periods; changes in libido (sex drive); and enlargement of uterine fibroid tumors. Side effects and risks increase because Premarin is an oral pill. A larger dose than that found naturally in the bloodstream is required because it must first pass through the stomach and liver, where much of the dose is lost to digestion.

HRT AND BREAST CANCER RISK

More troubling than the short-term side effects is the increased risk of breast cancer faced by women on HRT, a risk confirmed in 1995. That year, Harvard researchers reported the preliminary results of the ongoing Nurses' Health Study, involving 121,700 women.

Women in the study who took estrogen after menopause had a 32 percent higher risk of breast cancer than those who hadn't taken the hormone. In 1997, the British medical journal *The Lancet* confirmed that breast cancer risk increases after only one year of estrogen use, and that it increases thereafter by almost 2.3 percent per year. These findings were based on a review of about 90 percent of the worldwide epidemiological evidence, including fifty-one different studies.[10]

The Nurses' Health Study also dashed hopes that taking synthetic progesterone with estrogen (the combination called HRT) would counteract estrogen's effects in stimulating tumors in the breast, as it does for tumors in the uterus. Women on HRT actually had a greater risk of developing breast cancer than women on estrogen alone.[11] This result was confirmed in a nationwide study published in *JAMA* in 2000, including follow-up data from 1980 to 1995 for more than 46,000 subjects enrolled in the Breast Cancer Detection Demonstration Project. The investigators found a significant increase in the risk of breast cancer in women taking HRT during the previous four years.[12]

A second study, published in the *Journal of the National Cancer Institute* in 2000, reviewed data collected from 1,897 breast cancer patients who had not undergone hysterectomy and 1,637 matched controls. For each five years' use of HRT, the risk of developing breast cancer rose by 10 percent. Again, risks were substantially higher for women who used HRT than for those taking estrogen alone.[13]

An editorial accompanying the *JAMA* study emphasized the relationship between duration of therapy and breast cancer risk. Because the risk rapidly declined with cessation of HRT, the researchers concluded that short-term use (two or three years) was probably safe, but the safety of long-term HRT use needed to be reexamined.[14] That means using HRT only for the short time in a woman's life when she is experiencing hot flashes probably won't significantly increase her breast cancer risk, but staying on HRT for life to reap its supposed benefits for the heart, bones, and brain could. Women taking HRT for these benefits could be trading them for an increased risk of breast cancer.

Using HRT even for the brief period when you experience serious hot flashes, however, can be problematic. Increasing your estrogen intake raises your hot flash threshold. If you go below that threshold, your pituitary gland causes hot flashes. When you stop taking the hormone, you can thus wind up with more devastating hot flashes than the ones you started out with. HRT can also cause a gain in weight that many women then have a battle losing.

New Research Raises Even More Questions

HRT has been recommended for postmenopausal women to forestall not only heart disease but also Alzheimer's disease and osteoporosis. All these benefits, however, have been challenged by recent studies. As recently as 1995, the American Heart Association (AHA) advised that all women with heart disease should consider taking estrogen. In July 2001, however, the AHA came out with new guidelines that drastically reversed this position. It said healthy women should not take hormones after menopause to prevent heart disease, and those who already have heart disease should not start on hormones. The advisory was based on the results of several studies of the effect of HRT on heart disease risk, including the four-year Heart and Estrogen/Progestin Replacement Study (HERS). HERS found that for women with heart disease, taking oral estrogen plus progestin actually raised the risk of recurrent heart attack and death during the first year of use and lowered it only slightly thereafter.[15] The May 2002 findings of the 16,000-person Women's Health Initiative study, mentioned earlier, sealed the coffin on this approach to heart disease prevention.

New studies also question the benefits previously claimed for estrogen in reversing Alzheimer's disease. A study reported in *JAMA* in February of 2000 found that once the disease has set in, estrogen affords no benefit. The study involved 120 older women with mild to moderate Alzheimer's disease who were given either a low estrogen dose, a high estrogen dose, or a placebo every day for a year. No significant differences were found in tests of mental function, mood, memory, attention, language skills, or motor function. By the end of the study, those taking estrogen actually fared somewhat worse than the placebo group in a rating of dementia. The researchers concluded that the results of the study did not support the role of estrogen in the treatment of Alzheimer's disease.[16]

That leaves the issue of slowing bone loss with HRT. A review of twenty-two studies finding that effect, published in *JAMA* in 2001, concluded that the earlier studies were flawed and that there is no solid evidence that HRT benefits the bones. There was some benefit for women who started taking estrogen earlier than age 50; but no significant benefit was found for older women, the age group most at risk of fractures.[17] Another study, reported in November 2000, found that estrogen replacement drugs given to younger anorexic women to prevent bone loss had no effect on bone density.[18]

The good news is that *natural* progesterone *has* been found in some studies to counteract bone loss, evidently without risking breast cancer. Estrogen inhibits the osteoclasts, the cells that tear down old bone. Progesterone stimulates the osteoblasts, the cells that make new bone. Natural progesterone, used in supplement form, has been shown to actually put bone back on.[19]

The Plant Hormone Alternative

Both progesterone and estrogen are available as natural plant derivatives. Plants, like animals, produce hormones that regulate cell metabolism and growth. In fact, plant sterols are the basis from which many cheap, commercially available hormones are made. The plant progesterone products currently on the market come from Mexican yams and soybeans, which produce cholesterol derivatives called sapogenins that are closely related to human progesterone. Only slight processing, not requiring the use of chemicals, is necessary to extract the sterols of these plants and make them exactly match the chemical composition of the body's own hormone. What is left after boiling is pure progesterone in powder form.

As already noted, the problem with earlier attempts to use this natural progesterone in its pure form was that the liver converted it so rapidly for excretion that it couldn't be absorbed by the bloodstream or used by the body unless it was injected. An oral micronized pill was later developed, but like other oral hormones including Provera and Premarin, it has the drawback that it has to pass through the stomach and the liver, where much of the dose is lost. Adequate blood levels can, therefore, be sustained only with large doses.

These drawbacks were overcome in the 1970s by a technique developed by Dr. Ray Peat, by which the natural hormone could be suspended in vitamin E oil. This stable solvent allowed efficient absorption of the hormone either through the stomach or the skin.

Studies have shown that hormones are actually absorbed better through the skin than through the stomach, substantially cutting dosage requirements.

For many women, natural progesterone cream alone can control hot flashes, without the use of estrogen. Their bodies apparently synthesize estrogen from progesterone as needed. Research also shows that natural progesterone is as effective as synthetic progesterone in protecting against uterine cancer.[20] Substituting natural for synthetic progesterone allows most women on HRT to reduce their estrogen dose by at least half. After six months, many women who take natural progesterone are well past menopause and can give up estrogen altogether.[21]

Effective hormone creams containing 3 percent natural progesterone are available over the counter. ProGest by Transitions for Health is a particularly good product. The protocol varies depending on hormonal status and brand. In general, if you are still menstruating, rub ⅛ to ¼ teaspoon of the cream on the abdominal area each night for the fourteen days before your period, stopping the day or so before your period starts. For postmenopausal women, use ⅛ to ¼ teaspoon for twenty-five days out of the month. (Be conservative; very little is necessary to get an effect.) Relief from hot flashes can take up to several months, since the hormone gets to the blood by way of the fatty layer under the skin and builds up only gradually; however, herbal and homeopathic remedies can be used to reduce hot flashes while the progesterone is kicking in.

Over-the-counter natural estrogen derived from plants is also available. Preliminary research suggests that unlike animal and synthetic estrogens, plant estrogens are not associated with increased rates of cancer of the breast and uterus and may even afford protection against those diseases. Research also indicates that plant estrogens are as effective as pharmaceutical estrogen in increasing HDL ("good" cholesterol), lowering LDL ("bad" cholesterol), and causing arteries to constrict and dilate when they should.[22] No significant side effects have been reported for natural estrogen creams, except for an occasional skin rash in women who are allergic to them. Particularly effective natural estrogen products are made by Bezwecken, including OstaDerm, Osta B3, and OstaDerm V. They contain plant progesterone along with plant estrogen, allaying any risk of uterine cancer. Again dosages vary, but the general rule is to use ⅛ to ½ teaspoon as needed, once or twice daily. For creams applied vaginally (such as OstaDerm V), use three times weekly.

(Pharmaceutical estrogens are also available that are closer to the natural human hormone than Premarin. They include Estrace, Ogen, Ortho-Est, Cenestin, and the transdermal estrogens—Estraderm, FemPatch, and others. These products may contain fillers, binders, and preservatives. They require a prescription and are more expensive than over-the-counter natural estrogen products. Unlike Premarin, newer pharmaceutical estrogens have not been extensively studied, so their long-term beneficial or detrimental effects remain unknown.[23])

Natural hormones can safely and effectively duplicate the body's own hormones and functions, but because they only address symptoms, they are still not the ideal solution. Herbal and homeopathic remedies can stimulate the body's own production of hormones and address the underlying causes of hormone imbalance—usually an onslaught of physical and emotional stressors. We'll look at that naturopathic approach in the next chapter, after a discussion of the drug approach and its downsides.

3

GOING NATURAL: REMEDIES THAT CORRECT UNDERLYING IMBALANCES

According to a 1998 study in *The Journal of the American Medical Association* (*JAMA*), pharmaceutical side effects are the fourth leading cause of death in the United States, following heart disease, cancer, and stroke. Every two weeks, as many people die from the *proper* use of prescription drugs as died in the World Trade Center tragedy.[1]

The side effects of HRT result when the drugs don't duplicate the body's own hormones. HRT is a "supplementation therapy," which means it tries to artificially add substances the body lacks. Most drugs, however, fall into the "suppression therapy" category. They produce side effects because they chemically inhibit the natural reactions and functions of the body.[2] They target the coughing, sneezing, fever, diarrhea, and elevated blood pressure we think of as the problem, when in fact these symptoms represent the body's attempt to get rid of the problem—the foreign toxins, microbes, or chemicals that have built up in the tissues. When these reactions are deadened with drugs, toxins are left to accumulate in the body, resulting in unwanted side effects. The assumption behind suppression therapies is that the body has run amok as a result of forces beyond its control—heredity or environment or invading bacteria—requiring science to step in and fix it. The assumption behind supplementation therapies (vitamins, minerals, or hormones) is that the body is deficient in something, either because it is not properly making or assimilating that substance or because of dietary deficiencies or blockages.

"Regulation therapies" take a third approach. The assumption on which they are based is that the body can and will heal itself if allowed to respond as it was designed. Regulation therapies stimulate the body's own processes, unblocking energy pathways and "stuck" functions so the body can create its own hormones and otherwise do what it is designed to do.[3] Options in this category include homeopathy ("vibrational" remedies that retune the body energetically), acupuncture (stimulating the meridians or lines of energy running through the body with fine needles), herbal therapies that stimulate natural body functions, detoxification techniques that eliminate toxic buildup and remove blockages in the flow of blood and energy, and mind/body techniques that eliminate emotional blockages and address the consciousness element of disease.

The Eastern Approach: Linking Emotion and Disease

In Chinese medical theory, physical ailments are closely associated with emotions. Energy is said to circulate along five major meridians, or lines of energy: the urinary/bladder/kidney/adrenal; the gallbladder/liver; the lungs/large intestine; the heart/small intestine; and the spleen (pancreas)/stomach. ("Spleen" actually refers to the pancreas, which makes all of the digestive enzymes.) Each meridian system regulates not only specific physical functions but specific emotions as well. The liver's job, for example, is to cleanse the blood and move energy smoothly and evenly through it, but it also handles anger. The gallbladder's job is to help digest fats, but it also regulates decision-making. The lungs are associated with grief, the kidneys with fear, and the heart with joy and sorrow.

The Chinese believe that the *shen*, or spirit, resides in the heart. The heart is nourished by the blood, but it also needs emotional nourishment. When it is not being properly nourished emotionally, the *shen* cannot live inside but must live outside the heart, throwing off mental balance. The person becomes psychotic, manic depressive, or schizophrenic. People with heart problems, say Chinese doctors, are often holding on to excess sorrow. While everyone experiences joy and sorrow, body functions are impaired when these emotions are clung to and become overwhelming. When the blood is weak and isn't nourishing the heart properly, a woman can become anemic, have heart palpitations, and feel off balance, like she is "losing her mind." She can also have nightmares, insomnia, and fatigue.

If the gallbladder/liver meridian is out of balance, the heart doesn't get nourished and a heart attack may result. Seizures or tremors are also a liver problem. Energy can get congested in the liver not only from chemical toxins but also from holding on to anger. When this happens, Chinese doctors say the anger flies out of your mouth involuntarily—for example, you get upset with the store clerk or waitress, then feel bad because you overreacted. Moving the liver energy will help move the anger out.

Low back pain is thought to indicate kidney imbalance. The kidney energy (adrenaline) has been spent. Fear and stress increase the excretion of adrenaline.

Mid-back (waist-level) pain is said to be stomach-related. It can also be the result of not getting enough love (nourishment) or what you desire. It may, for example, strike soon after a major fight with a loved one.

John Diamond, M.D., confirmed the emotion/organ link by extensive testing with applied kinesiology (muscle testing). He found that each negative emotion—unhappiness, depression, anger, and so on—related to a specific acupuncture meridian, and that it unbalanced the life energy in the organs served by that meridian. He also found that an emotion-induced imbalance in the life energy could be corrected, at least in the short term, simply by saying positive affirmations. If repeated often enough and made into a lifestyle, this type of positive thinking could actually heal disease.[4]

Chinese doctors move energy and regulate body functions with herbs and acupuncture (using fine needles to stimulate the meridians crisscrossing the body). Western naturopathic doctors also use a variety of herbs. Homeopathy is another effective alternative. These remedies affect not only physiological functions but also the stress patterns that can unbalance them.

HERBAL REMEDIES

Herbs have been used for healing throughout recorded history. Many conventional drugs are extracted from plants, but naturopathic doctors maintain that the whole herb is more therapeutic than its isolated ingredients and is less likely to result in side effects. USDA ethnobotanist Dr. James Duke observed that while prescription drugs kill more than 100,000 people annually, herbs kill fewer than 100, and then it is usually through abuse or exceeding the recommended dosage.[5] For most people, herbal remedies are considered quite safe in recommended doses. For children and pregnant women, however, professional advice is recommended, since a few medicinal plants can cause bodily harm when taken in excess.[6]

Herbal remedies are available as pills, teas, drops, and distillations of various sorts. *Aromatherapy* consists of distillations of the essential oils of the plant. These oils carry the plant's important information and have been referred to as the "blood" or "life force" of the plant.

Gemmotherapy, another form of herbal therapy, is derived from the immature shoots of plants. Gemmotherapy remedies are said to contain more vital life force than other herbal options. The usual dosage of drops is once daily, although in severe cases they can be taken two or three times daily.

Note that many herbs and other natural remedies work by stimulating the body to do its own housecleaning. While toxic substances are being eliminated through the bloodstream, they can make you feel more tired and irritable than before the remedy was taken. This reaction soon passes, however, and the user is boosted into a higher state of well-being.

BACH FLOWER REMEDIES

Even safer than herbs are Bach flower remedies, vibrational remedies derived from flowers that are entirely nontoxic. Dr. Edward Bach, a British physician, categorized thirty-eight flowers, all of which work on different emotions of the body. Walnut helps during stressful life changes such as moving or changing jobs. Pine helps with feelings of guilt. Star of Bethlehem helps with shock. Rescue Remedy is a combination remedy that is very effective for relieving stress and irritability. Taken daily over several months, Bach flower remedies can effect profound emotional changes.

Bach flower remedies are a great start for a woman whose life is filled with day-to-day stresses. Just a dropperful of Rescue Remedy placed in an 8-ounce bottle of water in the mornings and sipped throughout the day can reduce stress and irritability, making your "crazed" existence feel more sane. Alternatively, put four drops of Rescue Remedy directly under your tongue, up to five times daily, or put a dropperful in a spray bottle filled with water and spray it around a hectic office.

HOMEOPATHIC REMEDIES

Also quite safe are homeopathic remedies. Where allopathic or conventional medicine suppresses symptoms, homeopathy encourages them, on the theory that they will stimulate the body to flush out toxins. The remedies consist of minute doses of natural substances—mineral, plant, or animal—that, if given to a healthy person in larger doses, would cause that person to experience the same symptoms that a sick person experiences from the illness. The principle is the same as for pharmaceutical vaccination, but vaccines are macro-molecules that can induce unwanted side effects. Homeopathic remedies are without side effects because they are extremely dilute—at some strengths so dilute that no molecule of the original substance is likely to be left in solution. Only its vibration remains.

Homeopathy's current renaissance in the United States is due in part to a series of studies that finally brought it some scientific validation. On September 29, 1997, the British medical journal *The Lancet* reported the results of an analysis of eighty-nine clinical trials of homeopathy. It found that the homeopathic medicines used in those studies had an average effect that was about two and a half times greater than placebos. For comparative purposes, in a similar analysis of twenty well-controlled studies of popular antidepressant medicines, the drugs were found to be only one and a third times as effective as placebos.[7]

Homeopaths can make deep, profound changes in people with single, high-potency doses of homeopathic remedies given over long periods of time. Many cases have been recorded in which serious or even fatal illnesses have been reversed and abnormal lab results have returned to normal in a few months—results that in Western medical practice would have been considered impossible. Treatment is individualized and is largely dependent on the practitioner's experience in selecting the correct remedy.

An increasingly popular alternative is for users to educate themselves and select their own homeopathic remedies. Combination remedies take a shotgun approach, including a range of likely homeopathic possibilities that helps take the guesswork out of the selection process. One proviso is that it is much easier for a practitioner to treat a problem at the onset. If time is lost in self-treatment with the wrong remedies, the practitioner will have a harder time of it. Another proviso is that homeopathic remedies given incorrectly *in high potencies* over a period of time can suppress the disease and make the condition worse, and so can any remedy given for a long period after symptoms have cleared. However, single remedies *in low potency,* and combination homeopathic remedies for minor ailments are quite safe and effective.

Homeopathy as Therapy for Emotional Trauma

Homeopathic medicine, like Eastern medicine, sees disease merely as a symptom of an underlying imbalance. The body is a mirror of what's going on in your life. Present symptoms often reflect past physical or emotional trauma. Rather than cutting out diseased organs or suppressing symptoms with drugs, which merely allows the disease process to continue, the homeopathic approach is to look at underlying issues and attempt to resolve them. Homeopathic remedies help your issues to come to the surface, where they can be dealt with rationally and dispassionately. Homeopathic *Ignatia,* for example, can help you deal with grief from a death or other major loss. *Phosphoric acid (Phosphorium acidum)* helps with depression from grief, with feelings of dullness, sadness, and indifference as if dead inside. *Colocynthis* helps with feelings of betrayal.

THE NEED FOR PROFESSIONAL ADVICE

Although homeopathic and herbal remedies are safe and many are available at health food stores, an experienced practitioner may still be required to help you in the selection of the right remedy. Often you can't "see the forest for the trees" in your own case. It may be a month or two, for example, before adrenal burnout from a period of unusual stress results in hormonal changes. You may think you are beginning menopause when the real problem is stress-induced hormone imbalance. A practitioner can spot the connection you missed.

Even when the "right" remedy has been determined, a qualified practitioner may be necessary to help you recognize and remove the layers of disease or imbalance that would otherwise prevent the remedy from working. The body may need to be cleared of toxins, pesticides, and chemicals; the diet improved; the lymph moved; and suppressed emotions cleared. This can take weeks or months; without this initial work, the remedy will not work. An experienced practitioner can run tests, take a history, figure out what is needed, and advise on dosages and length of treatment.

Dosages and Scheduling

Dosages for most homeopathic remedies needn't be as exact as for drugs. One pellet or three, five drops or ten will generally have the same effect—"kicking" the system back into balance—since the remedies work vibrationally rather than chemically. For most homeopathic remedies, use ten drops three times a day or according to label directions until symptoms subside, unless otherwise directed by a homeopath.

Two exceptions are homeopathic series therapy and detox drops. Series therapy consists of a box of ampules in different potencies to be taken in a particular order. The remedies should be taken at the rate of one ampule every three days for a month. For detox drops, the appropriate dose depends on how toxic you are. If you are very toxic, taking high doses can cause cleansing reactions, including body aches, headaches, nausea, and dizziness. To avoid them, begin with a single drop in water once a day and work up slowly. If you do experience cleansing reactions, drink plenty of water and take a bath to help eliminate toxins. A practitioner can help you determine your toxicity level.

When using any homeopathic remedy, you should be prepared for a *homeopathic aggravation*—a slight aggravation of symptoms that can sometimes take place before you feel better. This is not only normal but desirable: it indicates that the remedy is the correct one and that healing is beginning to occur. When improvement in symptoms is seen, the remedy should be discontinued. Homeopathic remedies exert subtle influences on the system. Their purpose is to encourage the body along its health-building path. When the body is healthy, it no longer needs the remedy. Prolonged use beyond that time may result in an aggravation of the symptoms the remedy was given to eliminate. If that happens, don't worry; the symptoms will disappear when the remedy is discontinued. If symptoms return after the remedy has been stopped, try a few more drops. If a practitioner is being consulted, it is best to return within two to three weeks to determine whether the remedy is still needed.

Use only 3X to 30X potencies, nothing higher, unless the remedies have been chosen by an experienced practitioner. "X" is the lowest potency, indicating dilution by 10; "C" indicates dilution by 100; "M" by 1,000. The highest dilutions are the strongest remedies, since their vibratory levels are higher.

Homeopathic theory holds that less is better. While requirements are very individual, the lowest potency and briefest course of treatment necessary to eliminate symptoms is best. The higher the potency, the deeper-acting the remedy. High potencies should be used only for chronic conditions. For acute conditions like rashes, you would use low potencies (6 or 30), unless the condition is both acute and very traumatic (as in auto accident injuries), in which case higher potencies would be appropriate but should be recommended by a homeopath.

Some brands of high-quality homeopathic remedies discussed in this book (including Deseret Biologicals, Molecular Biologics, Marco Pharma International, CompliMed, and Professional Complementary Health) are available only from licensed practitioners or by special order from homeopathic pharmacies. Other brands (Dolisos, Hyland's, Boiron, Bioforce, BHI, Nelson's, Longevity, and so on) are widely available in health food stores.

Other Rules for Using Homeopathic Remedies

Take homeopathic remedies away from food and drink—a minimum of fifteen minutes before or after eating or drinking anything except water. Your mouth should be clean and free of food, drink, toothpaste, gum, and so on. Avoid camphor, mint, menthol, and eucalyptus products, which can render the remedies ineffective, as can coffee or even coffee-flavored ice cream or candy. Homeopathic medicine should never be used along with steroid drugs, including hydrocortisone creams. Homeopathic remedies encourage the body to regain its original vitality. Steroids work by an opposing mechanism, suppressing the immune system's own efforts.

Avoid touching homeopathic remedies with your hands. When taking pellets, shake them into the cap of the bottle, then drop them into your mouth. They should be kept under the tongue until they dissolve. When taking liquid remedies, let the drops fall from the dropper or bottle into your mouth, taking care not to touch the dropper to your tongue or lips; or put the drops in a little water. Hold the liquid in your mouth for thirty seconds before swallowing, then wait at least thirty seconds before taking another remedy.

Store the remedies in a dark place away from perfumes, medications, foods, herbs, strong-smelling substances, and electronic equipment. If they go through a X-ray machine at the airport, they can still be used, but they may be less effective. If you are traveling, the best idea is to send them by mail.

OTHER WAYS TO DEAL WITH STRESS

Besides herbal and homeopathic treatment, stress can be relieved with physical therapies—heat or cold applications, massage, acupressure, water therapy, cranio-sacral therapy, yoga, tai chi, or qi gong. A number of counseling techniques are available for pulling up and releasing repressed negative emotions. Meditation is excellent. You can also break the stress cycle with a short period of fasting.

Most important is to heal your life by finding something you love and going after it. The ideal is to be doing work that you love; however, if you are limited to a job that just pays the bills, you can still incorporate things into your life that keep you looking forward to the day. Make time for what excites you—classes, friends, women's groups, gardening, reading, hobbies, or sports. This is the underlying principle of holistic ("wholistic") medicine—healing your life, making it whole and satisfying.

4

NUTRITIONAL BALANCE: SUPPLEMENTING NUTRIENT NEEDS AND CLEARING METABOLIC WASTES

D rugs can mask symptoms, and herbs and homeopathic remedies can stimulate body functions that have gone awry, but health will still elude you as long as there is an underlying lack of essential nutrients in the body. Health problems are increasingly being traced to nutritional deficiencies, which can be corrected only by supplying missing vitamins, minerals, amino acids, and other essential nutrients.

Supplements alone, however, won't resolve metabolic imbalances. In some cases, too many capsules and pills just add to the stress of an already-overloaded liver. Detox therapies may be necessary to clear out metabolic buildup and clear the digestive machinery so that ingested nutrients can be efficiently absorbed.

NUTRITIONAL SUPPORT

Few people these days eat a balanced diet of natural, unprocessed plant food. But even if more people did, they couldn't rely on this ideal fare to satisfy nutrient requirements completely. At one time, everything the body needed was furnished by foods from the earth. Today, however, the land seems as depleted as our bodies are. Back in 1936, a report presented to the U.S. Department of Agriculture concluded that our soils and the crops grown on them were so mineral deficient that the only way to prevent and cure the resulting deficiency diseases was by taking mineral supplements.[1] Since then, the situation has only gotten worse. Canning, irradiation, and other methods of processing, preserving, and extending shelf life have further decreased the biological value of our food by removing its natural antioxidants.

For most conditions, a wide range of nutritional support is required. It is the rare single nutrient that will cure a disease unless the disease happens to be due to a very specific deficiency. (Rickets, for example, is caused by a lack of vitamin D and can be cured by supplying that vitamin.) On the other hand, every person in a diseased state can benefit from a balanced vitamin and mineral supplement program.

Your Own Vitamin and Mineral Routine

It is important to get into a routine that will actually work for you. We commonly see people who spend large sums of money on a wide array of nutrients, then fail to take them. Spend your money on quality rather than on quantity. Supplements should be all-natural. Inexpensive vitamins are usually synthetic. Nutrients also need to be combined in proper balance and taken in an absorbable form. Particularly good brands are mentioned below.

It would be wonderfully convenient if you could find a single supplement that met all your daily needs, but few supplements have the necessary range of nutrients. Vitamins A, B, C, D, and E are all required, along with essential minerals. Calcium is of particular concern for women because of their increased risk of osteoporosis. It is usually in short supply and needs to be added separately. The recommended intake of calcium is 1,500 mg daily, but some of this requirement is met in the diet. If your diet contains substantial amounts of dairy products and green vegetables, you need only about 1,000 mg of calcium in supplement form, and even that may be too much because you may not be able to absorb it. Calcium that is not absorbed can settle in the joints and do more harm than good. A better approach is 500–1,000 mg of supplemental calcium accompanied by a product that will help increase calcium absorption. Good options are Calcium Absorption by Bioforce or Recalcify by Molecular Biologics (both homeopathic remedies), or Red Spruce (a gemmotherapy). For recommended forms of calcium, see "Osteoporosis" in Part Two.

If your liver is congested, you should also take green supplements (blue-green algae, Sun Chlorella, Ultimate Green, spirulina, liquid chlorophyll, or concentrated green vegetables). To protect your cells from rapid aging, antioxidants are excellent, including green tea extract, grapeseed extract, coenzyme Q_{10} (CoQ_{10}), and alpha lipoic acid (ALA).

PROBLEMS OF OVERDOSING AND NON-ABSORPTION

Although it's important to take the supplements you need, many women are dosing themselves with too many unnecessary vitamins and minerals. Breaking down all that excess further stresses the kidneys and liver. In many cases, healing turns not on putting more into the body but on removing a toxic load that is congesting the liver and overwhelming its resources. You need to know what you're taking and why you're taking it. If you think you may be overdosing on nutritional supplements, try going two weeks without them to give your metabolic system a rest.

In some cases, getting what you need either from your food or from nutritional supplements is impaired by the condition of the digestive system. Inadequate absorption of nutrients may result when the digestive tract is inflamed, subject to acid reflux, or infected with *Candida* or parasites. For alternatives for correcting these conditions, see "Digestive Problems," "Fungal Infections," and "Parasitic Infection" in Part Two.

Inadequate absorption may also result from insufficient digestive enzymes. Cooking, microwaving, and processing destroy enzymes found naturally in foods. As a result, food gets to the colon undigested, leaving poisonous residues for the liver to detoxify. When the liver becomes overloaded, toxins enter the blood, where they can evoke an aggressive autoimmune response. Proteins that are not broken down properly by pancreatic enzymes also evoke an autoimmune response.[2]

To aid digestion in the stomach, pancreatic enzymes that are not enteric coated may be taken with meals. Transformer and Tyler are good brands available in health food stores, but there are many others. Take one to three capsules with each meal or as directed by a health practitioner. Another alternative to aid digestion is to take apple cider vinegar and honey before meals (2 tablespoons of apple cider vinegar in water with 1 teaspoon of honey).[3]

Caution: Supplemental enzymes are not recommended for people with bleeding disorders, inflammation of the intestines, reflux, or ulcers.

AN OVERLOOKED NATURAL CURE

Another inexpensive and natural key to health that is often overlooked is plain, unadulterated water. In *Your Body's Many Cries for Water,* F. Batmanghelidj, M.D., links the major chronic epidemics of modern life to water dehydration. Our mistake, he says, is in thinking we have satisfied our need for water by satisfying our thirst with other beverages. We need half our body's weight in ounces of water per day—not coffee, tea, soft drinks, or juices, but plain (filtered or bottled) water. Thus, a 128-pound woman would need 64 ounces, or eight 8-ounce glasses of water. Dr. Batmanghelidj reports seeing many diseases reversed with this simple therapy, including high blood pressure, low back pain, asthma, allergies, and ulcers, among others. The regimen is also a good way to lose weight.

Wait a half hour before meals and two and a half hours after meals for your heavy water doses to avoid diluting your digestive juices. Increase your water intake gradually to make sure your kidneys are functioning properly. Output should increase proportionately with input.[4] Dr. Batmanghelidj's protocol includes getting sufficient daily exercise (for example, an hour's walk) to stimulate internal movement and healing. He also advises adding ½ teaspoon of salt to your diet daily for every ten glasses of water you drink. Note, however, that table salt has been heated to very high temperatures in processing and can be treated by the body as a foreign toxin. Unheated sea salt is better. Better yet is a product called Bio-Salt by Gilbert's Health Food Labs in England, a biochemically balanced mineral salt compound containing sodium chloride plus all the cell salts.

THE LIVER CLEANSE DIET

To improve the functioning of a congested liver, detox treatment may be required. A detox program that is easy to integrate into a woman's busy schedule is this three-week diet, specifically designed for cleaning the liver:

◆ Begin each morning with the juice of half a lemon squeezed into a cup of warm water.

◆ Eat only whole, fresh foods—no preservatives, coloring, or fillers (all found in processed foods). Emphasize green vegetables, the foods that stimulate the liver to release and process toxins. Limit protein to 30 grams a day.

◆ Drink at least 64 ounces (eight 8-ounce glasses) of distilled water while on the detox diet. (Distilled water isn't recommended for more than seven days when you're not on a detox diet.)

◆ Drink the juice of fresh mixed greens (parsley, celery, or carrot) at least twice a day. If you can't find these drinks or make them yourself, drink one ounce of chlorophyll in 2 to 4 ounces of water or juice daily.

◆ Throughout the day, drink unfiltered apple juice and one of the detox teas available at health food stores, containing herbs or spices that open the pores and encourage the release of toxins.

◆ Exercise or walk briskly at least twenty minutes a day.

HERBAL DETOX THERAPIES

Herbal supplements that can help detoxify the body are also available. Naturopaths and practitioners of Ayurvedic and Chinese medicine recommend many herbal formulas both for detoxification and to strengthen the immune system. If infections or parasites have been found, they can also be treated with herbal or homeopathic formulas. (See "Parasitic Infection," "Fungal Infections," and "Infection, Bacterial and Viral" in Part Two.) For toxic bowel syndrome and digestive tract disorders, herbal laxatives and high-fiber foods, such as psyllium seeds, can cleanse the digestive tract and promote elimination. Colonics (irrigation of the colon) are used to cleanse the lower intestines. Acidophilus and other friendly bacteria can be reintroduced into the system with nutritional supplements.[5] Milk thistle extract, called silymarin, is a powerful herb used for detoxifying the liver. Cayenne pepper is a good natural antibiotic and detoxifier.

SKIN BRUSHING

Another detox technique is skin brushing. The skin is a major organ of elimination, and new skin is made continually. Brushing with a natural bristle brush removes the top layer, leaving fresh new skin underneath. Healthy uncovered skin should dispose of two pounds of waste acids daily; however, the skin's elimination is hampered by garments, oils, lotions, and dirt and chemical buildup. To open the pores for proper cleansing, you need to stimulate the skin manually. Recommended procedure is to brush the entire body except the face with a natural bristle brush with a long handle. (Don't use a nylon or plastic bristle brush.) Use the brush dry before dressing or bathing in the morning. A special brush may be used for the face.[6]

FASTING

If you can afford several days just to indulge yourself, a short fast is a great way to purge the system and rejuvenate body and mind. Fasting is one of the oldest ways to detoxify the body; for eliminating metabolic wastes, it is still one of the best. Fasting is a period without food during which the body metabolizes waste products. Fasting expert Dr. Paavo Airola explains that after the first three days of fasting, your body lives on itself, burning and digesting its own tissues. However, it eliminates the dispensable tissue first. That means that diseased, aging, or dead cells; morbid accumulations; tumors; abscesses; and damaged tissues are the first to go. During this initial purge, the faster loses her craving for food. But when the nonessential tissues have been exhausted and the body is reduced to eating its own essential tissue, hunger suddenly returns with a vengeance. This is considered the physiologically correct time to end the fast.[7]

Many people avoid fasting because they get headaches and feel weak whenever they go without food for a few hours. But if they can go without food for a longer period of time, they will find that the headaches will pass and they will feel more energetic than before they stopped eating. The headaches and weakness are, therefore, not caused by lack of food. Fasting experts say these symptoms come because when we refrain from food, our bodies take the opportunity to go into detox mode and dump toxins. While these toxins are passing through the bloodstream, they cause symptoms to appear. As with all detox therapies, this healing crisis can make us feel worse before we feel better, but this is actually a sign that good things are happening.

We can control the speed of elimination of toxins and facilitate the body's ability to move them out by taking supplements and fresh-squeezed juices during the fast. When our air was pure, our water clean, our food free of pesticides and preservatives, and our remedies natural, we could safely fast on water. But today our environment has become so polluted and our bodies so laden with drugs, pesticides, and industrial wastes that long water fasts are considered dangerous. Cleansing can proceed so rapidly that the released toxins overwhelm the body. Dr. Airola recommends fasting on vegetable and fruit juices, and for no more than seven to ten days unless you are under medical supervision. A three-day juice fast is considered quite safe when undertaken at home, and it can provide noticeable relief of pain.

Dr. Airola believes that daily enemas are essential to speed the elimination of toxins. In *3 Days to Vitality,* Pamela Serure also recommends enemas. She observes that people don't want to think about this cleansing technique (which she refers to as the "E" word) until they try it. Then they find out how satisfying and relieving the experience can be.[8]

Dr. Bernard Jensen, in the fasting classic *Dr. Jensen's Guide to Better Bowel Care,* advises the use of coffee enemas to stimulate the liver to release toxins.[9] Although not recommended for habitual use, coffee enemas can be quite helpful during a fast. If you want to undertake a fast, these and other books commonly found in health food stores can guide you through it.

DETOXIFYING FROM CHEMICAL AND HEAVY METAL BUILDUP

Although fasting and special diets are excellent for clearing the body of backed-up metabolic wastes, they fail to eliminate those toxic metals and chemicals that are so new to genetics that the body has no established mechanism for removing them. Animal studies have shown that while fasting breaks down fat cells, the chemical toxins stored in these cells simply move from the fat into the muscles. When food is again eaten, they move back into the fat tissue.[1]

Women's bodies today are subject to toxic buildup from an alarming array of industrial chemicals and heavy metals. We come into contact with hundreds of them each week, ranging from the coloring and additives in processed food, to the pesticides in fruits and vegetables, to the chemicals used in refinishing furniture, to the formaldehyde used in painting. Toxic chemicals are present in new car upholstery, floor stains, wall coverings, and the deck outside your home. New furniture can be very toxic, particularly beds that are protected with flame-retardant sprays on which people typically spend eight hours a night. Swimming subjects you to chlorine toxicity. Pumping your own gas exposes you to additional toxins.

These toxic substances are likely to affect women more than men, either because our bodies are generally smaller and more easily affected, or because our livers are already subject to overload from the processing of hormones, or because of greater exposure. We are more likely than men to be exposed to the chemicals in beauty products and household cleaners, the pesticides in garden sprays, the acetaldehydes and chemicals in the fabric used in sewing and reupholstering, and the petroleum in petroleum-based lotions and creams, which may be absorbed through the skin and incorporated into body cells.

The fatty tissue in women's breasts is particularly efficient at storing toxins. The highest rate of breast cancer has been found in women golfers, evidently due to the pesticides sprayed on golf courses. An interesting finding is that breast cancer is eight times more likely to develop near where deodorant is applied than anywhere else on the breast. Aluminum is contained in most deodorants, and antiperspirants suppress sweating, trapping toxins inside.

Estimates by the United States Centers for Disease Control are that more than 80 percent of all illnesses have environmental and lifestyle causes. This shouldn't surprise us. DDT, a cancer-causing insecticide that has been banned for decades, is still regularly found in the fatty tissue of animals, birds, and fish. For each person living in the United

States, American agriculture uses nearly 10 pounds of pesticides annually on the food supply, and the further up the food chain we go for food, the more of these pesticides we consume. When we eat meat products, we are exposed to the full range of chemicals and additives used along the entire agricultural chain, including not only the pesticides and herbicides sprayed on the grains the animals ate, but also the synthetic hormones, antibiotics, and other chemicals with which they were injected.

One in four Americans is thought to suffer from some level of poisoning from the heavy metals used in industry and dentistry, including mercury, lead, aluminum, cadmium, and arsenic. Heavy metals that have accumulated in the brain have been linked to serious neurological disorders, including Alzheimer's disease, Parkinson's disease, and multiple sclerosis. The link has been established when victims recovered or improved after having the metals removed from their teeth and the residues removed from their tissues.[2]

Symptoms of toxic overload include unexplained fatigue, increased allergies, hypersensitivity to common materials, intolerance to certain foods, indigestion, aches and pains, low-grade fever, headaches, insomnia, depression, sore throats, sudden weight loss or gain, lowered resistance to infection, general malaise, and disability. Detoxification has been found to help people suffering from a wide range of chronic diseases and conditions including allergies, anxiety, arthritis, asthma, cancer, chronic infections, depression, diabetes, headaches, heart disease, high cholesterol, low blood sugar levels, digestive disorders, mental illness, and obesity. It can also help relieve immune system diseases that conventional medicine is unable to treat, including chronic fatigue syndrome, environmental illness/multiple chemical sensitivity, and fibromyalgia.[3]

HOMEOPATHIC DETOX REMEDIES

Homeopathic remedies are effective alternatives for reducing toxic chemical and heavy metal buildup. The detoxifying properties of homeopathic remedies were demonstrated in a laboratory study in which rats were given crude doses of arsenic, bismuth, cadmium, mercury chloride, or lead. Animals pretreated with homeopathic doses of these substances before and after exposure to the crude doses excreted more of the toxic substances through urine, feces, and sweat than did animals pretreated with a placebo.[4] For specific remedies, see "Multiple Chemical Sensitivity" in Part Two.

THE "NIACIN FLUSH"

A primary means of eliminating heavy metals from the body is sweating them out through the skin. A detox treatment called the "niacin flush" combines exercise and sauna or sweat therapy with high doses of the B vitamin niacin, which aids the process by dilating the capillaries. The face turns red and the skin turns hot as the niacin flushes out toxins. Documented results from a program using the niacin flush along with nutritional supplements attest that it has successfully detoxified hundreds of people from the adverse effects of legal and illegal drugs, radiation, and toxic chemicals, including the chemicals to which a group of firefighters were exposed.[5]

In a California study, participants undergoing this treatment experienced significant drops in blood pressure, improvements in vision, increases in IQ points, and lessening of the symptoms of a number of physical ailments, including asthma, allergy, migraine, and hypoglycemia. Participants also reported reexperiencing the smells and physical effects of drugs taken in the past. The program was followed daily for a period of three weeks. It involved twenty to thirty minutes of vigorous exercise (jogging, stationary bicycling, and rowing), followed by thirty minutes in the sauna, a five-minute cooling off period, then thirty more minutes in the sauna. Sauna times could be gradually increased to two hours. Niacin dosage began at 400 mg spread throughout the day. The dose was then increased gradually to as high as 6,000 mg, depending on tolerance.[6]

Note: The "niacin flush" can be quite intense. Test your tolerance gradually. At high doses, niacin should be taken only with medical supervision. Even 400 mg is a large dose; starting at 100 mg would seem more prudent. It's also important to balance niacin intake with a B-complex vitamin containing the other B vitamins.

CHELATION

Heavy metals can be eliminated from the tissues and arteries through chelation. A natural process in the body, chelation is the method by which minerals and metals are transported across the intestinal wall and throughout the body.

EDTA (ethylenediamine disodium tetra-acetic acid) is a chelating substance that has long been used conventionally as a treatment for lead poisoning. Its effectiveness as a treatment for blocked arteries was discovered accidentally in the 1950s, when N. E. Clarke, M.D., used EDTA to treat tenants in a World War II tenement house in Detroit who had been exposed to lead-based paint in the building.[7] In addition to having lead poisoning, the patients were all elderly, and many had cardiovascular problems. To Dr. Clarke's surprise, when the lead was chelated out of their arteries, their cardiovascular troubles were reduced dramatically.

Ray Evers, M.D., an early pioneer of intravenous chelation therapy, analyzed the heavy metal levels in his patients through hair analysis and twenty-four-hour urine tests. He found that the vast majority of them had some abnormality in heavy metal content, with lead and mercury usually highest. Elevated levels of lead were present in nearly all of his arthritis patients. Remarkably, chelation successfully relieved their symptoms. Dr. Evers also found that diseases of the cardiovascular system—the number-one cause of death in industrialized countries—were significantly alleviated with the therapy.[8]

Note: Some experts maintain that intravenous chelation should not be performed until all of the metals used in dental work are removed from the mouth. Otherwise, more metal may simply be pulled from the teeth into body tissues.[9]

Oral Chelation with Drugs and Herbs

Oral chelators are also available. Some require a prescription, including DMPS (Dimaval) and DMSA (Chemet). These drugs, however, can have serious side effects and require professional monitoring. Safer chelators are available over the counter or in the supermarket, either singly or as combination products.

The chlorophyll in plants is a natural chelator. Cilantro, a leafy green herb, is particularly effective.[10] The problem is finding a pure source. In the United States, most commercial cilantro has absorbed environmental toxins. Buy organic. An alternative source of chlorophyll that is more likely to be uncontaminated is the freshwater algae chlorella. The recommended dose is ½ teaspoon a day, up to 1½ teaspoons according to tolerance.

Alpha lipoic acid (ALA) is a very powerful antioxidant that can bind to toxic metals, increasing the liver's detoxification and metabolic enzyme production abilities. It is both water-soluble and fat-soluble, so it can travel to and permeate all the cells of the body, including the brain. You can get it from spinach, kidney, heart, skeletal muscle (beef), and broccoli, or you can buy it in a concentrated form as a supplement.[11]

The Bottom Line

Natural body-supporting treatment involves more than simply looking up your disease and finding the recommended pill. That approach works for drugs that suppress symptoms, but naturopathic doctors don't see symptoms as something to be suppressed. They regard symptoms as the body's efforts at cure. Healing is an ongoing process, in which discordant layers are located and harmonized one by one, until your life is balanced as a whole. With that in mind, let's move on to specific women's ailments and their best natural curatives.

PART TWO

AN A-TO-Z GUIDE TO COMMON WOMEN'S AILMENTS AND THEIR BEST TREATMENTS

The following guide presents a wide selection of common women's ailments in handy reference form. Each entry includes an analysis of conventional treatments and the natural remedies available from various disciplines, including homeopathy, herbalism, nutrition, and flower essences. The focus is always on remedies that work, as reported by real women known to the authors.

ACNE

Acne, or an outbreak of pimples, is the most common skin disorder in the United States. While not gender specific, it has a clear hormonal component. Acne often appears during the raging-hormone years of adolescence, and flare-ups tend to be worse for women the week before their menstrual periods.

Pimples result when sebaceous glands at the base of hair follicles get clogged with oil, causing inflammation and attracting bacteria. In response, white blood cells rush to the scene and fight the infection, making the surrounding area swell. Hormones can aggravate the condition, leaving teenagers, women about to have their periods, and women on oral contraceptives particularly susceptible. Other aggravating factors include stress, food allergies, and poor diet.

Cystic acne is a serious form of the disease that can result in permanent pits and scars. Heredity is a factor in cystic acne. The inherited trait may actually be an allergy to certain foods. Milk products are common culprits. Blemish problems may also be traced to certain drugs. In fact, drug-induced eruptions are among the most common skin disorders encountered by dermatologists. Even over-the-counter drugs can be responsible.[1]

CONVENTIONAL TREATMENT

Drug treatment of acne is problematic. Antibiotics have been a mainstay, but they have been so overused that they are no longer producing the results they once did. Several recent studies have shown that the bacteria that cause acne have developed strains resistant to both oral and topical antibiotics. Dermatologists have, therefore, turned to the stronger and more expensive minocycline, a semi-synthetic form of tetracycline sold under the name Minocin. But signs that it's also becoming resistant have been cropping up, and its side effects are even worse than those of its forerunners.[2] Among reported side effects are severe liver disease resulting in death, hepatitis, lupus, and other autoimmune diseases. Minocycline can also cause dizziness, inflamed and aching joints, and shortness of breath.[3] All antibiotics can also lead to *Candida* yeast infections—which may, ironically, provoke skin eruptions.[4] Despite medical reports of these hazards, many doctors still routinely prescribe minocycline to their younger patients.[5]

Birth control pills have also been used to treat acne because estrogen suppresses the production of oil by the sebaceous glands.[6] When the Pill was first used, it seemed to clear up complexions, but it contained quite high levels of estrogen. When doses were later lowered to safer levels, improvements in the complexions of women on birth control pills became much less common. Many women also noticed a rebound effect, that is, a worsening of acne, when they stopped taking the Pill. In fact, for some women, acne can actually be a paradoxical side effect of taking the Pill.[7] More serious side effects include blood clots, stroke, and heart attacks, as well as an increased risk of developing breast cancer, particularly at a young age.[8]

Accutane (isotretinoin) is another prescription option. One of a class of vitamin A derivatives called retinoids, which have revolutionized dermatology, Accutane can produce dramatic clearing of lesions in severe cystic acne that doesn't respond to conventional therapy. The problem, again, is its high risk of side effects and birth defects. In a study of

154 women who took the drug while pregnant, odds of having a child with major deformities turned out to be about fifty-fifty, and spontaneous abortions were common. Other side effects include drying and inflammation of the lips and skin, an increased sensitivity to sunlight, aches and pains in the muscles and bones, headaches, fatigue, irritability, and most especially, depression. The drug carries a warning: "Accutane may cause depression, psychosis and, rarely, suicidal ideation, suicide attempts and suicide." Charles Bishop, a fifteen-year-old who flew a small airplane into a Florida building in 2002, had been taking Accutane.[9] Specialists now recommend that the drug be used only on patients with deeply seated cystic or pustular acne that is unresponsive to any other form of treatment, and who have been carefully screened for contraindications by physicians who are thoroughly familiar with the drug.[10]

Mild acne can be treated with the topical cream Retin-A (tretinoin), a milder retinoid that is subject to side effects similar to Accutane's but in lighter form. Retin-A is likely to cause sun sensitivity, so its prescription should always come with warnings to use sunscreens.

Over-the-counter topical acne remedies have also proliferated, including a variety of creams and gels based on drying agents like benzoyl peroxide. However, the products are only marginally effective. They take four to six weeks to work, if they work at all, and when you stop using them, the acne comes back. They are also quite drying to the skin. Medicated cleansers are of questionable effectiveness because the medication washes off, and harsh facial scrubs and facial saunas can actually aggravate acne.

TRACKING THE CAUSE OF ACNE

Naturopathic doctors view the skin as an important organ of elimination. Drugs can suppress its eruptions, but the toxins the skin is trying to eliminate will only be driven further into the body, manifesting later as more serious diseases. Another problem with the suppression of skin eruptions by drugs is that the drugs must be used continually. When you stop using them, the problem comes right back. A lasting cure needs to rout out what triggers the acne in the first place. Likely suspects include dietary offenders, environmental toxins, and certain drugs.

To find out if food allergies are the problem in your case, try going on an elimination diet, that is, a diet free of anything made with wheat, corn, dairy, eggs, yeast, or refined sugars. If after two or three weeks your acne goes away, systematically add foods back in, one every couple of days.[11] If a food is definitely implicated by the return of symptoms, eliminate it from the diet for at least three months. It can then be tried cautiously. If no reaction occurs, it can be eaten in moderation.

There is no scientific proof that chocolate, nuts, or colas trigger outbreaks, but anecdotal evidence suggests that they do. Since these foods have no redeeming dietary virtues, cutting them out can't hurt. Eating less fat and more fruits and vegetables can also make your skin less oily. Freshly squeezed fruit and vegetable juices—particularly carrot and cucumber juices—help oxygenate the blood and the skin it feeds. Macrobiotic fare (whole grains, no milk, and no or few animal products) has been reported to work miracles on blemishes.[12]

Bad skin can also be the result of constipation. If toxins cannot escape through the rectum, they are excreted through the skin. For natural remedies, see "Constipation" on page 91.

Acne around the mouth can indicate digestive problems. For this, digestive enzymes can help, along with general nutritional support. Colostrum (the first mammary secretions of lactating cows) can also help reduce infection. Colostrum is now available in pill form in health food stores. Product strengths vary; follow label directions.

Natural Remedies

Herbal and homeopathic remedies can help eliminate acne permanently by encouraging the body's elimination of underlying toxins.

Chinese doctors believe that toxins build up in the blood and come out through the skin. A very effective Chinese patent remedy that works to eliminate this toxic buildup is Margarite Acne Pills. The remedy is available in different strengths. You can buy it at your local health food store or from reputable distributors on the Internet. Follow label directions for use.

Effective combination homeopathic acne products are also on the market, including Clear-Ac by Hyland's (available both as an oral tablet and a topical cream) and Nelson's Acne Gel. Again, follow label directions.

For acne traced to sensitivities to specific chemical and environmental toxins, a new line of homeopathic remedies formulated to eliminate particular target toxins can be quite effective. See "Multiple Chemical Sensitivity" on page 185 for specific remedies.

Tea tree oil has been shown to remove and stop the growth of bacteria on the skin. An Australian study showed that a 5 percent tea tree oil gel was as effective as 5 percent benzoyl peroxide in treating acne. Tea tree oil should be applied to all acne-prone areas, not just to lesions, to stop pimples before they get to the surface. There are no side effects, with the exception of rare allergic reactions or irritation in sensitive individuals.[13]

Helpful Tips

The following simple home measures can help keep acne symptoms under control:

◆ **Wash with ordinary soap and water.** Dr. Bronner's pure castile soap is good. Once or twice a day is sufficient, since washing your skin too often can actually worsen acne.

◆ **Use either no cosmetics or water-based cosmetics.** Avoid greasy hair dressings and wear your hair away from your face.

◆ **Do not pick at blemishes.**

RECURRING ACNE CLEARED

Nineteen-year-old Kelley was quite self-conscious about her complexion, which was severely stricken with acne. She began taking Margarite Acne Pills (six pills twice daily), and in two weeks her complexion began to clear. In three weeks, it looked great. After that, she needed it only during flare-ups, when her blood needed cleaning.

Helen was concerned about acne in her nine-year-old daughter, Ashley, who seemed too young for the problem. Ashley's acne became aggravated whenever she went swimming. The recommended treatment was a homeopathic remedy by Mediral called Chlorex, specifically formulated for eliminating chlorine from the system. The dosage for this remedy varies with the patient's toxicity level, but for Ashley, it was five drops three times a day until the acne went away, then as needed. The remedy cleared Ashley's acne, except on days that she swam. Helen started giving her daughter Chlorinex before and after swimming, and the results were dramatic. Ashley has had no further acne problems since then.

◆ **For a facial scrub, try oatmeal.** Make a paste of rolled oats and water; leave it on your face until it dries, then wash it off.

◆ **For a natural facial mask and moisturizer, try an apple.** Peel and core an apple and put it in a blender with a little lemon or apple juice. Smooth the mixture on your face. Leave it on for about fifteen minutes, then wash it off. Lemon juice may also be used as a natural astringent. A slice of raw tomato wiped on the face is good for oily skin. Cucumber works as a refining lotion to tighten pores.

◆ **If you feel you need a commercial product, use natural formulations.** Aloe vera products, widely available in health food stores, can provide quick relief from redness and inflammation. The best aloe product contains 100 percent aloe without additives.

◆ **If possible, spend some time at the beach.** Sunshine brings oil to the surface of the skin, and saltwater acts as an astringent and cleans out the skin. For sunscreen recommendations and cautions, see "Skin Cancer and Sunburn" on page 221.

◆ **To draw oil out of blemishes, apply a paste.** You can use healing clay (available at health food stores) or make a paste by mixing baking soda and water. Another idea is to use a dab of toothpaste and tea tree oil on the blemish.[14]

ACNE ROSACEA

Acne rosacea, sometimes called "adult acne," is an acnelike condition found most commonly in fair-skinned adults between the ages of 30 and 50. It may begin as a tendency to flush or blush easily, a ruddy complexion, or an extreme sensitivity to cosmetics, progressing to persistent redness in the center of the face, and gradually involving the cheeks, forehead, chin, and nose. Over time, it may become more pronounced and persistent, leaving pimples, visible blood vessels, and sometimes an enlarged nose (the "W. C. Fields look").

The cause of acne rosacea is not known, but a bacterial or parasitic infection is suspected. It is more common in women than men, but the reason for this is also unknown. Some cases have been associated with menopause.[1] The condition can be aggravated by cold or hot weather, stress, alcohol, and spicy foods. Heredity is also a factor.

CONVENTIONAL TREATMENT

Standard drug treatment combines the oral antibiotic minocycline with MetroGel applied topically to the skin twice daily. Both drugs come with hazards. MetroGel contains metronidazole, the same strong antibiotic found in Flagyl, a parasite remedy marked with the FDA warning: "Metronidazole is carcinogenic in rodents. Avoid unnecessary use."

Minocycline, a type of tetracycline, comes with side effects including skin sensitivities, pigmentation of the skin, and severe phototoxic reactions (reactions to the sun). Other reported side effects include severe liver disease resulting in death, hepatitis, severe arthritis, and the autoimmune disease lupus, apparently caused by the body's immune system turning on itself.[2] Minocycline can also cause dizziness, discoloration of the teeth, and inflamed and aching joints and shortness of breath.[3] In addition, all antibiotics can lead to *Candida* yeast infections—which may, ironically, provoke skin eruptions.[4] Hazards are compounded by the fact that these strong medications are being put on damaged and sensitive skin. The drug combination costs between $125 and $150 a month. If you discontinue treatment, your skin returns to the state it was in before starting on the medications.[5]

NATURAL REMEDIES

Some recent evidence points to the aspergillus mold as a cause of acne rosacea. Following this lead, author Dr. Walker has recommended the combination homeopathic remedy Aspertox by Molecular Biologics for more than a dozen women, with exciting results. The remedy completely cleared redness from the faces of all of them. The recommended dosage is ten drops three times daily until the complexion clears, then ten drops once daily for maintenance, then ten drops once daily only when the face is red.

Other homeopathic remedies that have helped clear facial redness include *Calcarea silicata* (*Calc sil*) and *Rhus toxicodendron* (*Rhus tox*) (in strengths of 6, 12, or 30, three pellets three times daily).

Safe nutritional remedies that can help include vitamin K cream (many brands are available) and oral antioxidants containing oligomeric proanthocyanins (OPCs). Pycnogenol is particularly good. The recommended dosage is 1 mg per pound of body weight.

A device made in Switzerland called a Bioptron Light Therapy machine very effectively eliminates the symptoms of acne rosacea, although it is expensive (about $400). The device is a rapidly blinking light that stimulates healing.

Other recommendations for alleviating acne rosacea include avoiding aggravating factors (stress, alcohol, and spicy foods); bundling up in cold weather and staying well ventilated in hot weather; eating right and exercising; and using a natural moisturizer. For some good natural home facial treatments, see "Acne" on page 31.

ACNE ROSACEA ELIMINATED WITHOUT DRUGS

Bunny, 52, had been told she would need to use topical MetroGel for the rest of her life to control acne rosacea, but she was worried that the drug would cause permanent damage to her face. To her relief, Bioptron Light Therapy, along with homeopathic *Rhus toxicodendron* and *Aspergillus* (Aspertox by Molecular Biologics) totally cleared the condition without drugs.

Ruth is a beautiful, rosy-cheeked, 40-year-old woman who looks much younger than her age. She was concerned, however, about her complexion because it had so much redness in it. Her dermatologist had told her that her face could get very inflamed and deformed and had urged her to use topical MetroGel. She consulted with Dr. Walker, who gave her *Calcarea silicata*. It helped, but she still had a few red blotches she was unhappy about. Dr. Walker then gave her homeopathic *Aspergillus* (Aspertox, ten drops three times daily). The remedy worked remarkably well, clearing up all remaining redness without drugs.

Sally, 40, also sought Dr. Walker's advice after her doctor prescribed MetroGel for her rosacea. She was leery of the drug but felt she had to do something about her condition. She was going on a trip where she would be meeting her boyfriend and she wanted to look her best. Dr. Walker recommended that she stop all perfumed soaps and use Nelson's Acne Gel, calendula lotion, and Aspertox. Sally, too, was delighted to report that these remedies cleared her complexion without drug treatment.

ADRENAL STRESS

The adrenal glands secrete adrenaline, the emergency hormone that wakes up the body and prepares it for action. Adrenaline is useful to an animal under attack requiring immediate action, but it can wreak havoc on the body of the modern woman who is on "red alert" all day long from the stress of her job, traffic, cell phones, and a busy lifestyle. Adrenaline is on the same hormone chain as the female hormones, so in times of stress, the body has to choose which to manufacture first. When additional adrenaline is secreted, other body hormones wind up in short supply.

There is some evidence that people with chronic fatigue syndrome, adrenal exhaustion, and anxiety syndromes have an abnormal response to adrenaline. Once they start secreting it, they can't turn it off. They can't sleep well at night, since adrenaline that hasn't been cleared keeps their systems in emergency mode. Then they are tired the next day, requiring even more adrenaline to get by, and so they become deficient in the female hormones. The cycle goes on this way until something is done to stop it.

CONVENTIONAL TREATMENT

These symptoms are conventionally treated with tranquilizers, sleeping pills, and SSRIs (selective serotonin reuptake inhibitors, the class of drug that includes Prozac). All these drugs have serious side effects (detailed under the "Insomnia," "Anxiety," and "Depression" sections), and they don't address the underlying problem—adrenal stress.

UNRECOGNIZED STRESS UNCOVERED AND RELIEVED

Mary Ann came to Dr. Walker for help after being diagnosed with symptoms of early menopause and given a prescription for hormone replacement therapy. Dr. Walker asked about her stress level, but Mary Ann denied being under any unusual stress. Dr. Walker persisted: How was her work? Her marriage? Who does the laundry and other household chores? Who pays the bills?

Soon Mary Ann's story changed. Her sister had been killed in a car accident six months earlier, and she had been left to deal with the whole family crisis herself. Her husband had lost his job around the same time and was very depressed. Still, she couldn't see what all that had to do with her hot flashes and her memory loss. When she came to understand that the unusual stresses in her life were the cause of her physical problems, she began to view her health problems differently. Supporting her adrenal system with Adrenal/Spleen by CompliMed (ten drops three times daily) and relieving her stress put her body back into balance and made her hot flashes go away.

NATURAL REMEDIES

Natural remedies can help support the adrenals and relieve adrenal stress. Animal extract adrenal complexes are available, but there is some concern that they may make the situation worse by increasing cortisol levels, and they don't seem to work well over the long term. Homeopathic and herbal remedies are preferred. Adrenal/Spleen, a combination homeopathic remedy by CompliMed, is particularly effective. Other good homeopathic options are Norepinephrine, Neuro I, and Neuro II by Deseret Biologicals. The dosage for all of these remedies is ten drops three times daily. Licorice root concentrate can also help, with the proviso that it may increase blood pressure. This herb is available in health food stores; follow label directions.

Most important for relieving adrenal stress is to take time to unwind, meditate, and regenerate. We often don't realize how much stress we're under during the day. We owe it to our bodies to slow down and relax. Exercise, a natural stimulant, can also help burn off old adrenaline residues.

ALLERGIES

An allergy is an inappropriate immune system reaction to some trigger in the environment (foods, pollen, dander, chemicals, and so forth). Symptoms may include skin rash, chronic coughs and bronchitis, diarrhea, migraine headaches, and colitis. Allergies have also been linked to a number of chronic degenerative and emotional diseases to which women are more prone than men, including chronic fatigue syndrome, fibromyalgia, candidiasis, parasitic infection, environmental illness, and multiple chemical sensitivities.[1] Women's immune systems seem to go on overload faster than men's; their livers have more to deal with, and their bodies are generally smaller and more easily overwhelmed.

One theory traces the underlying problem in allergies and other immune dysfunctions to an abnormal permeability of the gastrointestinal tract, lungs, and skin—meaning things seep into them more easily. Because of this condition, inappropriate food constituents, chemicals, and pollens are allowed into the blood, where they can trigger an immune reaction. Also called leaky gut syndrome, hyperpermeability of the intestinal tract can result from parasitic infection or from insufficient digestive enzymes.

Low stomach acid and low digestive enzyme levels impair digestion, weakening mucous membranes and allowing unwanted toxins to pass through the defense of the gut wall and into the bloodstream. Since poor digestion only partially breaks down food, the food particles passing through the gut barrier are unusually large. As a result, the immune system does not recognize them as food but thinks they are foreign invaders. System-wide immune reactions are set off, in which immune system cells called lymphocytes are produced in great numbers and sent on the rampage. Excess lymphocytes then wind up attacking weakened cells in normal body tissues.[2]

An increased incidence of allergies in industrialized countries has been linked to an increase in pollutants, chemicals, pesticides, and other allergy-provoking foreign substances. See "Multiple Chemical Sensitivity" on page 185.

CONVENTIONAL TREATMENT

Antihistamines have been available for the treatment of allergies since the 1940s, but the drugs only address symptoms without reaching the cause, and they can have unwanted side effects. A drawback of the older versions (Benadryl, Allerest, and Chlor-Trimeton) is that they produce drowsiness. A later-model antihistamine called terfenadine (Seldane) overcame this problem, but the FDA withdrew it from the market in 1997 when a rash of deaths was attributed to its use in conjunction with certain other drugs. Other antihistamines

(Claritin, Hismanal, Zyrtec, Allegra) are available and effective, but their modes of action are similar to Seldane's, making them potentially hazardous as well.[3]

Steroid-containing nasal sprays are also available for the treatment of hay fever (Vancenase, Flonase, and so on). The sprays are thought to reduce the serious systemic effects of steroids taken by mouth, since they come into contact only with the nose rather than with the whole body; however, their safety still remains to be established. The new steroid inhalers for asthma, which were also thought to be safer than steroids taken by mouth, have now been found to have some of the same side effects as oral steroids.[4] Other drawbacks of the sprays are that they take two to four days to work and can irritate the nasal passages.

For the treatment of hay fever, decongestants or decongestant/antihistamine combinations should be avoided, since they can cause a rebound effect and are potentially addicting if used for more than a few days. They are particularly hazardous for use with hay fever, which tends to last for longer periods of time.

Allergy Shots

Allergy desensitization injections are generally reserved for people with severe allergies, since they are a long and expensive commitment with an uncertain outcome. A typical course can take three to five years, and it may be a full year before any improvement is seen. The required once- or twice-weekly office visits have been called annuities for allergists. Whether the shots actually reduce or eliminate allergies has never been proven, since many young people outgrow their allergies without treatment. A study reported in *The New England Journal of Medicine* in January 1997 found that most children with asthma don't benefit from allergy shots.[5]

NATURAL REMEDIES

Homeopathic and herbal remedies can rebalance the body in a way that helps eliminate the underlying cause of allergies, including poor digestion, a weakened immune system, and parasites.

For poor digestion, supplemental enzymes can help. Insufficient digestive enzymes come from the cooking, microwaving, and processing that destroy enzymes found naturally in foods. Food gets to the colon partially undigested, leaving toxic residues that must be detoxified by the liver. When the liver becomes overloaded, toxins enter the blood, evoking an autoimmune response and the production of circulating immune complexes.

Pancreatic enzyme formulations have been shown to reduce autoimmune symptoms.[6] These enzymes should be taken on an empty stomach, not less than forty-five minutes before or two hours after meals. To aid digestion in the stomach, enzymes that are not enteric coated may be taken with meals.

Digestion can also be improved by eating enzyme-rich raw fruits and vegetables. For other suggestions, see "Digestive Problems" on page 104. *Caution: Supplemental enzymes are not recommended for people with bleeding disorders, inflammation of the intestines, reflux, or ulcers.*

Although a tendency to develop allergies is often hereditary, the allergies may not manifest themselves if the adrenal glands are producing enough cortisol. Adrenal/Spleen homeopathic drops by CompliMed, or Adrenal Liquescence by PCH, have helped many people with allergies. For both, take ten drops three times daily or according to label directions. Use particularly on stressful days.

Effective homeopathic remedies are available that can help desensitize the body to specific allergens. A number of companies make good combination homeopathic remedies identified on the label by allergen. CompliMed makes Mold/Yeast/Dust, Enviro-Pest, Enviro-Met, Enviro-Chem, and Dairy. Molecular Biologics also makes a remedy called Dairy, as well as Weeds and Grass, and Grains and Seeds, for grain and gluten sensitivity.

To reduce pesticide toxicity, homeopathic detox remedies such as Ex-Chem by Apex or Enviro-Pest by CompliMed can help. Directions for use of all of these products are on the labels. Avoid the offending allergens while undergoing homeopathic treatment. Combination homeopathic remedies are also available for people who don't know what they are allergic to, including Allerdrain and Aller-Total by Apex. To help in choosing the right remedy, a homeopath's advice is recommended, particularly if you are allergic to several different foods.

A new concept in allergy therapy is the theory of phenolics—meaning that people with allergies to several foods are allergic not to the foods themselves but to one or more chemical components common to them. Homeopathic treatment of a single phenolic can address multiple allergies. Malvin, for example, is a chemical found in red foods. If you're allergic to tomatoes, apples, and grapes, you may have a malvin allergy. If you're allergic to both wheat and dairy products, you may have a sensitivity to rutin, a chemical found in both types of foods. Deseret Biologicals makes a line of homeopathic remedies based on the phenolic theory. Again, it's best to see an experienced homeopath for guidance in your own case.

Substantial improvement from food allergies may also result simply by avoiding the common offenders—eggs, milk, nuts, soy, wheat, and nightshade vegetables (tomatoes, potatoes, green peppers, and eggplant). If you suspect a food allergy, try eliminating these foods until symptoms disappear, then add them back into your diet one by one. If a food is definitely implicated by the return of symptoms, eliminate it from the diet for at least three months. It can then be tried cautiously. If no reaction occurs, it can be eaten in moderation.[7]

For congestion, try hot tea made with natural decongestants such as fenugreek, anise, and sage (available as commercial preparations in health food stores). Garlic, onions, and hot and spicy foods can also thin out mucus.

A gemmotherapy that can help relieve allergies is Black Currant by Dolisos. Take fifty drops in half a glass of water each morning.

In *Your Body's Many Cries for Water*, F. Batmanghelidj, M.D., asserts that allergies and asthma (a chronic respiratory condition usually triggered by allergies) are diseases of water dehydration. He has seen many cases cured simply by increasing the patient's intake of pure water.[8] He says we need half our bodies' weight in ounces of water per day—not coffee, tea, soft drinks, or juices, but plain (filtered or bottled) water. Thus, a 128-pound woman would need 64 ounces, or eight 8-ounce glasses of water. Wait a half hour before meals and two and a half hours after meals for your heavy water doses to avoid diluting your digestive juices. Dr. Batmanghelidj advises adding ½ teaspoon of salt to your diet daily for every ten glasses of water you drink. (Unheated sea salt is preferred. Better yet is Bio-Salt by Gilbert's Health Food Labs in England, a biochemically balanced mineral salt compound containing sodium chloride plus all the cell salts.)

ALZHEIMER'S DISEASE

More than 4 million Americans have Alzheimer's disease, and women outnumber men with it by about two to one. A mental deterioration in the elderly that cannot be explained by normal aging, Alzheimer's disease now strikes half of all people over age 75. Nearly twenty times as many deaths were reported from it in the early 1990s as in the late 1970s.[1] Alzheimer's disease also accounts for 30 percent of nursing home admissions. Symptoms include gradual memory loss, disorientation, loss of language ability, and personality changes that can extend over a number of years.

Conventional research has focused on genetics, but the cause of Alzheimer's disease remains elusive. Although female hormones may play a role, the theory is controversial. Research has suggested that women who take estrogen are less likely to develop Alzheimer's disease, but a study reported in *The Journal of the American Medical Association* (*JAMA*) in February 2000 found that once the disease has set in, estrogen affords no benefit. The study involved 120 older women with mild to moderate Alzheimer's disease who were given either a low estrogen dose, a high estrogen dose, or a placebo every day for a year. No significant differences were found in tests of mental function, mood, memory, attention, language skills, or motor function. By the end of the study, those taking estrogen actually fared somewhat worse than the placebo group in a rating of dementia. The researchers concluded, "Overall, the results of this study do not support the role of estrogen in the treatment" of Alzheimer's disease.[2]

Other research has linked Alzheimer's disease to aspartame, a very popular artificial sweetener. Aspartame (NutraSweet) is a chemical poison that slowly kills neurons, and weight-watching women are more likely than men to use it.

Still other research has linked Alzheimer's disease to shingles and the herpes virus.[3] Shingles, like chicken pox, is caused by the virus herpes zoster. The homeopathic theory is that drugs given to treat these conditions (usually acyclovir) actually trap the virus inside the brain, precipitating Alzheimer's disease.

For the role that heavy metals may play in Alzheimer's disease, see the inset "Alzheimer's Disease and Heavy Metals" on page 41.

CONVENTIONAL TREATMENT

Conventional medicine has no cure for Alzheimer's disease. A drug called tacrine (Cognex) can slow deterioration somewhat, but it can also cause uncomfortable and dangerous side effects, and it is expensive and hard to administer.[4] Other drugs can ease pain, agitation, and paranoia, but conventional treatment for the most part consists simply of helping patients and their families cope with the disease.

One drug that seems to help is desferrioxamine, which removes aluminum from the body by binding with it. In a placebo-controlled trial, the drug was found to significantly reduce the rate of decline in the ability of a group of people with Alzheimer's disease to care for themselves.[5]

The success of desferrioxamine again points to toxic chemical and heavy metal buildup as a suspected cause of this elusive disease. Case studies indicate that if caught early enough, the disease process may be reversible by detox techniques that eliminate this buildup. Getting toxic chemicals and heavy metals out of the diet and the teeth is only half

ALZHEIMER'S DISEASE AND HEAVY METALS

Some evidence points to toxic chemical and heavy metal buildup in the brain as causal factors for Alzheimer's disease, a condition known to involve degeneration of nerve cells. The nerves become twisted and tangled, and hardened deposits of chemical plaque are found in the brain. The blood-brain barrier keeps most chemical toxins from entering the brain, but it also prevents those that do get in from getting back out. Thus, they continue to build up over the years, progressively blocking brain and nerve function.[6]

Aluminum, mercury, and lead are leading suspects. The link with aluminum has been demonstrated by accumulations of the metal found in the brains of patients who died of Alzheimer's disease. Pathological changes similar to those seen in Alzheimer's disease have also been observed after exposure to aluminum.[7] Earlier observations linking the metal to the disease were confirmed in a study of eighty-eight county districts in England and Wales, which found a definite connection between the incidence of Alzheimer's disease and average aluminum levels in the water supply.[8] The use of aluminum-containing antiperspirants and antacids has also been associated with Alzheimer's disease.[9]

Mercury was linked to Alzheimer's disease in humans in 1990, when University of Kentucky researchers found significant elevations of mercury in the brains of 180 Kentucky residents who were autopsied after dying of the disease.[10] Cats fed fish containing methyl mercury show Alzheimer's-like brain lesions, and humans who eat mercury-laden fish exhibit neurological symptoms, including memory loss, tremors, irritability, insomnia, numbness, and visual disturbances.[11]

The greatest human exposure to mercury seems to be the standard silver/mercury amalgam dental filling. Recent research has established that mercury from fillings is released into the body with chewing, and that it accumulates in brain tissue.[12] In studies of the cadavers of accident victims, those with a mere five amalgams had three times the amount of mercury in their brain tissue as cadavers without amalgams.[13] A later autopsy study done by the Mayo Heavy Metals Lab on an 82-year-old decedent with confirmed Alzheimer's disease found fifty-three times the normal level of mercury in the woman's brain. The "neurofibrillary tangle" characteristic of Alzheimer's disease was also found. The woman had multiple amalgams in her teeth. Other research shows that people with mercury fillings have higher levels of mercury not only in their brains but also in their urine and blood.[14]

the battle. They must also be eliminated from brain tissues. For this, chelation techniques may be effective.[15] The chelation process and available chelation alternatives are described in detail in Chapter 5.

NATURAL REMEDIES

Besides therapies to reduce toxins in the brain, a number of nutritional and herbal remedies have been found to help relieve the symptoms of Alzheimer's disease.

The herb ginkgo biloba has been shown to reduce mental decline in more than a dozen double-blind studies, including one reported in *JAMA* in October 1997. The world's oldest species of tree, ginkgo has long been known in traditional Chinese medicine to benefit mental function. It seems to increase blood flow to the brain, improving the supply of oxygen and glucose.

Traditional Chinese healers also maintain that a tea made from a plant called club moss (*Shen Jin Cao*) improves memory and failing mental capacity. A drug now undergoing testing for Alzheimer's disease called Huperzine A is a derivative of club moss. The tea version is currently available in the Chinatown sections of large cities.[16]

In April 1997, *The New England Journal of Medicine* reported that 2,000 IU of vitamin E daily is a simple home remedy showing benefits for those with Alzheimer's disease. The remedy was easy to administer, inexpensive, and had no unwanted side effects.[17]

Another nutrient found to help people with Alzheimer's disease is nicotinamide ade-

REMARKABLE RESULTS WITH HOMEOPATHY AND CHELATION

Pam, age 56, was referred to Dr. Walker after being diagnosed by several doctors with early onset Alzheimer's disease, a rare disorder. The person who referred her hadn't seen Pam in almost a year and said she appeared to have aged ten or fifteen years in that time. On the day Pam came in for consultation, Dr. Walker chanced to read about congressional investigations into NutraSweet and its link to Alzheimer's disease. When Pam was found to be severely chemically toxic and was asked about her NutraSweet ingestion, Pam's daughter's jaw dropped. She said her mother drank up to six diet cokes daily and added NutraSweet to everything she ate. Pam was advised to stop all NutraSweet intake and was put on homeopathic *Aspartamine* to clear aspartame residues from her body. She was also given homeopathic *Zinc,* a constitutional remedy specific to her symptoms, to help eliminate other heavy metals from her system. In a month, she was a different person. Her memory and personality had returned, she began driving again, and she was fully coherent. She continues to make progress to this day.

In *Beating Alzheimer's,* Tom Warren attests that his own diagnosed case of Alzheimer's disease was reversed after he had all of his teeth pulled and replaced with dentures. (His teeth contained twenty-eight mercury amalgam fillings.) He also had chelation treatments and took homeopathic remedies to remove heavy metals from his tissues, changed his diet, took heavy doses of nutritional supplements, and eliminated environmental toxins from his surroundings. Other cases he cites include that of a physician who recovered from Alzheimer's disease after the removal of thirteen teeth containing root canals.[18]

nine dinucleotide (NADH). NADH is present in all living things and plays a central role in cellular energy production. In one study, patients given 10 mg of this supplement a half-hour before breakfast for eight to twelve weeks showed significant improvement on an examination of mental state.[19]

An Italian study found acetyl-L-carnitine to be effective in slowing the progression of Alzheimer's disease.[20] In another study, Alzheimer's patients given 90 mg of zinc, 2 mg of selenium, and 6 g of evening primrose oil scored better on a battery of mental function tests than those in a placebo group.[21]

Alzheimer's disease patients tend to be low in vitamin B_{12}, even when dietary intake is adequate. Apparently, they have a problem absorbing the vitamin. For this deficiency, vitamin B_{12} shots can help.[22] Improvements have also been documented in Alzheimer's disease patients given coenzyme Q_{10}, iron, and vitamin B_6. Other studies have found improvements with various protocols using DMSO (dimethyl sulfoxide, a natural wood derivative).[23]

F. Batmanghelidj, M.D., documented a case in which Alzheimer's disease symptoms were reversed simply by increasing water intake to eight 8-ounce glasses a day. See Chapter 4 for details of this water treatment.

While all of these remedies could be of benefit, Alzheimer's disease is clearly a serious and complicated disease, for which professional medical help should be sought.

AMENORRHEA (PREMATURE CESSATION OF MENSTRUATION)

Secondary amenorrhea, or a premature lack of menstrual periods in a woman who has previously had them, is experienced by about 1 percent of women. Besides pregnancy, skipped periods can have a number of causes including emotional or mental shock, stress, and hormone imbalance. Overactivity of the adrenal glands or underactivity of the thyroid gland can cause it. So can birth control pills—for up to six months after they are discontinued. If hot flashes, breast atrophy, and decreased sex drive accompany the condition, it may be due to premature ovarian failure or early menopause. Menstrual periods may stop in women athletes during rigorous training schedules (a condition called athletic amenorrhea), or during excess weight loss or weight gain. Anorexia nervosa is often accompanied by secondary amenorrhea. Certain medications such as phenothiazines used for psychiatric disorders and some narcotics can also cause amenorrhea.

CONVENTIONAL TREATMENT

The medical solution is to give Provera (synthetic progesterone) in high doses, then discontinue it. Menstruation typically follows. Synthetic progesterone, however, can have significant side effects (detailed in Chapter 2). Another drug given for this purpose is the birth control pill.

NATURAL REMEDIES

The first step in natural treatment is to locate the cause of the problem. If hormonal imbalances are found, remedies to correct them can help. One homeopathic option is Hormone Combination by Deseret. The dosage is ten drops three times daily to balance the hormones, then ten drops once daily for maintenance. Constitutional homeopathic remedies specific for a woman's constitution and type can also help rebalance the body. Deseret and other companies make homeopathic progesterone and estrogen that can be of benefit.

ProGest natural progesterone cream is another option, which works like Provera but without the side effects. Women 35 to 40 years old need to use it for only a short period, perhaps for three or four days before menstruation. If it is then stopped abruptly, the period usually follows. For women in perimenopause, the number of days' use can be stretched to seven or fourteen, as needed.

Emotional, weight, and stress problems also need to be addressed, and correcting the diet is important. If iron is deficient, more iron-containing protein should be included in the diet. To locate and correct mechanical obstructions, see a physician.

AMENORRHEA CORRECTED WITH NATURAL REMEDIES

When Barbara stopped menstruating for a year at age 38, she was diagnosed by her doctor as being in early menopause. Depressed and unhappy with this diagnosis at such an early age, she decided to explore natural remedies. At Barbara's first exam, Dr. Walker discovered that her thyroid levels were very low and her stress level was high, affecting her hormone balance. After only a few months on Thyroid homeopathic drops (ten drops three times daily) and ProGest natural progesterone cream (¼ teaspoon daily for half of each month), Barbara's periods returned. However, they stopped again two months later. On her next exam, to her surprise and delight, she learned that she was not experiencing early menopause; she was pregnant! Her medical doctor was also quite surprised, when she dropped in to review his earlier diagnosis and to show off her healthy baby boy.

ANEMIA

Anemia is a condition in which body tissues get insufficient oxygen, either because there aren't enough red blood cells in circulation or because the blood is low in hemoglobin, an essential protein. Iron deficiency anemia occurs when the body lacks iron, a necessary constituent of hemoglobin. Normal, healthy women can become anemic just from menstruating, since iron is lost with menstrual blood. Iron deficiency anemia can also result from a lack of iron in the diet, something to which dieting women are susceptible. It may also result from a lack of other nutrients, including folic acid and vitamin B_{12}. Other causes of anemia include chronic blood loss from stomach ulcers or hemorrhoids, or from something that destroys blood cells or interferes with their production in the body. Some types of anemia (for example, sickle cell anemia) are hereditary.

Drugs and alcohol can also cause anemia. The daily loss of imperceptible amounts of blood in the stool from habitual aspirin use, as by arthritis victims, is particularly insidious because it produces no symptoms. This is a problem particularly for women, whom arthritis strikes nearly twice as often as men. Older people who already don't get enough iron, and women who lose iron through heavy periods, are at additional risk from heavy aspirin use. Besides iron, aspirin also increases your need for certain vitamins, notably vitamin C, vitamin B_1, and folic acid.

CONVENTIONAL TREATMENT

Anemia is usually treated with supplemental iron, but iron supplements aren't very effective in rebuilding the blood. They take a long time to be absorbed, can be constipating, and are highly toxic in overdose. Enteric-coated supplements cannot be effectively absorbed and should be avoided. *It's best not to take iron supplements unless directed to do so by a health professional.*

Anemia may also be treated conventionally with supplements of folic acid or other nutrients in which the patient's blood levels are low. Serious types of anemia, such as those caused by bleeding of the digestive tract, are conventionally corrected by surgery.

NATURAL REMEDIES

If iron supplements are definitely needed as confirmed by a health professional, ferrous gluconate is a good absorbable form. Floradix is an iron-containing herbal combination that is easily absorbed. Follow directions on the label. Hemaplex by Nature's Plus is another good option. Take one tablet daily.

Chlorophyll, the "blood" of plants, has a chemical composition very similar to hemoglobin and can help rebuild the blood. Chlorophyll is particularly abundant in green vegetables. Another alternative is supplemental chlorophyll (2 ounces in water two to three times daily), or "green" pills: spirulina, chlorella, or Ultimate Green by Nature's Secret. Dosages are on the label.

Excess soy in the diet can inhibit iron absorption, leading to anemia and iron deficiency in women.[1] It is best is to limit intake to one serving of a soy product daily.

The homeopathic remedy for anemia is *Ferrum phos* taken as a cell salt in a 6X potency three to four times daily. It will build the blood over a period of several months without causing constipation like most iron supplements. It also boosts the immune systems of people who suffer from chronic colds. Moreover, it is a good remedy for bleeding problems, including chronic nosebleeds and long, heavy menstrual periods.

The Eastern Approach

In Chinese medicine, anemia is referred to as "blood deficiency" and is diagnosed from a pale tongue or the faintness of the lines on the palm of the hand. Chinese doctors say there is not enough blood in these cases to "nourish the heart," so the *Shen* (spirit), which resides in the heart, is disturbed. The patient can't sleep, has nightmares, experiences heart palpitations, becomes pale, and loses her hair. The Chinese formula for correcting this condition in women is called Women's Precious Pills. Take eight pills three times daily or as directed on the label.

ANGINA PECTORIS

See HEART DISEASE.

ANOREXIA NERVOSA AND BULIMIA

Anorexia nervosa and bulimia are eating disorders that are psychological in origin but can have serious physical consequences. Both involve an obsession with weight loss. People with anorexia starve themselves, while people with bulimia engage in episodes of bingeing on large quantities of food, followed by severe food restriction and often vomiting, laxative abuse, or excessive exercising to prevent weight gain. Health risks include major disturbance of the blood chemistry and rupture of the stomach, which can cause sudden death. More common adverse effects are zinc deficiency and damage to the teeth resulting from stomach acid constantly washing over them. If the illness is severe, the victim may also become withdrawn, fail to make normal relationships, and become moody and intolerant. The greatest risks are from suicide or self harm as a result of emotional disturbances.[1]

CONVENTIONAL TREATMENT

Psychotheapy, nutritional support, appetite enhancers, antidepressants, and antianxiety drugs are the usual conventional treatments. For the downsides of the drug options, see "Depression" on page 95 and "Anxiety and Panic Disorders" on page 46.

NATURAL REMEDIES

For eating disorders, zinc therapy may help. After a few weeks of not eating, mineral deficiencies become the compelling reason for rejecting food. Without an optimum level of zinc in the body, food has no taste or tastes quite bad. A taste test with a zinc solution will reveal this deficiency. The anorexic person notes no disagreeable taste, while a normal person with sufficient zinc in the tissues will spit the solution out immediately. Metagenics makes a test called Zinc Tally, available from pharmacies or health practitioners.

If anorexia is due to anemia, an iron tonic can help boost the appetite for solids. Floradix is a good brand that is available in health food stores. Use as directed on the label.

A gemmotherapy called Lime Tree by Dolisos can help in cases of both anorexia and bulimia. Take fifty drops in water daily.

Platina 30C is a homeopathic remedy that can help in the case of a girl who believes she is overweight when others feel her weight is normal. The dosage is three pills three times daily or as needed.

For natural remedies for the anxiety associated with eating disorders, see "Anxiety and Panic Disorders" below.

ANTIBIOTIC OVERUSE

See INFECTIONS, BACTERIAL AND VIRAL.

ANXIETY AND PANIC DISORDERS

Ten percent of the American population suffers from anxiety disorders, which are significantly more common in women than in men. Explanations offered for the gender difference include the increased pressures of work and family on women today, the sexual and physical abuses to which some women are subject, and the roller coaster of female hormonal changes that can throw stressed women out of balance.[1]

General anxiety disorder is a pathological condition characterized by disabling apprehension, worry, irritability, and vigilance, initially manifesting about age 20 to 35. When anxiety progresses to full-blown panic disorder (unpredictable episodes of intense anxiety), physiological responses can result (rapid heartbeat, dizziness, trembling, and choking).[2] Other distressing signs and symptoms are dyspnea (shortness of breath), palpitations, headache, a sense of smothering, nausea, bloating, and a feeling of impending doom. Recurrent sleep panic attacks (not nightmares) occur in about 30 percent of people with panic disorder. Less obvious effects of chronic anxiety include weakened immunity, nervousness, indigestion, problems concentrating, sleeplessness, increased blood pressure, and chronic fatigue.

Other anxiety disorders include phobias—claustrophobia, agoraphobia (fear of open or public places), acrophobia (fear of great heights)—obsessions (obsessive-compulsive disorder, compulsive hand washing, counting rituals, mechanical impulses like turning a light switch off and on), hair pulling, nail biting, hypochondria, and eating disorders. (See "Anorexia and Bulimia" on page 45.)

CONVENTIONAL TREATMENT

Doctors are liable to approach anxiety disorders either by doing a very expensive psychological workup or by treating the problem lightly with comments such as "You're just anxious, dear," and sending the patient home with a prescription for a minor tranquilizer.[3] Both approaches may miss the real cause, and drugs have other downsides.

In the 1950s, the drugs of choice for anxiety were a class of prescription sedative/hypnotics called barbiturates (phenobarbital, amobarbital, and butabarbital), which produced an intoxication similar to that of alcohol. One problem was that moderate overdoses could be fatal. They became favorites of people with suicidal tendencies and were the drugs that killed Marilyn Monroe and Judy Garland.

The benzodiazepines, or "minor" tranquilizers, were considered a major advance over the barbiturates. Valium (diazepam) was the market leader for many years. In 1980, Valium was among the top five drugs prescribed in the United States. Originally thought to be nonaddicting, Valium now heads the list of drugs that cause dependence. Unfortunately, by the time the fallacy of this presumption became apparent, thousands of people were already hooked on it.

Meanwhile, the newer benzodiazepines—Xanax (alprazolam) and Halcion (triazolam)—had climbed to third and sixteenth among brand-name prescription drugs.[4] Halcion became the world's best-selling sleeping pill. But charges against these newer benzodiazepines, too, are mounting. Halcion has been linked to violent behavior and to seizures, amnesia, hallucinations, personality disorders, and other side effects.[5] As for Xanax, some researchers assert that it is potentially one of the most dangerous drugs on the market. It can cause powerful withdrawal symptoms, including severe convulsions. It and other benzodiazepines have also been linked to casualties ranging from highway fatalities to hip fractures from elderly patients tripping or falling out of bed.[6]

The newer benzodiazepines have shorter half-lives (an indication of the amount of time they stay in the body), but that means they can have more serious side effects when you try to break the habit. This syndrome can cause you to keep taking them when you'd rather quit.[7]

The latest craze in drugs for anxiety, depression, and a host of other ills are selective serotonin reuptake inhibitors (SSRIs)—Prozac and its relatives (Zoloft, Paxil, and others). Although SSRIs can prevent panic attacks, they won't stop them once begun. Xanax and Valium, on the other hand, can stop panic attacks, but these drugs are addictive and cause sedation. SSRIs can also have quite serious side effects, and they alter brain chemicals so that getting off them can be difficult and can lead to rebound panic. For a fuller discussion of SSRIs and their side effects, see "Depression" on page 95.

Caution: If you are on prescription antianxiety or insomnia drugs, switching to a different remedy should be done only under professional supervision.[8]

NATURAL REMEDIES

Natural Serotonin Stimulants

The natural, balanced way to decrease anxiety is to increase levels of serotonin, a neurotransmitter that makes us calm, mellow, and content. It can be increased by increasing its natural precursors, the amino acids L-tryptophan and L-tyrosine. Tryptophan, the most effective serotonin producer currently known, was used as a safe and natural alternative to pharmaceutical tranquilizers for nearly half a century. In 1989, however, it was removed from the market by the FDA following reports of some serious side effects and deaths from

TRACKING THE CAUSE OF ANXIETY AND PANIC ATTACKS

Drug treatment may miss the real cause of an anxiety order. Women with symptoms of sweating, chest pain, and accelerated heart rate are more likely than men to be misdiagnosed with anxiety disorder when they actually have heart disease, a condition for which postmenopausal women are at increased risk. Panic attacks can also be precipitated by an underactive or overactive thyroid. For testing for and correcting hormonal imbalances, see "Hypothyroidism" on page 150, "Hyperthyroidism" on page 148, and "Menopause and Perimenopuase" on page 174.

Other causes of panic and anxiety symptoms include excess consumption of caffeine, nicotine, alcohol, and common over-the-counter medications, including cold medicines containing antihistamines or decongestants, diet drugs, and pain relievers such as ibuprofen.[9] Anxiety may also be triggered by hypoglycemia or food allergies.

its use. The problem was ultimately traced to contamination in a manufacturing process involving genetic engineering used by a particular Japanese manufacturer.[10] Food sources of this amino acid include milk, pumpkin seeds, and turkey.

New on the market is a highly effective homeopathic serotonin enhancer called Serotonin by Deseret. It stimulates the body to produce its own serotonin and, like all homeopathics, is entirely safe. Many people have succeeded in weaning themselves off Prozac and pulling themselves out of their inexplicable depressions using this simple and inexpensive remedy. For seasonal depression or for depression with insomnia, use either homeopathic Serotonin by Deseret or Serotonin & Tryptophan by CompliMed. The dosage for both is ten drops three times daily.

The body's serotonin levels may also be raised by changing the diet. High-carbohydrate foods have been found to relieve depression, anger, tension, tiredness, and moodiness, apparently because they elevate serotonin levels.[11] Sugary foods should be avoided, however, since they can wreak havoc on the blood sugar level, and erratic drops in blood sugar can cause both depression and binging. The best carbohydrates are whole grains—oatmeal and other whole-grain cereals, whole-grain breads, rice, and potatoes.

Exercise has also been shown to increase brain concentrations of serotonin and norepinephrine.[12] Running is well known for the "runner's high." Note, however, that jogging carries certain risks as you get older, including blood clotting, which can increase the risk of strokes and heart attacks; flat feet; varicose veins; and uterine prolapse.[13] Walking, swimming, and low-impact aerobics are safer alternatives.

Homeopathic Options

For phobias and to bring out and eliminate the underlying cause of anxieties, constitutional homeopathic treatment from a qualified homeopath is often effective. Below are some homeopathic remedies that are good for alleviating specific anxieties. Take three pellets as needed.

- ◆ For dread of the future—*Argentum nitricum.*
- ◆ For a letdown or sad event—*Ignatia.*
- ◆ For anxiety from hot weather—*Pulsatilla.*

◆ For anxiety from the aftereffects of a fright (for example, a car accident)—*Aconite.*

◆ For anxiety that is worse when alone—*Arsenicum.*

◆ For anxiety that is worse at nightfall—*Phosphorus.*

◆ For "anticipatory anxiety" (nervousness before a speech or an exam)— *Gelsemium* 30X.

Botanical Alchemy makes an effective combination product line that includes the following:

◆ For held-in resentment—Transform Anger.

◆ For old emotional wounds, resentments against mates or ex-mates—Healing Heart.

◆ For menopausal women who have lost interest in sex, women who withhold sex out of resentment, and other sexual problems—Sexual Healing.

Also excellent for emotional imbalances is Energize by CompliMed. Take one tablet as needed. Cherry Plum and Rescue Remedy are Bach flower remedies that can calm anxieties without side effects. Take two to four drops up to four times daily as needed (under the tongue or sipped in your water bottle).

Herbal and Other Alternatives

Research shows that herbs can be as effective as prescription drugs for treating anxiety, without their dangerous side effects. St. John's wort is an herbal substitute for Prozac that many people find effective at a much reduced cost. Recommended dosage is 300 mg three to four times daily.

An herbal formula found to be effective without side effects is Skullcap Oats by Eclectic Institute. Use as directed on the label.

The Chinese feel that a stagnant liver can contribute to anxiety. *Xiao Yao Wan* (Relaxed Wanderer) is an Eastern herbal remedy that helps move liver stagnation. Another Chinese herbal remedy useful for anxiety and heart palpitations is *Bai Zj Yang Xin Wan.* These remedies are available from different manufacturers at Chinese drugstores or from acupuncturists.

A nutrient formula that can help is Stress X by Trace Minerals Research. Follow label directions.

For obsessive-compulsive disorder, a gemmotherapy called Lime Tree by Dolisos can help.

In some circumstances, simple relaxation can be as effective as drugs in alleviating anxiety. In a study of patients about to undergo surgery, acupressure (a form of massage) and relaxation/meditation tapes were found to work as well as or better than Valium. EMG biofeedback relaxation methods have also proven effective in relieving both anxiety and insomnia.[14] Music therapy and color therapy are other possibilities. Blue light is calming.

RESCUED FROM PANIC ATTACKS

Jennifer's chief complaint was severe depression. Homeopathic treatment seemed to aggravate the condition, bringing on panic attacks, but Dr. Walker saw that as a positive sign. Jennifer's emotions had been suppressed and were coming to the surface; she was finally feeling emotions she hadn't acknowledged previously. To help calm and relax her, Dr. Walker gave Jennifer Skullcap Oats (two droppersful three times daily), then Cherry Plum (three drops in water three times daily) to help her move through the reasons for the attacks. These remedies were followed by *Argentum nitricum* 200C daily for a week. Jennifer's attacks then stopped completely and she started making real progress in her life. She got out more and began doing things with friends. Her problems weren't all solved, but she was moving forward.

Kathy, a dog trainer, telephoned Dr. Walker in an acute state of panic after trying to discontinue the drug Prozac. Kathy was depressed and had been experiencing panic attacks for about a year. She had been on the drug since her symptoms had first appeared and said she was much better with it than without it, but she still had symptoms and wanted to be drug-free. A review of her symptoms indicated that her underlying problem was simply menopause. She was 42 years old with no previous history of anxiety or depression. She was given Rescue Remedy and Skullcap Oats, to be taken as needed for support while her underlying problem was being treated. In two days, Kathy called to say how much better she felt. A week later, she stopped by to say she no longer needed the Skullcap Oats. She felt terrific. Two months later, she reported that she had lost weight and felt better than she had for years. She had no depression or anxiety. She was convinced she had never needed the Prozac and that her real problem was hormonal changes induced by menopause.

ARRHYTHMIA

See IRREGULAR HEARTBEAT.

ARTHRITIS

Arthritis, or inflammation of the joints, strikes women far more frequently than men and is the most common and disabling chronic condition reported by them. Arthritis can destroy joint tissue, damage internal organs, shorten life expectancy, weaken the spine, and make bones brittle. Osteoarthritis affects 11.7 million women, representing three-fourths of all cases. Rheumatoid arthritis affects 1.5 million women, representing 71 percent of all cases. Osteoarthritis causes the breakdown of joint cartilage and leads to joint pain and stiffness. Rheumatoid arthritis is an autoimmune disease in which the immune system seems to turn against healthy body parts, especially the joints. Systemic lupus erythematosus, another autoimmune disease affecting the joints, afflicts 117,000 women. Juvenile rheumatoid arthritis affects 61,000 girls. Fibromyalgia, a complex arthritis-related disorder involving widespread pain in the joints and muscles, claims 3.7 million victims, of whom seven-eighths are women.[1] See also "Lupus" on page 170 and "Fibromyalgia" on page 113.

CONVENTIONAL TREATMENT

The conventional approach to arthritis is to suppress joint pain with drugs. Aspirin and other nonsteroidal anti-inflammatory drugs (NSAIDs) relieve pain by blocking the inflammatory process, but this approach comes with a price. NSAIDs are now credited with the most frequent and severe side effects of any drugs on the American market. A recent

Stanford study attributed 107,000 hospitalizations and 16,500 deaths yearly to them. If you regularly take NSAIDs, you are six times more likely to be hospitalized for ulcers and other gastrointestinal problems.[2]

In an effort to circumvent the ulcer problem, drug manufacturers developed the Cox-2 inhibitors. These "super aspirins" block the Cox-2 enzyme that drives inflammation, but they don't block the Cox-1 enzyme that releases the prostaglandins protecting the stomach. The drugs are quite expensive and don't suppress pain or reverse the ravages of the disease any better than older options, but their manufacturers claim that they have fewer side effects than other arthritis drugs.[3]

The FDA is not convinced by this claim. It approved Searle's Cox-2 inhibitor Celebrex as a good option to relieve arthritis pain but declared there is no proof that the drug is easier on patients' stomachs than other drugs. The FDA has required the same warning about side effects that appears on older painkillers.[4] Potential downsides of Celebrex reported in *The Proceedings of the National Academy of Sciences* include a reduction in beneficial prostaglandins and an increase in the risk of heart attack.[5]

Merck, the world's largest drug company, sought government approval for its own Cox-2 inhibitor, Vioxx, in the spring of 1999. Merck hoped to persuade the FDA that Vioxx is superior to Celebrex and does not need any warning label about gastrointestinal effects.[6] But as with Celebrex, while the drug was approved, the FDA has not permitted Merck to claim that Vioxx is less damaging to the gastrointestinal tract than traditional NSAIDs. The reviewing committee observed that the side effects of Vioxx, including swelling, high blood pressure, and elevated potassium levels, increase with increasing doses, suggesting the drug might not be safe for long-term use. The committee advised against its use for chronic pain and said that its use for acute pain should be limited to five days—the longest Merck had studied it for that purpose.[7] Limited to five days, Vioxx wouldn't be much help for arthritis sufferers, who need long-term relief. In July 2001, research was released showing that Vioxx patients ran four times the risk of heart attacks as patients taking the older arthritis pain relievers such as aspirin and ibuprofen. Whether this was because the Cox-2 inhibitors lack aspirin's beneficial ability to reduce blood platelet adhesion or because the drugs actually damage blood vessels wasn't clear. However, the FDA is now considering adding warnings to both Vioxx and Celebrex about cardiovascular side effects.[8]

Worse, in August 2001, the FDA reconsidered its opinion on Celebrex and concluded that it offers no proven safety advantage over older drugs in reducing ulcer complications. The research results originally published in *The Journal of the American Medical Association* (*JAMA*) were for only the first six months of the study presented to the FDA. In the second six months, more ulcer complications occurred in the Celebrex group, making the overall effect a draw. These results, it turns out, were actually known to the authors when the study was presented to *JAMA*; it was on the basis of that misleadingly favorable study that Celebrex proceeded to take the market by storm.[9]

Even if the Cox-2 inhibitors are not hazardous to the stomach (a matter that remains in dispute), there is a more fundamental problem with these drugs. All arthritis drugs, including the Cox-2 inhibitors, relieve joint pain merely by suppressing some stage of the inflammatory process, thus relieving pressure on the nerves. They do this by inhibiting the synthesis of prostaglandins that cause dilation of the blood vessels. The problem is that this dilation is necessary to increase the blood flow required for the repair of joint structures.

Studies have shown that suppressing inflammation not only does not cure arthritis but also actually speeds the course of the disease. Inflammation is a natural process by which the body tries to remove dead or damaged tissue cells and lays down the matrix for new cells to replace the old. It does this by a buildup of body fluids that serves to destroy or wall off toxins and injured tissue and carry immune system cells to the site of injury. When this process is interfered with, the already compromised joint simply deteriorates more rapidly.[10] Animal studies have shown that aspirin, indomethacin, and other NSAIDs promote the rapid breakdown of cartilage.[11] All NSAIDs can also cause sodium and water retention, which is thought to trigger changes in deteriorating cartilage.[12] And NSAIDs suppress the production of proteoglycans, a glycoprotein found in connective tissue. The stiffness and cushioning of cartilage is directly correlated with the content of these substances.[13]

When NSAIDs no longer work to suppress arthritic pain, corticosteroids (steroids) are prescribed. Steroids work by suppressing the immune system and thus inflammation, which is a normal immune response. Steroids like hydrocortisone, prednisone, and dexamethasone are powerful anti-inflammatories that are used by doctors to treat severe pain, but they can have correspondingly severe side effects. Long-term steroid use can also cause weight gain and facial fullness, hypertension, diabetes, osteoporosis, cataracts, intestinal bleeding, and increased susceptibility to infections. After taking steroids for prolonged periods, a serious condition known as adrenal insufficiency can develop if withdrawal isn't tapered very carefully to give the body a chance to recover its own ability to produce natural steroids. For rheumatoid arthritis, other strong drugs may be given, with even more serious side effects.

When all else fails, the conventional approach is to replace the joint with an artificial one. Joint replacements are major surgeries requiring long postoperative recoveries that can be painful, expensive, and expose the patient to serious hospital-generated infections. Surgery is an invasive procedure involving implantation of a foreign synthetic object that does not come with a lifetime warranty into the body. Artificial joints can last for years but not indefinitely; by the time the patient is ready for another replacement, he or she may be too old to sustain the major surgery involved.

Natural Remedies

Natural therapies are available that can safely and effectively relieve pain and, in some cases, actually reverse the course of the disease. They include nutritional supplements that help rebuild degenerating joints, detox therapies that eliminate any toxic buildup that is irritating the joints and causing inflammation, and therapies that tune up the body and release its own healing power.

Currently, the most popular nutritional remedies for arthritis are glucosamine and chondroitin sulfate. Derived from animal cartilage, these nutrients pass through blood to the joints, where they stimulate the production of new cartilage cells and reduce the action of enzymes that harm cartilage. Emer'gen-C, which contains 500 mg of glucosamine and 400 mg of chondroitin, is more bioavailable than other products because it is taken in solution, and it is relatively inexpensive. Take two to three packets daily.

Another cheap and readily available cartilage source is plain gelatin. Mix one or two packets daily in a glass of juice and drink. Gelatin is also available in capsules.

A close competitor in popularity for joint pain relief is MSM (methyl sulphonyl methane or $DMSO_2$), the major metabolite of DMSO, a solvent derived from trees. Stanley Jacob, M.D., who helped develop MSM as an arthritis remedy, asserts that it has proven in his clinical practice to be more effective in reducing the pain and inflammation of arthritis than glucosamine.[14] Dr. Walker recommends all three of these supplements—glucosamine and chondroitin sulfate to rebuild the joints, and MSM to relieve inflammation. Again, Emer'gen-C with MSM is a particularly bioavailable source, since vitamin C is required to properly metabolize MSM, and the product includes potassium. Recommended dosage is one to three packets daily.

Also good for relieving the pain of arthritis and fibromyalgia is S-adenosyl-methionine (SAMe), the activated form of the amino acid methionine. Researchers have concluded that SAMe, like glucosamine and chondroitin sulfate, may go beyond the symptoms of arthritis and actually slow the disease itself.[15]

A range of other nutrients is necessary for rebuilding the joints, including the minerals calcium, zinc, selenium, copper, and magnesium; and vitamins E, B_1, B_6, and B_{12}. Antioxidants can also help by reducing the formation of free radicals that can injure and irritate the joints. Combination products are on the market that allow the intake of many nutrients in one capsule. Arth-X Plus by Trace Minerals Research in Ogden, Utah, contains glucosamine sulfate and trace minerals along with a long list of other nutrients and herbs. Use as directed on the label.

Another way to get many of the nutrients needed for joint repair in one product is with green food drinks such as Green Magma, Barley Green, Kyo-Green, and Green Radiance.[16] Deep-green plants are constantly exposed to the high-energy rays of the sun, which they transform into chlorophyll. Chlorophyll protects plants from oxidative damage, is an excellent cleanser, and has anti-inflammatory properties. Chlorophyll or alfalfa can also be taken as a supplement.

Cod liver oil is good for arthritic joints because of its high content of vitamin D (necessary for the assimilation of calcium) and essential fatty acids (EFAs). The omega-3 fats in fatty fish like sardines, herring, and trout block prostaglandins that create inflammation. Fish oil capsules are available at health food stores.[17] Good plant sources of EFAs, including omega-3 oils, are also available, including soybean oil, walnut oil, and flaxseed oil. Also good for arthritic joints are evening primrose oil (2,600 mg at bedtime) and black currant seed oil (500 mg three times daily).

Arthritis can also result from too much acid in the body. Good products for changing the body's pH balance include AlkaLife and InnerLife. See Dr. Robert Young's book *The pH Miracle* and the discussion under "Fungal Infetions" on page 120.

HORSE TRAINER'S ARTHRITIS RELIEVED

Joan, a 57-year-old horse trainer, was so stiff with arthritis that she could hardly move. Riding was so painful that she dreaded going to work. The first week after trying AlkaLife, her pain disappeared. More than a year later, she says AlkaLife is her best friend. Terrified of going back to being debilitated by arthritis, Joan has a cupboard fully stocked with this natural remedy.

Ellen, one of the authors of this book, had a similar experience with InnerLight alkalizing greens and chlorine dioxide drops.

Herbal Remedies

Many herbs have been found to help relieve arthritis pain and inflammation. Curcumin, the yellow ingredient in curry powder and a component of turmeric, has been shown to be as effective as cortisone in suppressing inflammation, without its side effects.

Other effective anti-inflammatory herbs include capsaicin (found in hot chili peppers, sold as a topical cream over the counter under several names including Zostrix and Capsaicin), ginger, boswellia, devil's claw, and Chinese thoroughwax.[18] Liberal doses of garlic can also help. Arth-X Plus contains yucca, devil's claw, burdock root, chaparral, Mexican sarsaparilla root, capsicum, and hydrangea, along with other nutrients. A Chinese herbal remedy called Tintzat has been found effective in alleviating arthritis pain in the hands and wrists. For all of these products, directions for use are on the label.

Dietary and Digestive Approaches

For many people with arthritis, symptoms are brought on by certain foods. Robert Bingham, M.D., medical director at the Desert Arthritis and Medical Clinic in Desert Hot Springs, California, reports that approximately one-third of patients with rheumatoid arthritis are sensitive to the nightshades (potatoes, tomatoes, peppers, and eggplant). Studies have also linked rheumatoid arthritis to dietary fat and to food allergens including dairy products, wheat, corn, citrus, coffee, and chocolate. Osteoarthritis, too, has been linked to food sensitivities and allergies.[19]

One theory attributes the underlying problem to the destruction of enzymes in the modern diet. Cooking, microwaving, and processing destroy enzymes found naturally in foods. As a result, food gets to the colon undigested, leaving toxic residues that must be detoxified by the liver. When the liver becomes overloaded, toxins enter the blood, where they can evoke an aggressive autoimmune response and the production of circulating immune complexes. Deteriorating joints also produce corrosive proteins leading to the production of immune complexes, which lodge in the joints and cause irritation.

The problem is magnified in people with rheumatoid arthritis, who tend to be deficient in hydrochloric acid (secreted in the stomach) and pancreatic enzymes (secreted by the pancreas). When proteins are not broken down properly by the pancreatic enzymes specific for their digestion, large molecules are left that are treated by the body as foreign, evoking an autoimmune response. Supplemental enzymes can help reduce inflammation and joint pain. Pancreatic enzyme formulations split the corrosive protein products that lead to joint inflammation into smaller chains of amino acids, which can then be eliminated from the system. These preparations have been found to be at least as effective as NSAIDs and other anti-inflammatory drugs in treating a variety of conditions including arthritis, and their side effects are very low. The preparations that have been extensively studied have usually involved combinations of the enzymes bromelain and trypsin.[20] Good brands available at health food stores include Transformation and Tyler.

Pancreatic enzymes should be taken on an empty stomach, not less than forty-five minutes before or two hours after meals. To aid digestion in the stomach, enzymes that are not enteric coated may be taken with meals. *Caution: Supplemental enzymes are not recommended for people with bleeding disorders, inflammation of the intestines, reflux, or ulcers.* For other digestive aids, see "Digestive Problems" on page 104.

Detox Solutions

Another cause of arthritis pain may be heavy metal buildup in the joints. Ray Evers, M.D., a pioneer of chelation therapy for heart and arthritic conditions, analyzed the heavy metal levels in his arthritis patients and found elevated levels of lead in nearly all of them. Mercury and other heavy metals were also high. The link was confirmed when chelation successfully relieved the patients' symptoms.[21]

A series of French studies found that autoimmune diseases including chronic polyarthritis, an inflammatory disease that affects several joints simultaneously, can be triggered by heavy metal accumulations from silver/mercury amalgam dental fillings.[22] Arthritis symptoms have been relieved both by removing fillings and by removing or disinfecting root canals.[23]

Abram Hoffer, M.D., reports dramatic results in arthritis victims given vitamin regimens including high doses of niacin (2,000–3,000 mg per day).[24] Niacin, like chemical chelators, eliminates heavy metals from the tissues. For a detailed discussion, see Chapter 5.

Topical Remedies

DMSO cream, applied directly to the joints as needed, can give immediate relief. Like glucosamine, DMSO has been popular as a veterinary product for decades, with a proven track record for relieving joint stiffness in dogs and horses. Although it is controversial, one of the authors (Ellen) found that DMSO cream alone of all the remedies she tried gave overnight relief from her hip joint pain (using about one-half teaspoon as needed). A good rose-scented DMSO cream in an aloe-vera base is obtainable from DMSO Marketing Inc., (800) 367-6935.

Caution: DMSO should be used only on clean skin. One of its unique properties is that it carries other molecules with it into the cells. This property can be hazardous, since pesticides and other pollutants can be transported into the cells along with DMSO.

Users also claim good results with an MSM/herbal combination topical remedy called Blue Stuff. For ordering information, visit the Web site www.bluestuff.com.

Woodlock Oil, a Chinese patent formula, is another topical remedy that can temporarily alleviate arthritis pain. Effective homeopathic creams include Arthricin by CompliMed and Zeel by Heel (also available as a tablet). Natural progesterone cream rubbed into painful joints is also effective over a period of time (⅛ to ½ teaspoon once or twice daily).

Other Natural Therapies

Classic single homeopathic remedies for arthritis include *Rhus toxicondendron* (*Rhus tox*) and *Ruta graveolens* (*Ruta grav*). *Spinaflex* is good for arthritis of the spine or neck.

A number of studies have demonstrated acupuncture's effectiveness on arthritis. In one reported in the *Bulletin of the New York Academy of Medicine,* 109 people with arthritis of different types received acupuncture treatments. Eighty-one experienced either complete or partial improvement over a six-month period.[25]

Other nondrug therapies useful in the treatment of arthritis are physical and occupational therapy, including warm-water swimming and other exercise, heat treatments, and rest. Total bed rest, however, is no longer recommended, since it causes loss of muscle tone. Correcting anatomical problems like unequal leg lengths or abnormal foot positions can also relieve symptoms, and so can exercise that puts the joints through their full range of motion. For overweight people, weight loss is also important to relieve stress on the joints.

A folk remedy for arthritis that dates back for centuries is sunlight therapy. In a Russian study, a significant reduction in arthritis was found in miners given routine sunlight treatments. In another study, one group of children with severe arthritis was given cortisone while another group was given sunlight treatments. In the sunlight group, relief came more slowly than in the cortisone group, but it did come; and unlike cortisone, sunlight left the patient with no unwanted side effects. Resistance to infection also increased.[26]

Another folk remedy many arthritis patients swear by is copper bracelets. Why they work is uncertain, but an Australian study found that they actually relieve symptoms.[27] Good copper bracelets are available from Sergio Lub Jewelry, P.O. Box 3400, Walnut Creek, California 94598; (800) 279-5587; http://sergiolubjewelry.com.

ASPARTAME, ADVERSE REACTIONS TO

Aspartame is an artificial sweetener that is about 160 times as sweet as sugar. Available as NutraSweet, Equal, and other brands, it is now found in about 4,000 foods and many soft drinks. It is added for the purpose of reducing caloric intake while satisfying the sweet tooth. Labeled as a food and considered safe, aspartame is consumed by millions of people; however, it is by far the most dangerous of food additives, accounting for more than 75 percent of the food-additive-adverse reactions reported to the FDA. According to the Centers for Disease Control, 76 percent of all reports of side effects come from women.

Reported side effects include blindness, eye pain, tinnitus, intolerance to noise, decreased hearing, seizures, headaches, dizziness, confusion, memory loss, sleepiness, numbness in limbs, slurring of speech, tremors, depression, irritability, anxiety, nausea, diarrhea, hives, weight gain, aggravated low blood sugar, and fatigue.[1]

Those are the immediately noticeable side effects. Research suggests that aspartame ingestion can also trigger or worsen a number of chronic conditions, including Alzheimer's disease, brain tumors, multiple sclerosis, epilepsy, chronic fatigue syndrome, Parkinson's disease, mental retardation, lymphoma, birth defects, and fibromyalgia. (For a dramatic case seen by Dr. Walker, see "Alzheimer's Disease" on page 40.)

A major constituent of aspartame is aspartic acid, an amino acid that significantly increases the level of aspartate and glutamate in the blood. The excess glutamate and aspartate seep into the brain and slowly destroy neurons by allowing too much calcium into the cells, triggering excessive amounts of free radicals that kill the cells. However, this process is an insidious one. Seventy-five percent of the neural cells in a particular area of the brain are dead before any clinical symptoms of chronic illness are detected.[2]

The insulin imbalance created by habitual aspartame ingestion is also thought by some researchers to precipitate insulin resistance. When you eat sugar, the body produces insulin to burn as energy. If there is too much insulin, your cells become desensitized to it. Following aspartame ingestion, insulin is sent in but not actually used. The excess insulin therefore attacks the cells, which no longer respond normally to it. This condition, called insulin resistance, is a common feature of diabetes.

To add insult to injury, while aspartame does decrease the calorie count, it may actually contribute to weight *gain* rather than weight loss. When the taste buds detect incoming sweet material, they send a message to the thalamus in the brain: "Incoming sugar!" The thalamus then sends a message to the pancreas, which activates beta cells to put insulin into the bloodstream to metabolize the anticipated sugar onslaught and put it into the cells for storage. But because there is no sugar onslaught, the sugar already floating in the bloodstream is stored instead. The blood sugar then falls, and appetite for more energy-producing sugar increases. You can test this effect yourself by drinking a diet soda sometime when you aren't hungry. About fifteen minutes later, you are likely to feel hungry; in an hour, you are likely to be ravenous for food—particularly sugary food. Many people have other symptoms besides an increased appetite when blood sugar falls, including headaches, migraine, anxiety, weakness, somnolence, hyperactivity, seizures, and depression.

Natural Alternatives

It's best to avoid artificially sweetened foods and drinks, but sugared soft drinks aren't recommended either; they are high in both sugar and phosphoric acid, which pulls calcium from the bones. Pure water remains the healthiest thirst quencher. Honey, pure maple syrup, and natural fruit sugars, which contain chromium and other nutrients, are preferable to either aspartame or refined sugar. *Stevia rebaudiana,* an herb of the Chrysanthemum family, is ten to fifteen times sweeter than common table sugar in its natural form and, in extract form, is 100 to 300 times sweeter. Stevia doesn't affect blood sugar metabolism, however.[3]

ASTHMA

Asthma, a breathing disorder characterized by wheezing, difficulty exhaling, and often coughing, has doubled in incidence in the last twenty years. It strikes men as often as women, but women's asthma attacks are more severe and are more likely to result in hospitalization. Why isn't clear, but a hormonal component is suspected. Before puberty, boys are twice as likely as girls to be hospitalized with asthma; after puberty, however, women are hospitalized for it two and a half times as often as men.[1] Obesity has also been linked to asthma in women but not in men. Obese women have almost double the risk of developing asthma as non-obese women.[2]

Asthma is an autoimmune reaction that can be triggered by many things, including food allergens, exercise, cold weather, and environmental irritants like dust mites, mold, animal dander, and chemical odors. The high level of airborne pollutants in industrialized countries is a leading suspect. Exercise, stress, and intense emotions can also trigger it, as can certain drugs.

The exponential increase in asthma deaths in recent years is attributed in part to a huge increase in availability and use of aerosol preparations in metered-dose inhalers for dilating the bronchial tubes. The products afford a false sense of security in the face of a dangerous condition. All antiasthma medications can produce life-threatening reactions, and the likelihood of these reactions is multiplied by the increased use of the medications.[3]

CONVENTIONAL TREATMENT

Asthma drugs are sold under many brand names and can include sprays, pills, powders, liquids, and shots. They fall into two groups:

1. *Bronchodilators* are used mainly to relieve sudden asthma attacks or to prevent exercise-induced attacks. They work by relaxing the smooth muscles lining the airways, making them open wider and letting more air pass through.

2. *Anti-inflammatory drugs* are medicines that help to control inflammation in the airways and prevent asthma attacks from beginning. The drugs reduce swelling in the air tubes and decrease mucus, keeping the air tubes open so attacks don't start. Anti-inflammatory drugs include cromolyn, nedocromil, and corticosteroids (steroids).[4]

Steroid drugs are pharmaceutical copies of the steroid hormones produced by the adrenal glands. The problem with taking them in drug form is that they suppress the immune system. The adrenals quit making their own steroids, so when you need natural steroids to cope with stressful emergencies, they are no longer available.

Steroids come in injected, oral, and inhaler form. For asthma emergencies, systemic steroids such as methylprednisolone (the injectable form) or prednisone (the oral form) can be very effective. But they can also have serious long-term side effects, including cataracts, bone loss, weight gain, easy bruising, and emotional problems. They are, therefore, not for long-term use and are recommended only when all other treatments fail.

Steroid inhalers, on the other hand, are considered safe for long-term use because their medication is poorly absorbed. Thus, the potential for adrenal suppression has been considered low. In fact, inhalers have been thought to be among the safest and most effective treatments for asthma. However, new research has cast doubt on the safety even of these drugs. In 1997, a link between cataracts and oral steroid use was found, and inhalers were associated with a higher risk of glaucoma than steroid pills.[5] Moreover, research reported in *The New England Journal of Medicine* on October 4, 2001, linked the long-term use of inhaled steroids to bone loss that can lead to osteoporosis, a debilitating disease that is responsible for more than 1.5 million bone fractures yearly, mostly among women.[6]

Inhalers can also contribute to the development of fungal mouth infections. For this reason, use of a mouthwash is advised after each dose.[7] Do not use antiseptic mouthwashes for this purpose, however. Like antibiotics, antiseptic mouthwashes can wipe out friendly flora along with unfriendly ones, leading to the very fungal and yeast infections you're trying to avoid.

Another drawback of asthma drugs in general is that virtually all of them draw magnesium out of cells. Research shows that a magnesium deficiency can actually lead to an asthma attack. Numerous studies have also found that low magnesium levels cause abnormal and decreased immune function, which can increase the tendency for asthma.[8]

Natural Remedies

Nutritional and Herbal Approaches

Magnesium has been used successfully for the treatment of asthma ever since the 1930s. Popular health writer Julian Whitaker, M.D., states that a large dose of magnesium will relax the constricted muscles of the lung bronchioles and almost magically eliminate severe asthma attacks. Large doses of magnesium given intravenously are very safe in most cases, particularly in comparison with the dangers of currently used asthma medications, which can cause cardiac arrhythmias and can be toxic to the heart muscle. Magnesium given along with asthma drugs enhances their action and blunts toxicity. It can be tried as the first line of defense against most asthma attacks. For magnesium injections, you'll need to see a medical doctor; for preventive purposes, however, you can supplement your diet with 1,000–1,500 mg of elemental magnesium in divided doses throughout the day (taken with calcium to reduce diarrhea).[9]

Another nutritional remedy that can help relieve asthma problems without side effects is black currant seed oil, which works by reducing inflammation in the lungs, thereby opening them for easier breathing. Readily available in health food stores, black currant seed oil can help relieve any type of breathing problem, including asthma and emphysema, and is particularly useful for exercise-induced asthma. Recommended dosage is two 500-mg capsules three times daily. To relieve exercise-induced asthma, take two capsules before workouts.

A good combination herbal formula for supporting the lungs is Lung Complex by Enzymatic Therapy. Elecampane is another herb that helps build up the strength of the lungs; it is available from Eclectic Institute and other herbal sources. Follow dosages on the label.

Homeopathic Options

Asthma by BHI is a combination remedy that supports the lungs homeopathically. Take ten drops three times daily. Another homeopathic remedy that helps in cases both of

---

ASTHMA RELIEVED WITHOUT DRUGS

Sheila, 45, complained of exercise-induced asthma. She worked out regularly to help control her weight, but as her asthma worsened, she found she was breathless after a few minutes of regular exercise. She saw a physician, who recommended an inhaler, but Sheila was reluctant to take steroids. Frustrated because she was putting on weight without her daily workouts, she went to see Dr. Walker, who recommended that she take two 500-mg capsules of black currant seed oil before each workout. Sheila reports having had no asthma problems since she took Dr. Walker's advice.

Chole, 19, had a long history of asthma and recurring colds and chest infections. She wanted to attend college without constant illness and the need to rely on inhalers. Black currant seed oil in combination with a constitutional homeopathic remedy specific for her symptoms, taken over the space of a year, improved her asthma so that she could breathe normally. She now attends college and is off inhalers. She reports that she is doing well and has not had a cold or lung problem in the last two years. She continues to take black currant seed oil daily, increasing the dosage to two pills three to four times daily if she feels her lungs are getting "tight."

asthma and emphysema is Lung RegenRx by Apex. It aids regeneration of the lung and improves cellular oxygenation.

Some allergic asthma has been traced to contact with cockroaches. For this problem (which can be diagnosed by a homeopath), the appropriate homeopathic remedy is *Blatta* 6X or 30X taken three times daily.

For other constitutional therapy specific to your body and personality type, see a homeopath.

Treating the Emotional Factor

Chinese doctors believe asthma can be the result of suppressed anger or grief. A typical case is an older woman who suddenly becomes a widow. She is so busy with the funeral and other arrangements that she has no time to grieve. Within a year of her husband's death, she begins to have lung problems: coughing, congestion in the morning, and frequent colds and flu that may turn into pneumonia or bronchitis. Homeopathic remedies like *Ignatia* can help release this "grief trapped in the lungs." Because the emotional trauma is deeply embedded in the system, a strength of 200X is recommended, under the guidance of a homeopath.

Other Nondrug Alternatives

Acupuncture can help alleviate asthma. A Chinese study published in 1989 reported a disappearance or decreased frequency of asthma attacks in 88.9 percent of cases treated.[10] Acupuncture once a week is recommended, or more in the case of acute attacks.

Learning to breathe properly from the diaphragm and to empty the lungs completely on exhalation is very important.[11] Biofeedback techniques can help. Twenty minutes daily of controlled breathing exercises learned through biofeedback have reduced asthma symptoms.[12]

Exercise is a natural adrenaline stimulant that can produce direct nervous stimulation to the nose.[13] Twenty minutes a day is good. Rest when short of breath.

F. Batmanghelidj, M.D., reports some remarkable asthma cures with water therapy.[14] He says we need half our bodies' weight in ounces of water per day—not coffee, tea, soft drinks, or juices, but plain (filtered or bottled) water. Thus, a 128-pound woman would need 64 ounces, or eight 8-ounce glasses of water. Wait a half hour before meals and two and a half hours after meals for your larger water doses, to avoid diluting your digestive juices. Dr. Batmanghelidj advises adding ½ teaspoon of salt to your diet daily for every ten glasses of water added. (Unheated sea salt is preferred. Better yet is Bio-Salt by Gilbert's Health Food Labs in England, a biochemically balanced mineral salt compound containing sodium chloride plus all the cell salts.)

For other natural remedies and preventive approaches, see "Allergies" on page 37.

ASTHMA RELIEVED HOMEOPATHICALLY

Bunny, age 54, had had severe asthma for years. She was constantly wheezing from congestion and required three different inhalers to manage her condition. Dr. Walker recommended *Kali carb* 30C (homeopathic potassium carbonate), a constitutional remedy matching Bunny's symptoms. To the amazement of her medical doctor, Bunny's condition improved so much after she took *Kali carb* that she no longer needed the asthma inhalers.

CHRONIC LUNG CONDITION RELIEVED WITH HERBAL AND HOMEOPATHIC REMEDIES

Barbara's husband died suddenly of a heart attack when she was 62 years old. It was so unexpected that no arrangements had been made. She knew nothing about their finances; her husband had always handled them. With that to consider and her family coming from out of town for the funeral, she hardly had time to mourn; even if she'd had the time, however, her relatives wouldn't have let her express her grief. Whenever Barbara started to cry, someone found something to keep her busy or talked with her to "cheer her up."

Months later, Barbara was hard at work in a new job. Her life wasn't going well, but she kept plugging on. She never cried, but she found herself staying up all night "thinking." Meanwhile, she had developed a chronic asthmatic cough and was coming down with colds every three weeks or so. When her lung problems turned into pneumonia, she sought advice from Dr. Walker. After a course of the herb elecampane to build up her lungs and homeopathic *Ignatia* 200X to release her grief, her cough went away and she was fine . . . but only after she had had a good cry!

ATHEROSCLEROSIS

See HEART DISEASE.

BACK PAIN AND SCIATICA

Back pain isn't gender-specific, but women's back pain tends to last longer than men's, and more women than men in the youngest and oldest age groups suffer from it. Men are more likely to suffer from the acute back pain that comes on quickly as the result of a sudden motion or injury. Women's back pain is more likely to be the result of chronic strain from long-standing activities such as domestic work and child care, carrying heavy objects, gardening, and vacuuming. Chronic back pain comes on slowly and can last for months or years. Its cause may be hard to trace, as it can be the result of a dysfunction in the body somewhere other than where the pain is actually felt.[1] Menstruation can trigger back pain, and pregnancy and child care can increase a woman's vulnerability to it. About half of all pregnant women experience back pain.[2]

Back pain often leads to sciatica, which results from compression of the sciatic nerve at the base of the spine. Sciatica is characterized by pain radiating through the buttock down the back of the thigh and leg, sometimes to the foot. Many of the remedies good for back pain can also help relieve this condition.

CONVENTIONAL TREATMENT

Back surgery is considered when pain is serious and unremitting or is getting worse. According to U.S. government data, however, many of those who suffer from back pain fail to benefit from surgery, and it always entails risk, with a chance of permanent damage and impaired mobility.[3] For less serious back pain, rest and painkillers are usually prescribed. While bed rest has traditionally been recommended, however, experts are now saying that recovery is liable to be quicker if you can keep moving. A physiotherapist may use mobilization techniques along with ultrasound, laser, or heat treatment. Nonsurgical treatment can include anti-inflammatory and muscle-relaxant drugs, traction, a collar or surgical corset, painkilling epidural anesthetic injections, antidepressants, or TENS (a mild form of electrical nerve stimulation done with a machine you can use at home).[4]

NATURAL REMEDIES

Studies have shown that chiropractic is more effective than conventional medicine for relieving back pain.[5] Other physical therapies that can help include massage, acupressure, and body work. Losing weight can also help. A sizeable belly can pull the back out by the "fulcrum effect." This effect is particularly obvious during pregnancy. Pregnant women should talk to their doctors before doing any kind of aggressive therapy for back pain.

Exercises are also important for maintaining low back strength.[6]

The emotional connection to back pain was shown by Dr. John E. Sarno, who attested in *Healing Back Pain: The Mind-Body Connection* that his patients experienced dramatic relief from back discomfort simply by releasing emotional trauma and tension.

Oriental doctors also hold that some back pain has emotional and dietary roots. If it is due to a serious anatomical injury or dislocation, it should always hurt. But some back and shoulder pain comes and goes. Chinese doctors say that if a condition can be better some of the time, it can be made better all of the time. Back pain that comes and goes may originate, not in the backbone, but in the gallbladder. If you have recurring pain between the shoulder blades (under the bra strap) for which nothing seems to help, yet there are periods when you feel fine, the pain may come from suppressed emotion or a gallbladder-stressing diet. Changing the diet and taking homeopathic remedies that balance the emotions can help. Specific remedies to relieve gallbladder stress are discussed under "Gallbladder Disease and Gallstones" on page 120.

Acupuncture can also help. Under Eastern medical theory, energy flows in a set pattern through meridians, or energy patterns, all over the body. When the energy becomes weak in a meridian system, things fall out of place. When the energy weakens in meridians that go down the spine, the vertebrae have a tendency to slip out. They can be manually pushed back into place (as by chiropractic adjustment), but physical or emotional stress will cause them to slip out of place again. Acupuncture can balance the energy down the meridian to strengthen the muscles and pull the vertebrae into place naturally. Often, when an acupuncture treatment is completed, the back will adjust itself, "cracking" spontaneously into place with bending. While this may occur after a single treatment, a series of weekly treatments is still usually necessary to strengthen the meridian system.

A Chinese patent remedy that effectively helps relieve back pain is Sciatica Pills. Another remedy that is good for strengthening the low back over a period of time is Specific Lumbaglin. These remedies are available over the counter in Chinese pharmacies. Take two capsules three times daily for one week, then one capsule three times daily for maintenance.

Homeopathic remedies can also help relieve back pain. Good combination products are Sciatica/Back Pain by CompliMed (ten drops three times daily) and Sciatica by BHI (one pill every fifteen minutes as needed for acute pain, then three times daily for maintenance). Sciataide by B&T is also good. For upper back pain, try Spinaflex by CompliMed or Back and Neck Aide by B&T. These remedies are available in health food stores or from homeopathic practitioners. Follow directions on the label or from your practitioner.

BACK PAIN RELIEVED WITHOUT DRUGS OR SURGERY

Dr. Walker's secretary, age 52, was having such severe back pain that she found it hard to walk and even harder to sit for long periods. Replacing her desk chair with a more ergonomic one was tried but did not help. Dr. Walker gave her *Gnaphalium* 30C, a homeopathic specific for low back pain (three pills three times daily), along with the Chinese patent remedy Specific Lumbaglin (two pills three times daily for the first box, one pill three times daily for the second box). Within three days her pain was significantly relieved, and after a month she had no back pain at all. She felt so strong, in fact, that she proceeded to wallpaper her whole house.

BALDNESS, FEMALE-PATTERN

See HAIR LOSS.

BLADDER INFECTION, IRRITATION, AND INFLAMMATION (CYSTITIS)

Bladder infections plague one in three women sometime during their lives. They are the second leading cause of lost workdays for women and are responsible for millions of doctor visits annually. Symptoms include the need to urinate frequently, a sense of urgency, painful burning, and sometimes bleeding on urination. Women are far more likely to get the condition than men, apparently because a woman's urethra is shorter than a man's and is close to the anus and vagina. Most bladder infections are caused by the bacteria *Escherichia coli* normally found in the intestines. Improper wiping is a possible route of infection, but lack of estrogen can affect internal flora and contribute to bladder infections as well.

Inflammation or irritation of the bladder can also result from food allergies, chemical sensitivity, bruising during intercourse, and vaginal *Candida*. Another cause is excessive acidity of the urine and other body fluids. The fluids in women's reproductive and urinary tracts are acidic to create a hostile environment for germs, and these fluids may be even more acidic during menstruation. The more acidic the urine, the more irritation a woman is liable to feel.[1]

Interstitial cystitis is a symptom complex involving painful urination for which no infecting agent shows up on bacterial cultures. At one time, it was thought to be a merely psychosomatic condition of hysterical women. But the approximately 450,000 sufferers of interstitial cystitis, who urinate dozens of times daily and experience lower abdominal pain and other distressing symptoms, have succeeded in raising public awareness of the ailment enough to prompt research by the National Institutes of Health.[2] The psychological element in nonspecific cystitis has been overplayed, but there is some evidence that emotional factors can trigger it.

Honeymoon cystitis is a term used for bladder infections acquired by young women new to sexual activity, either because their organs aren't used to the stimulation or because bacteria get pushed back into the urethra. Viagra cystitis is a modern-day variant of this syndrome that strikes older women unaccustomed to frequent intercourse. Bladder infection has been linked to frequent sexual activity in another way. High numbers of urinary tract infections have been noticed among women who use diaphragms for contraception. When refittings did not solve the problem, researchers finally traced the link to a popular spermicide called nonoxynol-9 that was being applied to the contraceptive device. A 1996 study found that women were three times as likely to get urinary tract infections if they used condoms with nonoxynol-9 more often than once a week.[3] The spermicide evidently kills not only sperm but also the friendly bacteria residing in the urinary tract, leaving it susceptible to invasion by unfriendly bacteria.

CONVENTIONAL TREATMENT

Antibiotics are the usual medical treatment for inflammation of the bladder, but they only help if bacterial infection is present, and for many women with cystitis, no infection shows up on bacterial culture. For other women, drugs may work in the short term but the cystitis keeps coming back. Antibiotics also have significant downsides. (See "Infections, Bacterial and Viral" on page 158.)

When antibiotics aren't effective, other medications may be prescribed. Elmiron, which is believed to create a protective coating over the bladder lining, helps about one-third of patients. Soothing medicines may also be used in the bladder, including anesthetics, the anti-inflammatory DMSO, and hydrocortisone, but again only about one-third of patients respond.[4] Elavil, an antidepressant, is often prescribed to relieve chronic pain.

Another drug now being sold over the counter for relieving the distress of bladder infection is a painkiller called Uristat. Its manufacturer, ironically, is Ortho Pharmaceuticals, the same company that makes one of the popular contraceptive creams containing nonoxynol-9, linked to urinary tract infections.

NATURAL REMEDIES

Cranberry juice, an old wive's remedy for bladder infections, has been shown in clinical studies to actually reduce cystitis pain and recurrences. In a study reported in *The Journal of the American Medical Association* (*JAMA*) in March 1994, researchers at Harvard Medical School showed that women who drank ten ounces of cranberry juice each day were 58 percent less likely to develop bladder infections. The juice not only acidifies the urine, inhibiting bacterial growth, but also engulfs the infecting bacteria and prevents them from becoming attached to the cells lining the urinary tract. Pure juice should be used, since "cocktails" can contain as little as 2 percent of it. The bitter cranberry taste can be alleviated with cold seltzer or natural sweeteners. Cranberry extract is available in capsule form.

A combination of parsley and celery juices can also help, by acting as a natural diuretic that flushes the body. You can make your own juice from the fresh raw vegetables at home using a vegetable juicer.

It is particularly important to drink eight to ten 8-ounce glasses of purified water daily to flush out the bladder, dilute toxins, and prevent bacteria from going back up the urethra and causing infection. Begin this routine at the first sign of symptoms. Keep sipping water every twenty minutes or so. Add ½ teaspoon of calcium ascorbate powder (vitamin C) to the water every three to four hours to boost the immune system. You can also drink chamomile tea to flush the body. Avoid acidic foods (fatty foods, onions, citrus and tomato juices, alcohol, and anything containing caffeine), peppermint and spearmint, and meat and dairy products, all of which make the urine more acidic. These simple measures can often alleviate cystitis attacks without the need for antibiotics.[5]

If antibiotics are taken, follow them with *Lactobacillus acidophilus, Bifidobacterium bifidum,* or *Lactobacillus bulgaricus,* "good" bacteria that protect the digestive tract from invasion by *Candida albicans* and other unwanted microorganisms. Lost beneficial bacteria can be replaced with these cultures. Some experts recommend yogurt, but not all yogurts contain live bacterial cultures, and yogurt itself is a fermented food. Acidophilus supplements in liquid or capsule form are better than yogurt. For other suggestions for combatting *Candida* infection, see "Vaginitis and Vaginal Infections" on page 240.

Homeopathic and Herbal Remedies

Homeopathic doctors maintain that antibiotics don't cure urinary tract infections but merely suppress their symptoms. Homeopathic remedies draw the problem to the surface and help the body eliminate it. For bladder infections, homeopathic *Cantharis* is excellent. The recommended dosage for treating intense burning before, during, and after urination is three pellets of *Cantharis* 6X or 30C four times daily. *Sarsaparilla* 6C to 30C is also effective.[6] The dosage is three pellets four times daily. This is also the homeopathic remedy for "honeymoon cystitis."

These single homeopathic remedies work when taken at the onset of a bladder infection (on the first or second day). However, a combination of homeopathic and herbal remedies is more effective after the problem has gone on for several days. Depending on what's available in your local health food store, take either Bacticin by CompliMed or *Tao Chin Pien* (a Chinese herbal combination), along with Bladder Irritation by Natra-Bio or Uri-Control by BHI, following this schedule:

◆ Bacticin: ten drops every fifteen minutes for the first hour, then once every hour for four hours, and then four times daily until the infection is completely gone, *or*

◆ *Tao Chin Pien:* four pills twice daily for five to ten days.

◆ Bladder Irritation: ten drops every fifteen minutes for the first hour, then once every hour for four hours, and then four times daily until the infection is completely gone, *or*

◆ Uri-Control: one tablet every hour for the first four hours, then one tablet four times daily until the infection is completely gone.

Natural Relief from Painful Urination

For bladder irritation caused by excess acidity in the fluids surrounding the urethra and vagina, baking soda can help. Baking soda is an alkaline substance that helps neutralize acid. Bathing in it, particularly when menstruating, can ease discomfort. For a soothing sitz bath, add ¼ cup of baking soda to a hip-high tub of water. For a full-tub bath, use ½ to 1 cup of baking soda. Soak daily for fifteen to twenty minutes as needed.

An old home remedy for calming an inflamed bladder is to mix ¼ teaspoon of baking soda with a half glass of water and drink it twice daily. A more modern alternative is a

BLADDER INFECTION CYCLE BROKEN

Wendy, age 54, had suffered recurring bladder infections for years, despite repeated courses of antibiotics. Bouts of burning and overfrequent need to urinate occurred monthly, though the cycle was not related to her periods, which she no longer had. Dr. Walker recommended homeopathic *Cantharis* to be used when Wendy felt symptoms coming on. She used it four or five times over the course of a year and has had no recurrences now for several years.

Connie, age 33, complained that she had had bladder infections repeatedly for the past six months, though previously she had never had them. Further questioning revealed that her mate, an older man, had begun using Viagra six months earlier. He had started wanting sex two or three times a day, every day. It used to be only once every week or ten days. She broke into tears as she told her story; she had a monster on her hands. She wasn't interested in more sex but couldn't tell him. He was a wealthy and powerful man and they had been together for four or five years but weren't married. Before, she had wanted to get married. Now she was having second thoughts. Dr. Walker surmised from Connie's bout of tears that the emotional component, not bacteria, was keeping her ill. Homeopathic *Sarsaparilla,* used to balance the emotions, succeeded in relieving the problem. Connie talked to her boyfriend and they worked it out.

product called AlkaLife, a patented, concentrated alkaline supplement that increases the pH of water, changing ordinary water into an alkaline solution. The product is available at health food stores or pharmacies. Follow directions on the label.

Helpful Tips

◆ Empty the bladder frequently. Holding the urine can increase bladder infections.

◆ Empty the bladder after intercourse.

◆ Avoid the use of spermicidal jellies or diaphragms. Even diaphragms used without spermicides can bruise the neck of the bladder and increase susceptibility to infection.

◆ Wear underwear with cotton crotches.

◆ Wipe from front to rear.

◆ Avoid hot tubs, which can further irritate the bladder.

◆ Use sanitary napkins rather than tampons, and change them frequently.

BLOATING, GAS, AND EDEMA

An uncomfortable sense of bloating can come either from the retention of water (edema) or from gas in the stomach. Salt is well known to cause water retention in tissues. Estrogen can also have this effect. The cells puff up, creating the appearance of smoothing out wrinkles in the face. In the stomach, however, the result can be unwanted puffiness and bloating. Bloating from estrogen imbalance is common in women before menstruation, during menopause or perimenopause, and on conventional hormone replacement therapy.

Bloating that comes from gas may be due to parasites. Women who have gas and bloating after eating are often found to have this problem. Parasites inhibit the digestive enzymes; undigested food ferments, releasing gas. *Candida* also feed on parasites and can cause gas.

Specific food sensitivities may also underlie the feeling of bloating and distention after eating. This problem, too, is traced to poor digestion, allowing food to rot or ferment and produce gas.

A cause of excess belching is air swallowing. Stomach gas consists primarily of oxygen and nitrogen, which come from swallowed air. Increased air swallowing can be caused by eating too rapidly, gulping, stress, gum chewing, poorly fitting dentures, postnasal drip, dry mouth, and carbonated soft drinks.

CONVENTIONAL TREATMENT

Diuretics, or water pills, are often recommended to relieve fluid retention.[1] However, the drugs work by forcing the kidneys to release body fluid, and along with the excess water, potassium, and other important minerals and chemicals are lost, throwing off electrolyte and mineral balance. That's why most diuretics are prescription-only drugs. In fact, premenstrual syndrome is the *only* condition for which over-the-counter diuretic use is approved, and that's only because the pills are intended for use only a few days each month.

NATURAL REMEDIES FOR BLOATING DUE TO WATER RETENTION

Unlike diuretic drugs, which release fluid prematurely from the kidneys and can cause the loss of vital potassium, natural diuretics can put the whole system back in balance, causing the release of built-up fluid at the cellular level all over the body.

Dandelion is a very powerful natural diuretic that has been shown to work as well as the popular drug Lasix (frusemide) in relieving edema or bloating. It is an excellent natural source of potassium, making it a safe, balanced way to relieve water retention.[2] It comes in standardized capsule form. Take one 400-mg capsule three times daily with food or as professionally prescribed. Pregnant women should not use this herb without the supervision of a qualified practitioner.

Homeopathic remedies can also help relieve bloating, but whether the problem comes from water or gas must first be determined. For bloating from water retention, a homeopathic remedy called Mededema by CompliMed is quite safe and effective. One by Dolisos called Zinc-Nickel-Cobalt can also help eliminate excess water bloat. (For bloating from gas, see page 68.)

Natural progesterone cream is another alternative for reducing water retention and bloating without side effects. ProGest by Transitions for Health is particularly recommended. Use ⅛ to ½ teaspoon as needed.

Other suggestions for relieving bloating from water retention include avoiding salt and salt-rich foods that cause you to retain water, and drinking less.

BLOATING TRACKED TO PARASITES AND ELIMINATED

Eve, age 48, said that her stomach was flat in the morning, but by evening, it was so bloated that she looked pregnant. She also complained of stomach gurgling, gas, and belching. Testing indicated parasites. Treatment was with the homeopathic remedies *Lamblia* and *Frangula*. (See "Parasitic Infection" on page 212.) Within two months, all of Eve's bloating was gone and her stomach was flat. She also felt much better and had more energy.

NATURAL REMEDIES FOR BLOATING DUE TO GAS

For intestinal gas, charcoal is a natural remedy that dates back to the time of Hippocrates. One quart of charcoal will absorb *eighty* quarts of ammonia gas. One downside of chronic charcoal use in capsule form is that it can interfere with the absorption of nutrients and other drugs.[3] This side effect can be avoided with homeopathic remedies for gas and bloating. Try the combination homeopathic remedies Vermicin by CompliMed or Gasalia by Boiron.

For bloating caused by parasites, use Copper-Gold-Silver by Dolisos or Nestmann. Dolisos and CompliMed products are available at health food stores. Nestmann products are available from practitioners or homeopathic pharmacies. Follow directions on the label or from your practitioner.

An herbal remedy for bloating from overeating is peppermint tea.

BLOOD PRESSURE, HIGH

See HIGH BLOOD PRESSURE (HYPERTENSION).

BLOOD SUGAR, LOW

See HYPOGLYCEMIA.

BONE LOSS

See OSTEOPOROSIS.

BONE SPURS AND PLANTAR FASCIITIS

Bone spurs are abnormal growths on the ends of the bones that can cause excruciating pain when they press on nerves and muscles during activity. Like osteoporosis, they are the result of calcium loss, and they particularly afflict older women. When the body is deficient in calcium, it begins to leach calcium from the bones. In many women, this happens in the heel of the foot or some other weak area of the body. As the calcium is being leached, it forms eruptions—the bone spurs—which typically develop on the feet, spine, or

BONE SPURS ELIMINATED

Nancy was skeptical. A woman of about 60, she had bone spurs on her neck that were distressingly painful. She just couldn't believe that an herbal protocol would cure the condition. She came back to the store five or six times to study the Metagenics literature before she finally made her purchase. She returned six weeks later, pleased to report that her neck was fine; the remedy had indeed worked.

For eight other women who had suffered for extended periods with bone spurs on their feet, Dr. Walker recommended SAMe. All reported dramatic relief after a month's treatment.

neck. Their formation on the spine and neck is linked to the vertebrae shrinking with age; the bone compensates for the expanding spaces between the vertebrae by growing bony protrusions. When bone spurs occur in the upper neck, the condition is called cervical osteoarthritis. Bone spurs in the feet can be from wearing the wrong kind of shoes in combination with low serum calcium levels.

Bone spurs are sometimes confused with plantar fasciitis—inflammation of the fascia (thin sheets of connective tissue holding muscles, joints, and organs together) on the bottom of the feet. Plantar fasciitis can be caused by pressure put on the foot by the arch in certain athletic shoes.

CONVENTIONAL TREATMENT

Conventional treatment is with anti-inflammatory painkillers (such as aspirin and ibuprofen); devices to take pressure off the nerves (such as orthopedic collars, back braces, and foam rubber shoe pads); or surgery. But these aren't actually cures, and even surgery doesn't reach the underlying problem, since the spurs are liable to grow back.

NATURAL REMEDIES

The problem underlying bone spurs is a low level of calcium in the body or an inability to use calcium properly. Helpful natural remedies are available. Calcium Absorption by Bioforce is a homeopathic remedy that aids calcium absorption. Take ten drops three times daily. A bioavailable supplemental calcium is also recommended. Good choices are Cal Apatite by Metagenics (one to two tablets one to three times daily) or Bone-Up by Jarrow (two tablets one to three times daily).

Other homeopathic remedies effective for bone spurs on the feet include *Hekla lava* 30C (two pellets three times daily), and *Calc fluor* and *Calc phos* 6X or 12X as cell salts (four pellets three times daily). One of these three will usually eliminate bone spurs in a month or so. It's also important to make sure your shoes are comfortable and fit properly.

For stubborn bone spurs on the spine, Metagenics makes a combination protocol designed to be taken over a six-month period consisting of Collagenics Intensive Care Formula and Arthrogen (niacinamide and NAC). This protocol has worked when conventional treatment failed. Follow directions on the labels.

S-adenosyl-methionine (SAMe), the activated form of the amino acid methionine, is another nutritional remedy that has proven remarkably successful in relieving bone spur pain on the feet. It is widely available from a variety of companies at health food stores. Take 400 mg one to three times daily.

Plantar fasciitis, once contracted, is hard to cure, but a strong massage on the feet three times in one week has been reported to work.

BOWEL DISORDERS

Most women suffer an occasional bout of diarrhea or constipation. For some women, however, bowel disease is continual and quite debilitating.

Irritable bowel syndrome (IBS) strikes women three times as often as men and is among the most common gastrointestinal disorders for which women seek medical attention. IBS is a cluster of symptoms that includes abdominal discomfort, bloating, constipation, diarrhea, or constipation and diarrhea alternately. Mucus in and around the stool is also common. Symptoms usually begin in the teens or early adulthood and are often worse during the first few days of the menstrual cycle. Patients are often depressed and may have suffered physical or sexual abuse.[1]

Inflammatory bowel disease (IBD), or spastic colitis, is a similar but more severe condition, which has been diagnosed in younger women more frequently over the past few decades. The cause of the disease is unknown. Twice as many women as men report it, and the condition adversely affects hormonal function and menstruation. While premenstrual syndrome (PMS) includes gastrointestinal symptoms, for women with IBD, this gastrointestinal discomfort is much more severe. Ibuprofen and other nonsteroidal anti-inflammatory drugs typically recommended for the relief of menstrual pain can make the situation worse, since the drugs themselves cause intestinal inflammation. Some women with IBD have irregular menstrual periods, and some report having no menstrual periods for months at a time. Once disease symptoms are under control, periods usually return. Part of the problem may be nutritional, an inability to absorb sufficient nutrients from food. If fat stores are insufficient, the body won't be able to produce adequate estrogen, the hormone that sets menstruation in motion.[2]

Celiac sprue is another condition involving chronic diarrhea, abdominal pain, and bloating. In this case, the cause is known—a sensitivity of the small intestine to gluten. Gluten is a protein found in most cereal grains but not in corn and rice. Women with celiac sprue often have trouble conceiving. The primary treatment is to avoid gluten-containing foods. New hybrids of wheat have been blamed for an increase in the disease.

See also "Constipation" on page 91 and "Digestive Problems" on page 104.

CONVENTIONAL TREATMENT

Chronic inflammation of the bowel can cause such debilitating symptoms during menstruation that doctors sometimes recommend eliminating menstruation altogether, using short-term injections of contraceptives or hormonal therapy. For severe bowel disease, immunomodulating drugs may be used. Steroids may also be used, but prolonged steroid use can have serious side effects, including weight gain and facial fullness, hypertension, diabetes, osteoporosis, cataracts, intestinal bleeding, and increased susceptibility to infections. Some doctors also prescribe antidiarrheal drugs, but the drugs don't address the underlying problem and can have side effects of their own.

NATURAL REMEDIES

A first step in treating bowel disorders is to consider parasites, an often-overlooked suspect in conditions involving chronic diarrhea and intestinal upset. Parasites are thought to thrive particularly where there is decreased acid in the stomach or some underlying immune suppression. A key diagnostic factor is a sudden onset of symptoms, often after traveling outside the country or after a bout with food poisoning or stomach upset. Typically, onset is also during a time when the sufferer is under unusual stress. When the host is anxious, nervous, or stressed, parasites become activated. For women who fit that profile, homeopathic Giardia Lamblia Remedy by Deseret is effective. Lamblia and BE, vibrational remedies by Kroeger Herbs, also work well. For other suggestions, see "Parasitic Infection" on page 212.

A homeopathic remedy effective for diarrhea is *Podophyllum* 30C. Take three pills as needed up to three times daily.

Constitutional homeopathic remedies specific to the patient are also effective. For the neat and organized "type A" personality, *Arsenicum album* 12c or 30C is a good choice (three pills as needed up to four times daily). See a homeopath for recommendations in your own case.

Also useful for treating flare-ups are minerals including magnesium and calcium, and natural herbal preparations including dong quai (willow bark), black cohosh (black snakeroot plant), ginseng tea, chamomile tea, primrose oil, and extracts from red clover or yams. A practitoner should be consulted to ensure that the amount or method of preparation won't increase discomfort.[3]

Extremely important is dietary modification. Women with celiac sprue must avoid all gluten products, and women with chronic diarrhea should consider avoiding those products. All dairy products (milk, cheese, ice cream, and so on) should be stopped, and cold food and raw foods are best avoided. Fatty foods are hard to digest and should be kept to a minimum, while fiber intake should be increased.

BREAST CANCER

See CANCERS, HORMONAL.

BREAST PAIN AND TENDERNESS, BREAST LUMPS, AND FIBROCYSTIC BREASTS

Breast pain and tenderness can have a variety of causes. They include breast fibrocysts (swollen, fibrous breast tissue) and other non-fibrous breast lumps, which come and go particularly in women in menopause or perimenopause. Other causes of breast pain are swelling and irritation caused by erratic hormone levels during pregnancy, nursing or menopause; and injury to the breasts.

BREAST LUMPS DISAPPEAR IN TWO DAYS WITH NATURAL TREATMENT

A woman was concerned about a lump in her breast that her boyfriend discovered. She had consulted a gynecologist, who had scheduled her for a mammogram and thought she would need a biopsy. She then sought a second opinion from Dr. Walker, who said she might simply have low thyroid levels. The woman acknowledged that she had had several tests done in which her thyroid level was low, although it was still within the normal range. Dr. Walker explained that the "low normal" range was often too low, and gave her liquid iodine and the homeopathic remedy Thyroid. The woman called later to report that the first day she took these remedies, she had more energy than she'd had for years, and that by the second day, her breast lump was gone. No biopsy was required.

Dr. Walker subsequently suggested these remedies to seven other women with breast lumps. In each case the lumps went away, though the time varied from three days to six weeks.

CONVENTIONAL TREATMENT

The medical concern with breast pain and breast lumps is the possibility of breast cancer. Breast fibrocysts are usually benign and will go away of their own accord without causing problems, either when the hormonal changes of menopause have subsided or with appropriate dietary change. But the fear of cancer is so great that doctors are liable to advise immediate diagnostic procedures followed by surgery, no matter what they find on testing.

Note: While most breast lumps are harmless and will go away with simple nondrug treatments (fewer than 0.2 percent of fibroid tumors are found to be malignant),[1] that remains a possibility. Consulting with a doctor is therefore advised.

NATURAL REMEDIES

Hormone researcher John Lee, M.D., coauthor of *What Your Doctor May Not Tell You About Menopause*, observes that breast fibrocysts and painful breast swelling are common when estrogen levels are high in the estrogen-dominant phase of perimenopause. Fibrocysts are characterized by an overgrowth of fibrous tissue and a higher level of circulating estrogen, indicating a hormonal imbalance. Dr. Lee maintains that fibrocysts can be both prevented and treated with natural progesterone, estrogen's antagonist. In his clinical experience, these breast lumps usually disappear after two or three months of natural progesterone treatment. Supplementing with natural progesterone before menopause can prevent fibrocysts from developing, and supplementing with it after menopause is an effective way to protect against bone loss while avoiding the risk of fibroid development that accompanies higher levels of estrogen. "Very few things in medicine are this easy to treat," he ob-

MASTITIS RELIEVED WITH NATURAL REMEDY

A young mother complained of severely cracked nipples and mastitis (inflammation of the mammary glands). She was given *Bryonia* orally along with Calendula lotion to be applied topically to the nipple. After only one day of treatment, she was happy to report that the problem was nearly cured.

WINDSURFING INJURY RELIEVED WITH HOMEOPATHIC REMEDY

Beth's entire breast was black and blue after it was hit while windsurfing, although the accident had seemed minor at the time. Treatment with *Bellis* cleared the condition very quickly.

serves. "It is staggering to consider the many women who suffer needlessly from these problems."[2] The brand found to be most effective by Dr. Lee, as well as by these authors, is ProGest by Transitions for Health. Chapter 2 explains how ProGest is used.

In Chinese medicine, breast lumps and breast tenderness generally reflect liver stagnation and hormone imbalance. The liver's job is to clean the blood. When it becomes congested, it cannot clear hormones properly, so they build up. Besides food and toxic chemical overload, congestion can come from the suppression of emotions, especially suppressed anger. To clean the liver, Chinese doctors use a patent herbal remedy called *Xiao Yao Wan* (available in Chinese pharmacies or from acupuncturists). Once the liver stagnation is moved with this remedy, lumps have been known to go away virtually overnight. Dosages are on the box, but it's best to see a practitioner for recommendations.

Breast lumps have also been correlated with low thyroid hormone levels. Homeopathic remedies that stimulate the thyroid can help. Thyroid by CompliMed is excellent (ten drops three times daily). Supplementing with iodine can also help, either as liquid kelp or in foods, including seaweed and sea cucumbers. (Many brands are available; follow label directions.) Women with breast lumps should also decrease their intake of soy products, which can suppress thyroid levels. (See "Hypothyroidism" on page 150.)

For breast pain during lactation, other homeopathic remedies can help. Below are some alternatives for specific conditions (directions are on the label):

◆ For relief if breast-feeding is painful (three pellets ten minutes before breast-feeding)—*Phellandrium 9C.*

◆ For a minor abscess in the breast—*Hepar sulph 30C.*

◆ For the early stages of an abscess in the breast, when the skin is red and hot—*Belladonna 30C.*

◆ For mastitis—*Bryonia 30C.*

◆ For cracks around the nipples—*Graphites.*

Homeopathic calendula cream may also be used topically. To relieve painful engorgement, the mother should persist in nursing until the baby drains the engorged milk from her breast.

A common concern of women, whether or not clinically justified, is that physical injuries to the breast may precipitate breast cancer. To allay this concern, a woman undergoing blunt trauma to that area should take *Bellis,* the homeopathic remedy for blunt trauma particularly to the breast. This common remedy is available in health food stores; follow label directions.

BULIMIA

See ANOREXIA NERVOSA AND BULIMIA.

CANCER, CERVICAL

Cervical cancer is now considered a sexually transmitted disease, based on a demonstrated causal association with human papilloma virus (HPV), a viral infection that can be passed during sexual contact and can lead to genital warts.[1] The virus suppresses the immune system, increasing cancer risk. While not all women with cervical cancer have a history of HPV, most do. Having unprotected sex and many sexual partners (or having sex with men who have had many sexual partners) increases the risk. Smoking and poor nutrition are other risk factors. About 12,800 new cases of cervical cancer and 4,600 deaths from the disease are now predicted annually.[2]

A CAUTION ABOUT PAP SMEARS

A word of caution is necessary concerning the value of the routine Pap (Papanicolaou) smear for detecting cervical cancer and sexually transmitted disease. In 2000, after analyzing nearly a decade of data, researchers from the Centers for Disease Control concluded that women who got annual Pap smears received no benefit over those tested less frequently, and that the tests could be causing harm by increasing the risk of unnecessary treatment and anxiety.[4]

One of the most common and popular laboratory tests, the Pap smear is also one of the most unreliable. In one study, experts disagreed on whether cancer cells were present in about 40 percent of the cervical smears examined. In another study, in about two-thirds of the cases studied, two Pap smears taken at the same time from the same woman showed different results.[5]

Dr. James McCormick of Trinity College, Dublin, observes that not only is the test unreliable but there are also no randomized controlled trials showing that it saves lives. The closest attempt was a trial in Canada, where mass cervical screening was done in British Columbia but not in the rest of the country. Deaths from cervical cancer did drop in British Columbia, but they also dropped in the rest of the country, and to the same extent.[6] In the United Kingdom, on the other hand, the death rate has not dropped despite 40 million Pap smears. Ironically, deaths from cervical cancer were rare to start with. An American study reported in 1990 concluded that the overall cost of extending one person's life by one year by annual Pap tests was then $930,000.[7]

Particularly for virginal women, women over age 65, and women at no risk of exposure to sexually transmitted disease, screening for cervical cancer can do more harm than good. John Littell, M.D., writing in the November 15, 2000 issue of *American Family Physician*, observes that the purpose of the Pap smear is to screen for sexually transmitted disease and allow women to take part in the medical decision-making process. "The insertion of a vaginal speculum into the vagina of a virginal woman (or, for that matter, many postmenopausal women with atrophic vulvovaginitis) is certainly not a benign procedure," he says.[8]

A study reported in 2000 from the University of California, San Francisco, looked at Pap smear results from 2,561 women with a mean age of 67 who had normal baseline smears. One or two years later, 110 of these women had abnormal smears, but only one woman actually had a cervical lesion. The other 109 (about 4 percent of those screened) underwent follow-up biopsies and other interventions unnecessarily. The study authors warned that false-positive testing can cause undue stress on a patient, needless concern, and unnecessary medical procedures. Given these adverse effects, they said, health-care providers should be cautious about applying tests that have a high likelihood of yielding false-positive results. The authors noted that a woman who has a long history of normal Pap smears and who is over 50 years old has a very low risk of developing new cervical disease.[9]

CONVENTIONAL DIAGNOSIS AND TREATMENT

Conventional treatment of cervical cancer is with chemotherapy and radiation. For a fuller discussion of chemotherapy and radiation and cautions, see "Cancers, Hormonal" below.

For detecting cervical cancer and sexually transmitted disease, the conventional recommendation has been that all women should receive Pap smears at the onset of sexual activity or at eighteen years of age. For Pap smear cautions, see page 74.

NATURAL PREVENTIVE REMEDIES

Cancer cannot legally be treated by homeopaths, but homeopathic remedies are useful for clearing the underlying HPV infection and for prevention. The traditional remedy is *Thuja*. Deseret series therapy for HPV is even more effective. Series therapy consists of a box of ampules of the remedy in different potencies to be taken in a particular order. The remedies should be taken at the rate of one ampule every three days for a month. For some dramatic case historics, see "Genital Warts" on page 125.

Alternative therapies that can be administered by physicians include high doses of oral folic acid (10–20 mg daily) and vitamin A injected into the cervix.[3]

For prevention, having only one sexual partner is recommended.

CANCERS, HORMONAL

Breast cancer, ovarian cancer, and uterine cancer are hormone-related cancers that are of particular concern to women. Cancer cannot legally be treated by alternative practitioners, putting its treatment beyond the scope of this book. But because it is such a serious health concern for women, we do want to include some research to help you with a treatment decision. It is important that you exercise your critical faculties and not be pushed into a course of treatment based on the advertising claims of drug companies to physicians. Chemotherapeutic drugs are highly toxic poisons that were developed from the nerve gases used in World War II. They destroy the immune system and can cause secondary cancers that show up many years after "successful" chemotherapy.[1] Whether or not you opt for conventional treatment, natural remedies can help by supporting the body's own efforts at healing. However, natural remedies need a viable immune system to work and will be more effective if done before chemotherapy and radiation, if they are to be done.

CONVENTIONAL TREATMENT

Conventional treatment begins with diagnosis with a breast mammogram or vaginal Pap smear, followed by a biopsy (excision of tissue for examination) in suspicious cases. Chemotherapeutic drug treatment, radiation, and/or surgery follow in cases confirmed to be malignant. All of these procedures are controversial. The Pap smear is diagnostic only of cervical cancer, which is now considered to be caused by a sexually transmitted disease. Its limitations are discussed under "Cancer, Cervical." Other conventional cancer procedures are discussed below.

MAMMOGRAPHY

Doubts about the value of mammography first surfaced in 1991, when the *Times* of London published an article titled "Breast Scans Boost Risk of Cancer Death." Its opening line: "Middle-aged women who have regular mammograms are more likely to die from breast cancer than women who are not screened, according to dramatic new research." The study reported the results of the Canadian National Breast Screening Study (NBSS), the largest study of its kind carried out anywhere in the world. The NBSS was the first randomized, controlled clinical trial to separate the effect of mammography from the physical examination of the breast. In all other major trials, dating back to the 1960s, participants were given either mammography plus breast exams or mammography alone. The NBSS tracked 89,835 Canadian women age 40 to 49 during the period 1980–1988. Half were given mammograms every twelve to eighteen months. The other half were given only a single physical exam. To the surprise and chagrin of the researchers, at the end of the eight-year period, deaths among the group getting regular mammograms were "significantly higher" than in the group getting none.[2] When the study was published in November 1992, the odds of dying of breast cancer if you had been screened were reported to be 36 percent greater than if you had not.[3] On September 20, 2000, the thirteen-year follow-up results were published for the NBSS, involving nearly 40,000 women in their fifties. Again, no benefits were found for those receiving annual exams, and any design flaws criticized in 1992 were carefully refuted.[4] The data confirmed that mammography is no more effective than a careful breast exam by a trained professional in detecting breast cancer in women *either* in their forties or their fifties.

In 1999, a study published in *The Journal of the American Medical Association* (*JAMA*) concluded that mammography offers very little life-extending benefit for women over age 69.[5] And a Swedish study reported the same year found no significant benefit for women age 50 to 69. The breast cancer death rate dropped only 1 percent between 1989 and 1996 for women in that age group, despite regular mammography screening. The results were called "a shocking disappointment," since an accumulated 25 to 30 percent mortality reduction had been predicted based on the findings of eight earlier randomized controlled clinical trials conducted worldwide previously considered the "gold standard" for information about mammography.[6]

As for those eight trials, in January 2000 the British medical journal *The Lancet* published a new analysis concluding that six of the trials were flawed in a way that exaggerated mammography's benefit; and the two remaining studies (including the NBSS) found no benefit for mammography. The conclusion of *The Lancet* analysis was that "Screening for breast cancer with mammography is unjustified. . . . [T]he data show that for every 1,000 women screened biennially throughout 12 years, one breast-cancer death is avoided whereas the total number of deaths is increased by six."[7]

Mammography is controversial for another reason. Breast cancer incidence has reportedly increased 30 percent since the 1970s when it came into vogue, and disturbing new research blames mammography itself for at least some of the apparent increase. Mammography and biopsy are detecting "precancerous" conditions that would not otherwise have turned into active cancers. That would make both the apparent incidence and the apparent cure rate go up, since the easiest cancers to cure are the ones that aren't really cancer. The disturbing part is that 30 percent of breast cancer "victims" may have been victims only of their unnecessary treatments: biopsy, surgery, radiation, and chemotherapy. Even the National Cancer Institute has conceded that mass screening may be responsible for the alarming increase (or apparent increase) in breast cancer incidence.[8] The suspicion was strengthened by a study at Fred Hutchinson Cancer Research Center in Seattle finding that the apparent increase in breast cancer could be explained by early detection alone.[9]

John Gofman, M.D., Professor of Molecular and Cell Biology at the University of California at Berkeley, asserts in a 1999 book *Radiation from Medical Procedures in the Pathogenesis of Cancer and Ischemic Heart Disease* that mammography and other diagnostic X rays have contributed to the cancer epidemic in another way: medical radiation itself substantially increases cancer risk. His detailed review of the evidence suggests that this may actually be the most important cause of cancer deaths in the twentieth century.[10]

CONVENTIONAL CANCER TREATMENT

Ironically, mammography *has* been found to be effective as an early cancer detection technique. The Canadian study found that it detected cancers earlier than physical examination alone and was more sensitive in finding smaller cancers and *in situ* carcinomas.[11] NBSS director Dr. Anthony Miller blamed the failure of mammography to save lives not on the procedure itself but on the cancer treatment that followed the diagnoses. "Studies in animals suggested that removal of the main tumour and radiation of the immediate area affected the body's immune system so that tumours elsewhere grow faster," he said. "You may find the cancers earlier (with mammography), but the women are still going to die. *Modern treatment does not work for these early cancers.*"[12] It was, of course, the early cancers that the cancer establishment has said modern treatment does work for. The late cancers, the ones that have spread to other areas of the body, are known to be much harder to cure. It was to catch the early cancers that billions have been spent on mass screening for early detection.

The statistics cited in support of cancer treatment in general are often misleading. While the National Cancer Institute (NCI) consistently claims gains in the cancer cure rate, the General Accounting Office has accused the NCI of regularly manipulating data in order to "artificially inflate the amount of 'true' progress."[13] In 1997, statistician Dr. John Bailar III, former editor of the *Journal of the National Cancer Institute,* compared the most recent cancer mortality rates with those in 1970, just before the National Cancer Act released billions of dollars for cancer research. Overall, he found, the odds of dying of cancer are 6 percent *higher* today than they were in 1970.[14] While some battles in the cancer war have been won, they have been primarily against uncommon forms of the disease, accounting for less than 2 percent of total cancer deaths. For the major killers—including not only the hormonal cancers of the breast, ovary, and prostate but also cancers of the lung and colon—deaths have either stayed the same or increased, despite the intervention of the world's most costly and sophisticated cancer technology.[15]

In an eye-opening 1995 book *Questioning Chemotherapy,* Dr. Ralph Moss documented the ineffectiveness of chemotherapy for prolonging life or improving its quality in the case of most cancers. He noted that the FDA defines an "effective" drug as one that achieves a reduction of 50 percent or more in tumor size over twenty-eight days. That means that to be "effective," a drug needn't be proven to extend life or improve its quality. After reviewing thousands of studies for more than fifty types of cancer, Dr. Moss concluded that in most cases the drugs do neither.[16] In a January 2001 update confirming his earlier statistics, Dr. Moss observed that cancer drug ads are often misleading. An ad for the cancer drug Arimidex, for example, claimed "56.1 percent survival" for breast cancer patients treated with it. What the ad was actually referring to was the two-year survival rate compared to an older drug, Megace. The median time to death for women on the newer drug was 26.7 months compared to 22.5 months for Megace, a difference that did not reach statistical significance. In either case, the patients lived only about two years after treatment, hardly the common definition of "survival."[17] And the "control" group involved another toxic drug, not natural treatment or no treatment.

Surgery and radiation have also not been proven in controlled trials to extend life. They didn't need to be, since they were grandfathered in before the FDA's "effectiveness" requirement.[18] Radiation can effectively shrink tumors in critical situations (when the tumor is pressing on an artery, airway, vital organ, or nerve), but long-term studies have found that it can actually shorten overall survival.[19]

As a last resort in serious breast cancer cases, oncologists have turned to bone marrow transplants.[20] In an article in the October 18, 1998, issue of *The New Yorker* titled "Healing Hell," Jerome Groopman, M.D., called this procedure both "the most powerful weapon in the growing arsenal against cancer" and "the most devastating treatment that the human body could be subjected to." Preliminary results reported in April 1999 of long-awaited international studies on bone marrow transplants, however, were called "a bitter disappointment." The therapy Dr. Groopman called conventional oncology's most powerful weapon against cancer was found to be no more effective in prolonging life than conventional chemotherapy, which is also only marginally effective for metastized breast cancer.[21]

Among breast cancer drugs, the market leader is currently tamoxifen (Zeneca's Novaldex), a synthetic estrogen compound that acts by blocking natural estrogen from binding with receptor sites in breast tissue. Roughly 1 million American breast cancer patients are now being treated with tamoxifen, but the drug is not a cure and comes with significant side effects, including troublesome hot flashes and a significantly increased risk of blood clots, serious thromboembolic events, and uterine cancer.[22]

Tamoxifen was recommended not only for treatment but also as a preventive measure for women at high risk for developing cancer of the breast, after it was shown to help prevent breast cancer recurrences in women already treated for the disease. But recruitment into a tamoxifen prevention trial at the University of Pittsburgh beginning in 1981 was temporarily halted following a finding that more than ten times as many women contracted cancer of the uterus in the tamoxifen group as in the control group. Despite those findings, the National Cancer Institute continued to spend millions of taxpayers' dollars giving the drug to cancer-free women already in the study, to see if it would keep them from developing the disease.[23] A nine-year Swedish study reported in 2001 confirmed the uterine cancer risk, finding a more than fivefold increase in its incidence in women given tamoxifen, and in 1998 the World Health Organization labeled the drug a carcinogen. Zeneca kept it off the official carcinogen list only by aggressive lobbying of California state regulators.[24]

Natural Remedies

As an alternative to synthetic estrogen blockers, hormone researcher John Lee, M.D., proposes using estrogen's antagonist, natural progesterone, to keep estrogen levels in check. He maintains that 80 percent of breast cancer could be prevented simply by keeping hormone levels in balance in this way. He cites a 1995 study involving premenopausal women scheduled for breast surgery, finding that cell proliferation in those who used natural progesterone cream was far less than in those who used placebo or estrogen creams.[25]

Estrogen's principal function is to encourage cellular proliferation and growth. Estrogen causes the proliferation of pre-embryonic cells that produces the growth of the fetus. Normal pre-embryonic cells are found not only in the ovaries but in other parts of the body, where they are thought to be involved in regenerating damaged or aging tissue. Wherever the body is damaged, estrogen is also found in great concentrations, in both men and women. It seems to serve as a stimulus to cellular growth and repair.[26] Most primary tumors occur where there is cell renewal due to irritation or trauma. When the repair is done, the growth should stop, as in benign tumors. Alternative practitioners maintain that cancer results when the normal regenerative growth gets out of control.[27] This occurs when estrogen becomes dominant over its antagonist progesterone, resulting either from increased estrogen intake or decreased progesterone production.[28] Stress and emotional trauma deplete progesterone supplies, allowing estrogen to be dominant and tumors to grow. Estrogen can also become dominant when supplied in hormone replacement therapy, in meats from animals fattened with hormones, or by the estrogenlike substances in pesticides and other environmental chemicals.

The obvious solution is to increase the supply of progesterone, either with natural progesterone creams or with homeopathic and herbal remedies that help the body rebalance hormone levels. For remedy alternatives, see Chapters 2 and 3 and "Breast Pain and Tenderness" on page 71.

Concerning alternatives to mammography, the Canadian National Breast Screening Study found that a careful manual breast exam performed by a trained nurse practitioner is not only as effective as a mammogram but is also safer and much less expensive. The researchers cautioned that most manual breast exams performed in a doctor's office are not as thorough as those in their study. They stressed the importance of proper training of medical personnel to perform a proper exam. Another alternative is breast screening by thermography, which measures the infrared heat radiating from the body. Where mammography can detect a tumor only after it has been growing for years and reaches a certain size, thermography can detect potential problems much earlier because it can image the early stages of angiogenesis. Angiogenesis is the formation of a direct supply of blood to cancer cells, a necessary step before cancer cells can grow into tumors.[29]

Many good books are available on the subject of alternative treatments for cancer.[30] Some of these treatments are currently being studied by the NCI's Office of Cancer Complementary and Alternative Medicine. Many alternative treatments are available only in other countries. If you want to take an active role, you could petition your congressperson for more funding for research into cancer treatment alternatives, or for a patients' rights bill allowing the pursuit of alternatives without having to go abroad for them. For further discussion of the legal and medical issues, read *Forbidden Medicine* by Ellen Brown.[31]

CHALLENGING CANCER INDUSTRY MARKETING CLAIMS

Dr. Candace Pert, a neuroscientist and research professor at Georgetown University School of Medicine, has extensively studied the receptors on cells and the man-made substances that can cause cancer by binding to them. Noting that breast cancer has increased at the rate of 2 percent a year since 1946, she says the evidence is overwhelming that environmental toxins, including herbicides, pesticides, and plastics, are the principal culprits. Plastics mimic estrogen and attach to its receptor sites on cells. Genetics explains less than 5 percent of cancer cases, and then it has to do only with how the body handles toxins.[32]

In *Mother Jones,* Monte Paulsen points out that the companies that stand to profit most from massive cancer prevention and treatment campaigns are some of the same companies responsible for these environmental toxins. Breast cancer strikes more than 180,000 women annually in the United States. Paulsen calls it "not only an epidemic, but also a market opportunity." Cancer drugs are particularly lucrative, generating $8.5 billion annually. Zeneca, which does a $470 million per year business in tamoxifen, is also the founder and sole financial sponsor of National Breast Cancer Awareness Month. Zeneca also does a $300 million business in a carcinogenic herbicide called acetochlor, and it has been named in a lawsuit brought by federal and state governments for allegedly dumping DDT and PCBs into the Los Angeles and Long Beach harbors. Zeneca's promotional literature urges, "Early detection is your best prevention . . . get a mammogram *now.*" About 24 million mammograms are performed yearly in the United States, 90 percent of them on asymptomatic women. General Electric does more than a $100 million business annually in mammography machines, while Du Pont makes much of the film used in those machines. General Electric and Du Pont also compete for the distinction of having the highest number of EPA Superfund hazardous waste sites.[33]

Challenging the marketing claims of Zeneca's National Breast Cancer Awareness posters, several massive recent studies found that mammography does not increase the survival rate from breast cancer *at any age.*[34] Other studies have found that the claims made for conventional cancer treatment are misleading. Dr. Pert warns, "One should be skeptical and look very carefully at the data before undergoing any cancer treatments. It's amazing how few cancers are really effectively treated by the current regimens, and they may literally do more harm than good. Testicular cancer and some lymphomas are cured by chemo, but for breast cancer, the data's not there. If you look at the experiments that got these treatments to be standard of care, they don't have a control group that has NO chemo, let alone a control group that has [non-drug] interventions."[35]

CANDIDIASIS

See FUNGAL INFECTIONS.

CARDIAC ARRHYTHMIAS

See IRREGULAR HEARTBEAT.

CARPAL TUNNEL SYNDROME

Carpal tunnel syndrome is a disorder characterized by pain, tingling, or numbness in the wrist, hands, and fingers, particularly at night. It results when swollen or inflamed ligaments put pressure on adjacent nerves. Compression of the nerves of the wrist can, in turn, cause painful elbows or shoulders. This syndrome is reported to have grown to

THE AUTHOR'S OWN EXPERIENCE WITH CARPAL SYNDROME

As an obsessive-compulsive overachieving law student, Ellen, a coauthor of this book, spent her days furiously scribbling notes. Soon, she noticed that her writing hand was getting numb. When she got pregnant after graduating from law school, both of her hands became numb, especially at night. She sought medical advice, but this was in the 1970s when carpal tunnel syndrome was an obscure condition, and no one seemed to know what it was. A neighbor with the same problem finally suggested wrist splints, which Ellen wore to bed every night for the next seventeen years. Then, when she turned fifty, she was suddenly able to sleep without them. She concluded this was because her estrogen levels had dropped relative to her progesterone levels, the combined result of menopause and of the natural progesterone cream (ProGest) she had been applying to her abdominal area every night for several years.

nearly epidemic proportions worldwide, a phenomenon attributed largely to the explosion in computer use.[1] While stress on the ligaments aggravates the condition, there is also a hormonal component. The incidence of carpal tunnel syndrome is particularly high among pregnant and menopausal women, and topical natural progesterone can, in many cases, relieve the condition.

CONVENTIONAL TREATMENT

Wrist splints can relieve symptoms and are particularly useful while sleeping. Pain relievers are also often prescribed. In extreme cases, surgery may be performed. But none of these remedies addresses the underlying cause. Even surgery may need to be repeated every few years.

NATURAL REMEDIES

Acupuncture, chiropractic, massage, ultrasound, and yoga can help relieve pain by increasing circulation. Avoiding unnecessary repetitive stress is another obvious precautionary measure. Homeopathic remedies can also help. If the right wrist is worst, the appropriate remedy is *Viola odorata* 30. If both wrists are equally affected, the remedy is *Actea spicata* 30. Take two pellets of either remedy three times daily.

For many women, however, the underlying problem is hormone imbalance. Estrogen causes water retention in the tissues. The resulting edema (swelling) can impinge on the nerves. Dr. Walker has seen carpal tunnel syndrome reverse itself in a matter of weeks in more than thirty women, with the regular nightly application of natural progesterone cream (ProGest) directly to their wrists. Progesterone is estrogen's antagonist and works to normalize hormone levels.

CELIAC SPRUE

See BOWEL DISORDERS.

CHARLEY HORSE

See MUSCLE CRAMPS AND SPASMS.

CHLAMYDIA

Chlamydia is the most common treatable sexually transmitted disease. An estimated 4 million new cases occur each year, but most go unreported, largely because the disease can be without symptoms. This is also one reason for its spread, since it may be hard to detect in either your partner or yourself. When there are symptoms, they include difficult or painful urination, a yellowish vaginal discharge, bleeding between periods or after intercourse, and pain in the pelvic area during intercourse. In men, symptoms include difficult or painful urination and penile discharge. Untreated chlamydia can lead to pelvic inflammatory disease, resulting in infertility, ectopic pregnancy, and sometimes death. Chlamydia bacteria can also be responsible for a chronic eye inflammation called trachoma, which is one of the world's leading causes of blindness. Because 60 to 80 percent of genital chlamydia infections in women may be asymptomatic, screening is important. In one randomized trial, screening high risk women and treating those found to be infected reduced the incidence of pelvic inflammatory disease by about half in twelve months.[1]

CONVENTIONAL TREATMENT

Penicillin has been so overused that chlamydia has developed a resistance to it, so drug treatment is usually with tetracycline antibiotics. But even they may fail, often due to reinfection by an untreated sexual partner.[2]

NATURAL REMEDIES

Staufen, a German company, makes an effective homeopathic series therapy called Chlamydia for this condition. Series therapy involves a series of potencies, taken one ampule every three days for a month. The result is to push pathogens out by strengthening the immune system. Comparable series therapy is now available in the United States from Deseret. To avoid spreading the infection while undergoing treatment, condoms should be used.

CHLAMYDIA PREVENTION

Condoms, diaphragms, and spermicides containing nonoxynol-9 may help reduce the spread of chlamydia. However, nonoxynol-9 is a synthetic estrogen mimic that can have other side effects. A 1996 study found that women were more than three times as likely to get urinary tract infections if they used condoms with nonoxynol-9 more often than once a week.[3] The spermicide evidently kills not only sperm but also the friendly bacteria residing in the urinary tract, leaving it susceptible to invasion by unfriendly bacteria. The safest course remains abstinence or careful selection of partners. Anyone who is sexually active should get regular checkups by a physician.

CHOLESTEROL, HIGH

Cholesterol serves necessary functions. It is the precursor from which all hormones are made. Without sufficient cholesterol, your female organs will not have the hormones they need to operate efficiently. The resulting imbalances can subject you to the whole range of female symptoms discussed in Chapter 1. But women tend to avoid the dietary fats from which cholesterol is made because they are fattening and because elevated cholesterol levels have been associated with an increased risk of heart disease.

In an October 2000 article in the *Journal of the American Dietetic Association* titled "Over-the-counter Statin Medications: Emerging Opportunities for MDs," researchers stated that up to 59 percent of the adult population may have at least mildly elevated cholesterol levels under the current stringent standards, which define it as anything above 200 mg/dl and HDL cholesterol below 35 mg/dl.[1] Some authorities have set the standard as low as 180 mg/dl. The question is, does cholesterol at these levels really pose a risk? In 1994, Yale researchers reported in *The Journal of the American Medical Association* (*JAMA*) that it does not appear to, at least for the elderly. Tracking 997 Connecticut senior citizens for four years, the study found that people with the worst cholesterol profiles had virtually the same rates of heart disease and death as those with the best profiles.[2]

Insufficient cholesterol can result in weak sexual organs, precipitating hysterectomies and other surgeries, and in problems handling stress. Women lacking sufficient cholesterol to make the stress hormone cortisol are less able to cope with crises. Several studies have found a threefold increase in suicide, homicide, or other violent deaths among people taking cholesterol-lowering drugs.[3] Statin drugs have been linked to an increased risk of depression and impaired brain function.[4] And because cortisol reduces inflammation, decreased cortisol levels could mean increased inflammation, contributing to arthritis (inflammation of the joints) and other inflammatory diseases. The drugs have also caused cataracts and birth defects in animals.[5]

Rather than eliminating cholesterol artificially with drugs or by drastic fat-free diets, a safer approach is to eliminate "junk food" fats while retaining healthy dietary fats for which the body can make its own cholesterol (such as fish oil, evening primrose oil, olive oil, and flaxseed oil). Serum cholesterol can be kept at safe levels with nutritional and herbal remedies.

CONVENTIONAL TREATMENT

The line of drugs known as statins (Mevacor, Lipitor, and others) is recommended to treat the high cholesterol epidemic. The drugs can cost up to $200 per month, a very lucrative proposition for drug companies.[6] The drugs have become so popular that a prominent medical authority recently predicted that half the population of the United States could eventually wind up on them.[7]

The statins were heavily promoted after studies found that using them to lower only mildly elevated cholesterol reduced the odds of a "coronary heart disease event" by 30 percent. There is, however, a little-noted wrinkle in the data: heart attack risk goes down, *but the overall risk of death does not.* In October 2000, The *British Medical Journal* published the results of a meta-analysis of studies on the effects of primary prevention with lipid (fat)-lowering drugs on coronary heart disease events, coronary heart disease mortality, and all-cause mortality. The researchers concluded, "Drug treatment reduced the odds of a coronary heart disease event by 30% *but not the odds of all cause mortality.* When statin drugs were considered alone, no substantial differences in results were found."[8]

One increased risk for people on the drugs may be of cancer. A 1996 *JAMA* article reported that statins can cause cancer in laboratory animals. The authors concluded, "[L]ipid-lowering drug treatment, especially with the fibrates and statins, should be avoided except in patients at high short-term risk of coronary heart disease."[9]

The drugs can have other side effects and risks. Bayer's statin drug Baycol was withdrawn from the market in August 2001 after thirty-one deaths were reported from a severe adverse reaction called rhabdomyolysis, resulting in muscle cell breakdown and release of the contents of muscle cells into the bloodstream. Symptoms of the condition include muscle pain (especially in the calves and lower back), weakness, tenderness, malaise, fever, dark urine, nausea, and vomiting. Cases of fatal rhabdomyolysis have been reported more often with Baycol than with other statins, but all of them have been associated with this adverse muscle reaction. All work the same way: they lower cholesterol levels by blocking a specific enzyme in the body involved in the synthesis of cholesterol. Statins still on the U.S. market include Mevacor, Pravachol, Zocor, Lescol, and Lipitor.[10]

NATURAL REMEDIES

Natural remedies can produce significant cholesterol-lowering effects without side effects or risks. One option is red rice yeast extract, a form of yeast similar to the yeast consumed in high quantities by the Chinese for thousands of years. Researchers from the UCLA School of Medicine reported in *The American Journal of Clinical Nutrition* in February 1999 confirmed that when combined with a low-fat diet, red rice yeast extract reduces cholesterol levels by an average of forty points in twelve weeks.[11]

Red rice yeast extract is contained in Cholestin, an herbal product that was pulled off the market by the FDA in 1998 because it contained mevinolin, a substance chemically identical to the patented cholesterol-lowering statin drug lovastatin (Mevacor). However, the company that produced Cholestin did not process the red rice yeast extract in any way. The extract was simply crushed and put into capsules. (For this reason, it also lacks the side effects of lovastatin.) Joseph Mercola, M.D., maintains that Merck should not have been allowed to patent a naturally occurring chemical.[12] The ruling did not stick and Cholestin came back on the market, but a June 2001 ruling in the FDA's favor has again put the market longevity of Cholestin and other red rice yeast extract products in doubt.

In the meantime, a red rice yeast extract called Cholestene is currently available from HPF, a company that has not yet been contacted by the FDA. Cholestene comes as 1,200 mg capsules. The recommended dose is two capsules twice daily. Another inexpensive option is Solaray Red Yeast Rice, available from the Vitamin Shoppe at VitaminShoppe.com.

Also quite effective in lowering cholesterol levels is an Ayurvedic remedy called guggul (*Commiphora mukul*). Doctor's Best Brand Guggul and Jarrow's Opti-Gugul are excellent options available at health food stores. Results are seen within a month to six weeks. Directions are on the label.

Niacin and the Detox Approach

Another alternative to the statins is high-dose niacin. Until 1997, when a major drug study was reported involving lovastatin, high-dose niacin was the only conventional cholesterol-lowering drug found to actually increase overall survival.[13] Besides being more effective than the other remedies, it was only one-tenth their cost. Why? Because niacin isn't really a drug. It is vitamin B_3.

One theory explaining cholesterol buildup in the arteries is that it is a defense mechanism to protect the arteries from toxic onslaught by heavy metals, pesticides, and other poisonous chemicals. That theory could explain why niacin works so well in lowering cholesterol and increasing survival. The "niacin flush"—the red face and skin you get when you take large quantities of the vitamin—indicate that your capillaries are ejecting toxins. Niacin opens the capillaries, increases circulation, and normalizes cholesterol.

Niacin's remarkable ability to release toxic buildup from tissues was demonstrated in a California study in which participants taking it in high doses along with sauna therapy to sweat out toxins experienced significant drops in blood pressure, improvements in vision, increases in IQ points, and lessening of the symptoms of a number of physical ailments,

DANGEROUSLY HIGH CHOLESTEROL STABILIZED WITH NATURAL HERBAL PRODUCTS

Pamela, in her late forties, was not the type of person you would expect to have high cholesterol levels. She was very athletic, ate right, and rode her bike and windsurfed regularly. But no matter what she did, her cholesterol lingered in the 280 range. Opti-Gugul by Jarrow brought it down to 185 within a month.

Jane, age 62, was prescribed cholesterol-lowering drugs after her cholesterol was found to be 260 mg/dl. Guggul reduced her cholesterol, too, to safe levels without drugs.

Mary, age 61, was depressed and nervous about her very high cholesterol levels, which averaged 320 mg/dl. To her relief, her cholesterol dropped to 190 after only a month on red rice yeast extract (two capsules twice a day).

including asthma, allergy, migraine, and hypoglycemia. The program was followed daily for three weeks. It involved twenty to thirty minutes of vigorous exercise (jogging, stationary bicycling, and rowing), followed by thirty minutes in the sauna, a five-minute cooling off period, then thirty more minutes in the sauna. Sauna times could be gradually increased to two hours. Niacin dosage began at 400 mg spread throughout the day. The dose was then increased gradually to as high as 6,000 mg, depending on tolerance.[14]

Caution: Although niacin is available without a prescription, you should talk to your doctor before taking high-dose niacin for high cholesterol levels to determine a correct dosage for you.

Dietary Alternatives

The safest, cheapest, most natural solution to high cholesterol levels remains dietary and lifestyle modification. In Dr. Dean Ornish's landmark program, cholesterol levels were lowered significantly in people who ate a low-fat vegetarian diet, quit smoking, walked one hour three times a week, and reduced stress by daily yoga and meditation. The only animal products allowed on the diet were nonfat milk and yogurt.[15] (See "Heart Disease" on page 135 for details.)

Another nutritional approach is to fortify your diet with soy products. A study reported in *The New England Journal of Medicine* on August 3, 1995, found that eating 47 grams of soy protein daily (about the amount in ¾ pound of firm tofu) lowered cholesterol by a full 20 percent in people whose levels were initially too high. Soy protein also significantly reduced LDL or "bad" cholesterol and triglycerides, both of which are primary heart disease risk factors. The effect was attributed to the phytoestrogen compounds called isoflavones.[16] In a 1997 meta-analysis of thirty-eight studies in which other variables were controlled, soy protein intake averaging 47 grams per day was associated with a 9.3 percent reduction in serum cholesterol and a 12.9 percent reduction in serum LDL cholesterol. Both were statistically significant. For people in good health, the reviewers suggested seven servings of soy protein a week, providing an average of 8 to 10 grams of soy protein daily. This could be obtained from an 8-ounce soy beverage daily; two soy muffins daily; two servings of tofu four times weekly; four soy burgers weekly; or one tablespoon of isolated soy protein stirred into a drink daily.[17]

For people with coronary heart disease, the reviewers suggested tripling that amount, but other studies suggest this may be too much. Excess soy can impair thyroid hormone levels and can inhibit iron absorption, leading to anemia and iron deficiency in women.[18] It is best is to limit soy products to one serving daily.

Another natural cholesterol-lowering foodstuff is plant fiber. The most effective type is the soluble fiber in fruits, vegetables, and oat bran. Unlike insoluble fiber, which remains coarse and gritty in water, soluble fibers dissolve to form a gel. All plant foods are rich in both types of fiber, but some contain more of one than the other. Insoluble fiber, the kind in wheat bran, increases stool bulk and promotes bowel function. Soluble fiber, the kind in oat bran, forms a gel that traps cholesterol-rich bile acids. These bile acids would otherwise be recycled by the body. When they're trapped and eliminated, the body has to use other cholesterol to make more bile acids, and serum cholesterol is reduced.[19]

Soluble fiber is also the kind found in bulk laxatives like Metamucil containing psyllium. In one study, volunteers with an average serum cholesterol level of 250 mg/dl were given a teaspoonful of Metamucil three times a day. After eight weeks, their cholesterol levels had dropped an average of 35 mg/dl, or 14 percent. This result was comparable to results with a low dose of the popular cholesterol drug Mevacor or with the prescription cholesterol-lowering bile-acid resins Questran and Colestid. In fact, psyllium works in much the same way as bile-acid resins. It binds bile acids in the intestines and prevents them from being reabsorbed. The advantages of psyllium are that it's easier to swallow, and its side effects are limited to occasional mild stomach cramps and gas.[20]

Cholesterol levels can also be lowered by eating common edible plant fibers, including the pectin found in apples and other fruits and vegetables. The mechanism is the same as with bile-acid resins. In combination with calcium, pectin binds readily to bile acids, rendering them useless as digestive enzymes. The liver senses there is a shortage of bile acid and compensates by extracting cholesterol molecules from the blood. These molecules are then modified into bile molecules. The result is a drop in serum cholesterol.[21]

CHRONIC FATIGUE SYNDROME

Chronic fatigue syndrome (CFS) is a disorder that affects as much as 7 percent of the American population, and two out of three sufferers are women.[1] Besides a debilitating, chronic exhaustion not relieved by rest, symptoms can include sore throats, painful or swollen lymph nodes, muscle and joint pains, headaches, sleep disturbances, and impaired short-term memory and concentration. Women with CFS report feeling sick all the time, have chronically swollen glands, and toss and turn at night, rarely getting a good night's sleep. Although they are enormously tired, they can look healthy and energetic, subjecting them to the further burden of being branded hypochondriacs.

CONVENTIONAL TREATMENT

No conventional therapy has proven effective in curing CFS in controlled clinical trials with prolonged follow-up.[2] At one time, CFS was assumed to have a viral cause and was described as chronic Epstein-Barr virus syndrome or chronic mononucleosis. Its designation was changed to chronic fatigue syndrome (CFS) or chronic fatigue/immune depression syndrome (CFIDS) after researchers concluded its cause was unknown.[3] The invading viruses originally thought to cause the disease were merely taking advantage of an immune system weakened from some other cause.

NATURAL REMEDIES

Although the cause of CFS is officially unknown, there are a number of alternative theories, and a number of effective natural remedies.

Homeopaths maintain that the suppression of the immune system resulting in chronic fatigue can be a direct result of antibiotic use. The drugs don't actually eliminate bacteria but merely push the invaders deeper into the system. Multiple stresses induce an abnormal immune system response. CFS is a slow breakdown of the immune system, which allows bacteria, viruses, and fungal parasites to be accepted by the body rather than rejecting them through acute illness. The typical CFS history involves an episode of extreme stress, such as a car accident, combined with a course of antibiotics. A healthy person who comes in contact with a bacteria or virus will get a healing response—runny nose, thick mucus, cough, headache, and so on—but people with CFS are too sick and their immune systems are too suppressed to react.

Bruce Waller, M.D., a medical doctor in Artesia, California, had remarkable success treating CFS homeopathically. He maintained that CFS is the end result of a deep suppression of the immune system, preventing the body from fighting its bacterial, viral, or parasitic invaders. As a result, it is liable to have a number of them cohabiting with it at any one time, producing layer upon layer of disease. Cure requires clearing these layers away one by one. Dr. Waller addressed each layer individually, treating each for about a month before moving on to the next.

Dr. Waller used homeopathic remedies, but other practitioners have eliminated layers of the disorder with other natural treatments. The following are some of the layers that may require "peeling":

Mononucleosis is a bacterial infection reported in the histories of perhaps 60 percent of CFS patients. The infection appears to be one of the first assaults to their immune systems.

Brucella, a bacteria found in cattle, causes muscle aches and pains, inflammation, aching joints, and swollen lymph glands. The joint and muscle pain of CFS is often found to be from this bacteria.

Peptostreptococcus, a bacteria normally found in the sinuses and throat, is the cause of repeated sinus infections in CFS patients. Each course of antibiotics pushes the bacteria deeper into the sinuses and makes the next infection deeper and heavier.

Coxsackie is a virus that resides in the spine, usually causing hip pain or pain along the spinal column. With trauma, it moves to the brain. The trauma is often a car accident, but it can also be a fall or head trauma. The result is foggy thinking and headaches. People with Coxsackie infection may have such difficulty trying to express their thoughts that they break down and cry. Although they have something they desperately want to say, they can't pull their thoughts together well enough to say it.

Giardia lamblia and other parasites contribute to the constant gas, bloating, and indigestion problems of CFS patients. Their immune systems are so run down that they easily pick up parasites. Parasites can puncture the digestive tract, allowing macromolecules to slip undigested into the bloodstream, where they strain the immune system.[4]

Candidiasis is another CFS symptom reflecting an overwhelmed immune system. Correcting an underlying pH imbalance can correct both candidiasis and CFS. See "Fungal Infections" on page 116.

Chemical hypersensitivity syndrome can complicate CFS. Poor oxygen absorption by fatigued muscle tissue results in an abnormal sensitivity to chemicals and environmental toxins—perfume, paint, carpets, and so on. (See "Multiple Chemical Sensitivity" on page 185.)

Allergies to foods, molds, chemicals, and a long list of other triggers are other possible underlying factors. The practitioner should also look for pneumonia, herpes, Lyme disease, toxic dental work, and exposure to environmental toxins.

See specific disease categories for remedies for these underlying conditions.

DENTAL FILLINGS AND CFS

CFS symptoms have been resolved not only by doctors but also by dentists. In *Toxic Metal Syndrome*, Drs. Casdorph and Walker assert, "[C]hronic fatigue/immune suppression

CHRONIC FATIGUE SYNDROME RELIEVED WITH HOMEOPATHIC REMEDIES

Rebecca, age 35, had had CFS for the past four years. She had to quit her job as a nanny because she was just too tired to do the work. The first assault to her immune system was evidently mononucleosis, which she had had as a teenager. This was followed by several bouts of sinus problems for which she took antibiotics. After a car accident in which her back was injured, she developed CFS. Homeopathic series therapy for Rebecca's sinus condition and for mononucleosis cleared up the condition. The first remedy used was Peptostrep. The second was Mononucleosis.

Bunny, age 54, said she hadn't been well since her daughter was killed nearly a decade earlier. Besides CFS, she had asthma and severe edema in her lower legs. Getting her well took an entire year of homeopathic remedies for a variety of problems, including colds, flu, and anxiety. Today, Bunny says she feels better than she has for years.

Christy, age 34, had suffered from CFS for more than seven years. She could barely work, and she had a 4-year-old child to take care of. Her glands were swollen, she had a great deal of trouble sleeping, and she was very depressed. She had exhausted her financial resources on a very expensive course of treatment that had focused on candidiasis, but her problems ran much deeper than that. She had a prior history of mononucleosis and of sexual abuse. For the latter, she was treated homeopathically with *Staphysagria* for held-in resentment, anger, and fear. For the mononucleosis, she took the homeopathic series therapy Brucella, then Mononucleosis. Christy had ups and downs during the treatment, but when it was over, she was delighted by how much better she felt. She was sleeping well, had gotten her energy back, and could get her projects done without strain. Four years later, she remains well.

syndrome (CFIDS) is directly connected to amalgam fillings. . . . Positive response against CFIDS is experienced by the patient and witnessed by the dentist within two weeks of amalgam removal."[5]

Sherry Rogers, M.D., another specialist in the field, explains that heavy metals cause fatigue because they sit in the enyzmes on the membrane and inside the mitochondria where energy is synthesized inside cells. Heavy metals displace essential minerals such as zinc, magnesium, manganese, copper, and iron, so the enzymes can no longer function normally.[6]

Dissimilar metals in the mouth can also create a "battery effect" that interferes with the body's own electromagnetic field, creating fatigue and other symptoms.

Replacing the metals in the teeth, however, requires careful protocols. What the dentist uses for a replacement material is important. Plastic composite materials can be as hazardous as metals, though in a different way. For a thorough discussion of this subject, read *The Key to Ultimate Health* by Ellen Brown and Richard Hansen, D.M.D.[7]

CLUSTER HEADACHES

See HEADACHES.

COLD SORES AND CANKER SORES

Two of the most common infections of the mouth, cold sores (fever blisters) and canker sores (aphthous ulcers) are not serious conditions but can mar a woman's appearance and make her feel self-conscious. Canker sores are small, painful ulcers on the inside of the mouth, usually lasting five to ten days. Cold sores are most likely to appear on the outside of the mouth and lips, although they can show up anywhere on the skin or on the gums. Canker sores are not considered contagious, while cold sores are. Cold sores may be accompanied by fever, swollen neck glands, and a general achy feeling. Canker sores are rarely accompanied by fever or other signs of illness. The cause of canker sores is unknown, but suspected triggers include stress, nutritional deficiencies, immune system defects, and allergy or sensitivity to some food, such as tomatoes, chocolate, and citrus fruits.

Cold sores are caused by the herpes simplex virus. After the initial outbreak, the virus usually stays dormant in the skin until something causes resistance to be low, such as a cold, sunburn, shock, dental or sinus infections, or menstrual problems.[1] There are two principal strains of herpes simplex virus, type 1 and type 2. Type 1 is the usual cause of cold sores, but type 2 (which is normally limited to the genital region) may also produce cold sores on the face. Touching cold sores can result in spreading the virus to new sites on the body or to other people, so it's important to keep hands off the infected area and to avoid kissing. Once oral herpes has been contracted, the virus remains in a nerve near the cheekbone, and outbreaks can recur. Like with genital herpes, oral herpes outbreaks have been linked to emotional stress, as well as to fever, illness, injury, and overexposure to the sun.

CONVENTIONAL TREATMENT

Antiseptic powders and ointments may be used to prevent secondary infections, and various lotions and powders can relieve pain and itching and hasten drying. However, there is no pharmaceutical "cure" for these skin eruptions, and the drugs used on them can have side effects. The antiviral drug acyclovir (Zovirax) may be used topically for cold sores, but the blisters tend to recur.[2] Zovirax comes with potential side effects, including nausea and vomiting, diarrhea, headache, and skin rash. It is not intended for canker sores. For canker sores, steroids, such as hydrocortisone cream, are typically recommended. These too can have harmful side effects, however, and they suppress the body's own efforts at cure. (See "Skin Problems" on page 222.)

NATURAL REMEDIES

Cold sores and canker sores will go away by themselves and usually need no treatment at all. However, if the sores are particularly bothersome or recurring, there are natural remedies that can relieve discomfort and speed healing.

The most well-known natural alternative for cold sores is the amino acid lysine. Dosage is 1,000 mg every four hours at the outset, or 500 mg two to three times daily to prevent recurrences. Although lysine works and is safer than Zovirax, it still addresses only the symptoms.

Homeopathic remedies not only can heal cold sores but can also prevent them from coming back. Homeopathic Calendula and Hypericum Ointment by Boiron clears up the blisters quickly, while *Natrum muriaticum* (*Nat mur*) 6X keeps them from recurring. The recommended dosage of *Nat mur* is four pills four times daily at the onset of symptoms. Although the cold sores may seem at first to be recurring more often but healing faster, in a few months they should be gone for good. For stubborn cases, a single dose of Herpes

RECURRING COLD SORES ELIMINATED

A woman complained of recurring cold sores. As soon as one cleared up, the next one appeared. She was delighted to report that topical Calendula and Hypericum Ointment, along with homeopathic *Pulsatilla* (a constitutional remedy specific to her), cleared the condition permanently.

An 8-year-old girl was miserable with recurring cold sores. She broke out with them every couple of weeks. Conventional treatment couldn't break this cycle. What did was the homeopathic remedy *Nat mur* 6X. The dosage for her was four pellets up to three times daily as needed.

simplex homeopathic nosode may also be given. (A nosode is a homeopathic remedy made from a disease product.)

Other effective homeopathic options include Cold Sores by Natra-Bio and Cliniskin H by CompliMed (also good for genital herpes). Natural topical remedies that can aid in healing cold sores include herbal Goldenseal and Propolis Cream by Eclectic Institute, Lic-gel by Scientific Botanicals, and Erpace by Dolisos. Follow label directions.

Homeopathic *Borax* 6X helps rapidly heal canker sore blisters. Take three pills three times daily. Another homeopathic remedy that heals canker sores and takes the pain out of them is *Hydrastis* MT (mother tincture), diluted at the rate of one part to ten parts distilled water. Rinse with the liquid, then spit it out.

If you are prone to canker sores, avoid acidic and spicy foods, and any foods to which you may be allergic.

COLITIS, SPASTIC

See BOWEL DISORDERS.

CONGESTIVE HEART FAILURE

See HEART DISEASE.

CONSTIPATION

Constipation is defined as an irregular retention of or delay in bowel movements. The bowel habits of normal women may vary from three stools a day to only one in four or five days.[1] Infrequent movements are not uncommon but not necessarily healthy. Julian Whitaker, M.D., asserts that virtually everyone in the United States is constipated, at least compared to people in the African bush, whose stools are wet, bulky, and occur several times a day.[2]

Insufficient dietary fiber or water can cause constipation, but so can stress and emotional upsets. Trying to juggle the car pool, the children's schedules, and PTA and luncheon meetings can make a woman so "uptight" that elimination is impaired. In Chinese medical theory, the large intestine is an organ that retains not only physical toxins but also trapped emotions. Women with long-term constipation are said to be "holding on" to old resentments, anger, or grief, not wanting to "let go." Other factors contributing to constipation in women are pregnancy and menopause.

Constipation can also be triggered by drugs. Common offenders include codeine, antihistamines, diuretics, antispasmodics, narcotics, sleeping pills, antidepressants, tranquilizers, iron supplements, cholesterol-lowering drugs, and antacids containing aluminum or calcium compounds.

In unusual cases, constipation may be caused by actual blockage of the intestines, as occurs in certain cancers of the bowel or bowel adhesions.

CONVENTIONAL TREATMENT

Among the many causes of constipation, ironically, is laxative use. Laxatives diminish your natural muscle reflexes, so peristalsis (intestinal movement) occurs only with stronger and stronger stimulation. Laxatives can also irritate and inflame the lining of the bowel, cause anal fissures and hemorrhoids, and deplete your body of important substances, including water, calcium, potassium, and magnesium. Water loss causes dehydration, calcium loss weakens the bones, and potassium and magnesium loss weakens the muscles and heart.

Laxatives particularly to be avoided are the stimulant, lubricant, and saline varieties. Ex-Lax, the stimulant type, forces evacuation by stimulating the nerves controlling the bowel muscles. The FDA concluded that Ex-Lax was so unhealthy that it pulled the popular laxative off the market in 1997, but it is now back in reformulated form.

Lubricant laxatives coat the stools with mineral oil or olive oil. Saline laxatives, including Epsom salt and Milk of Magnesia, pull water into the bowels. These laxatives are not only irritating but can also upset the body's mineral balance if used long term.

The best pharmaceutical products are the bulk-forming and stool-softening varieties that encourage normal bowel function. The bulk-formers (like Metamucil) generally contain psyllium seed, while the stool softeners (like Doxidan) generally contain docusate.

NATURAL REMEDIES

Wheat bran can aid constipation by softening stools, preventing straining, increasing the weight of stools, and speeding intestinal transit time.[3] But relying on pure wheat bran can be hazardous, since it irritates the delicate lining of the intestines and can inhibit mineral absorption. Fortunately, the same laxative effect can be achieved by eating whole foods containing fiber. Raw vegetables, raw and dried fruits, and most beans and whole grains are high in fiber and create a heavy intestinal mass that travels quickly through the intestines. The standard prescription for constipation given by Dr. Julian Whitaker is two carrots and two apples per day, totaling about 16 grams of dietary fiber. Peristaltic contractions squeeze bulk along the digestive tract, the way you squeeze toothpaste out of a tube. Without bulk, there is nothing to squeeze, and bowel function halts.[4] Rhubarb is also a good natural laxative. One suggested recipe is three stalks of rhubarb blended with a cup of apple juice, ¼ peeled lemon, and a tablespoon of honey.[5] Foods to reduce or avoid are those devoid of fiber, particularly animal foods (especially cheese) and refined foods (especially sugar).

Beneficial bacteria (acidophilus and bifidus) in yogurt or capsule form can also aid elimination. In a study of bedridden elderly people, stool frequency improved after they ate bifidus-supplemented yogurt. When the yogurt was withdrawn, stool frequency again

REGULARITY RETURNS WITH NATURAL REMEDY

Ruth, a 40-year-old first-time mom, had had bouts of constipation before pregnancy, but after she had the baby she seemed to be constipated continually. Because she was breast-feeding, she dared not take the usual cascara and other natural laxatives she was used to, since they might give her child diarrhea. *Gres rose* worked to keep her regular without affecting the baby. She doesn't need it on a daily basis but keeps it on hand for when she does.

Peggy acknowledged that she had been constipated a good portion of her life. She often would not have a bowel movement for several days at a time. After she began taking wineberry (fifty drops in water in the morning), she was excited to report that she became quite regular and had a bowel movement daily.

became poor, demonstrating that supplementation needs to be long-term and continuous.[6] Many brands of beneficial bacteria are available at health food stores. Take as directed on the label.

Greens and green-type nutritional supplements can facilitate bowel movements by helping to clean the liver and adding fiber. Green supplements include chlorella, spirulina, and blue-green algae. Taking spirulina or chlorella twice a day typically results in normal bowel movements in about four days.

Aloe vera juice is another effective aid to regularity. Drink one cup each morning before breakfast.

For chronic constipation, homeopathic remedies can help. Cholenest by Nestmann is a combination homeopathic remedy that is good for minor constipation and disturbance in fat digestion. BHI also makes a good homeopathic combination called Constipation. Anti-Constipation Drops by Professional Complementary Health is a third option. Take ten drops three times daily.

Gres rose is a lithotherapy (a homeopathic remedy made from a mineral) that helps relieve constipation.

Wineberry is a gemmotherapy that helps with hard, dry stools by remoisturizing the intestines and balancing hormones. Take fifty drops in half a glass of water in the morning.

Sankaijo is a Japanese patent remedy that works for many women. Take one to six pills in the morning and again at night, increasing the number until a firm bowel movement daily is achieved. Then, decrease the dose by one tablet each week. The bowel movements should stay the same even when weened off the pills entirely.

Helpful bowel cleansing products include Perfect 7 by Agate and Ultimate Cleanse by Nature's Secret. Cascara is a time-honored remedy good for occasional use.

Also important, of course, is to avoid haste, allow time for nature to take its course, and respond when it calls.

CORONARY HEART DISEASE

See HEART DISEASE.

COSMETIC SURGERY, RECOVERY FROM

See SURGICAL TRAUMA.

CRAMPS, MENSTRUAL

See MENSTRUAL PROBLEMS.

CYSTITIS

See BLADDER INFECTION, IRRITATION, AND INFLAMMATION (CYSTITIS).

CYTOMEGALOVIRUS

Cytomegalovirus (CMV) is a common sexually transmitted virus in the herpes family. It generally causes no symptoms, but it can result in severe infections and even death in infants of infected mothers, who may not even know they have the disease. CMV has also been linked to Epstein-Barr virus–associated infectious mononucleosis, characterized by fever, malaise, myalgias, and arthralgias, and abnormal liver tests. CMV infections have been found in the gastrointestinal tract, liver, lungs, and nervous system. A major concern with CMV, like with mononucleosis, is that the disease can impair the immune system and develop into chronic fatigue syndrome.

CONVENTIONAL TREATMENT

Conventional medicine has no effective cure for CMV. A strong antiviral drug with serious potential side effects is used, but only in severe cases involving AIDS patients.

NATURAL REMEDIES

The German company Staufen makes an effective homeopathic remedy specifically for CMV called Cytomegalie. Dosages and directions are on the label, but a qualified practitioner should be consulted to rule out or correct underlying problems. CMV is complex and is usually the result of multiple assaults to the immune system. Stress, trauma, poor diet, and toxins all contribute to breaking down the body's resistance, allowing the virus to flourish.

DANDRUFF

See HAIR LOSS.

DEPRESSION

The World Health Organization ranks depression as the most disabling disease affecting women. Clinical depression affects an estimated 15 million Americans, and two-thirds of them are women. One in five women and one in ten men will experience at least one major episode of depression in their lives. In a third of sufferers, the condition will be chronic.

Why women experience depression more frequently than men was explored in a study reported in 2001. The findings suggested that women more often get caught in a cycle of despair and passivity because they have a lower sense of control over important areas of their lives, have more chronic strain, and are more prone to "rumination" (chronically and passively thinking about feelings).[1]

Hormonal imbalance is another obvious suspect. Premenstrual, perimenopausal, and menopausal women are notorious for being moody and depressed. The stress hormone cortisol, the sex hormones estrogen and progesterone, and thyroid hormone come from the same hormone chain and compete for hormone precursors. When stress levels are up, progesterone and thyroid hormone levels drop, causing moodiness and feelings of gloom.

Unlike the ordinary depression that comes with a bad day at the office or at home or that signals menstruation, "melancholic depression" is a chronic stress response in which the brain of the depressed person won't turn off, and sleeping and eating become difficult. The stress signals of a depressed woman's brain go into chronic worry mode, triggering physiological reactions that keep the body in a state of hyperarousal. A noise in the night wakes her and her problems immediately come flooding in, setting off the red alert that makes further sleep impossible. Controlling these responses through sheer willpower and positive thinking can elude the most strong-minded person.

Besides lowered mood, symptoms of depression may include feelings of guilt, worthlessness, or hopelessness; loss of energy, appetite, or sex drive; headache; and disturbed or excessive sleep. Related disorders include panic attacks, bipolar disorder (alternating manic and depressed phases), and seasonal affective disorder (caused by too little sunlight in winter months).

CONVENTIONAL TREATMENT

Amphetamines have been used for fifty years to give people with depression a "lift." But controlled trials have failed to establish that the drugs relieve depression significantly better than placebos. Amphetamines were later replaced with other drugs, including the monoamine oxidase inhibitors (MAOIs) and the tricyclic and other antidepressants. However, in some cases, the newer antidepressants actually posed a greater risk to health than the amphetamines, especially for the elderly and the medically ill.[2] People on MAOIs need to watch their diets and avoid foods rich in tyrosine, including alcohol, cheese, red meat, and yeast extract.

Prozac (fluoxetine) ushered in a new line of antidepressants called selective seroto-nin reuptake inhibitors (SSRIs) that were considered a significant advance. Other popu-lar SSRIs include Zoloft, Paxil, Luvox, Effexor, and Celexa. Serotonin is a mood-elevating neurotransmitter, a natural "upper" that mediates depression. The drugs don't actually produce serotonin but are serotonin "enhancers." They act by inhibiting a natural process, the reuptake of serotonin by the neurons. SSRIs are being used to treat not only depression and anxiety but also addiction, bulimia, overweight, and a host of other ills. Some 30 million Americans have taken serotonin enhancers, and many of them were not clinically depressed but were among the "worried well."[3]

The number of prescriptions written for antidepressants has doubled since 1985 be-cause SSRIs are considered so much safer than the old-line antidepressants.[4] But while they are less likely to result in high blood pressure or loss of balance, the tradeoff may be something worse. Serious side effects can include sleeplessness, nervousness, nausea, anx-iety, a loss of sexual interest and ability to perform, memory loss, impaired concentration, bipolar disorder, diabetes, multiple sclerosis symptoms, mania, chronic fatigue, severe rebound depression, symptoms of Cushing's syndrome (puffiness in the face), inability to handle stress, looking or feeling pregnant, and mood swings.[5] Too much serotonin can trigger a condition known as "serotonin syndrome," which involves lethargy, confusion, flushing, sweating, and muscle jerks. In severe cases, serotonin syndrome can be fatal. Withdrawal from the drugs may also be difficult, producing disturbing symptoms de-scribed as "a bad case of the flu."[6]

The most serious concern, however, is that psychotropic drugs unbalance brain chemicals. Brains exposed to high doses of serotonin enhancers show the same abnormal-ities as those exposed to high doses of a class of drugs called serotonin releasers that in-cludes the street drug Ecstasy (MDMA).[7] Serotonin is the same brain chemical that LSD and other psychedelic drugs mimic to produce their hallucinogenic effects.[8] While the first reaction to SSRIs may be one of euphoria, this feeling soon degenerates into a sort of "dead zone" in which users say they are neither happy nor sad, just numb. The drugs oblit-erate anxiety and depression by numbing the whole system. Numbness, of course, is bet-ter than suicide or institutionalization, but when enough time has elapsed that the underlying issue (for example divorce or death) could be dealt with in the ordinary course of events, women report having trouble getting off the drugs. Their nervous systems have adapted to that stimulus and go into a deeper-than-normal depression and imbalance without it. Worse, like in the tale of Dr. Jekyll and Mr. Hyde, suppressed impulses can emerge unbidden, particularly when withdrawal from the drug is attempted. Some 3.5 percent of patients who weren't suicidal before treatment with Prozac get that way on the drug, and homicides have been blamed on it, generating a spate of lawsuits.[9]

A number of notorious cases have made the news in which SSRI users have killed people indiscriminately either soon after starting on the drugs or soon after going off them. Eric Harris, one of the killers involved in the Columbine High School massacre that resulted in thirteen deaths, had recently stopped taking Luvox. Kip Kinkel, the Ore-gon school killer, had been on Prozac. Reginald Payne killed his wife and then committed suicide after taking Prozac for eleven days. In 2001, the first-ever court verdict was awarded against an antidepressant, in a case brought by the relatives of Donald Schell. Schell murdered his wife, his daughter, his granddaughter, and himself after two days on

Paxil. The jury found the drug 80 percent responsible and awarded the family $6.4 million.[10] In August 2001, a class-action lawsuit was filed against Paxil's manufacturer Glaxo-SmithKline PLC, alleging the company concealed evidence of the drug's addiction potential. The thirty-five plaintiffs allegedly suffered from symptoms ranging from electriclike shocks to suicidal thoughts after discontinuing use of the drug.[11]

Caution: If prescription antianxiety or insomnia drugs are already being used, discontinuing or switching remedies should be done only under professional supervision.

NATURAL REMEDIES

Natural Serotonin Stimulants

The natural, balanced way to increase levels of serotonin is with its natural precursors, the amino acids L-tryptophan and L-tyrosine. Tryptophan was used as a safe natural alternative to pharmaceutical tranquilizers for nearly half a century, until it was removed from the market in 1989 in response to reports of some serious side effects and deaths following its use. However, the problem was ultimately traced to contamination in a manufacturing process involving genetic engineering used by a particular Japanese manufacturer.[12] Food sources of this amino acid include milk, pumpkin seeds, and turkey.

New on the market is a highly effective homeopathic serotonin enhancer called Serotonin by Deseret. It stimulates the body to produce its own serotonin and, like all homeopathics, is quite safe. Many people have succeeded in weaning themselves off Prozac and pulling themselves out of their inexplicable depressions using this simple and inexpensive remedy. For seasonal depression or for depression with insomnia, homeopathic Serotonin & Tryptophan by CompliMed may be used. The dosage for both is ten drops three times daily.

The body's serotonin levels can also be raised by changing the diet. High-carbohydrate foods have been found to relieve depression, anger, tension, tiredness, and moodiness, apparently because they elevate serotonin levels.[13] Sugary foods should be avoided, however, since they can wreak havoc on blood sugar levels. Erratic drops in blood sugar can cause both depression and binging. The best carbohydrates are whole grains—oatmeal and other whole-grain cereals, whole-grain breads, rice, and potatoes.

Exercise has also been shown to increase brain concentrations of serotonin and norepinephrine.[14] Running is well known for the "runner's high." But jogging also carries certain risks as you get older, including blood clotting, which can increase the risk of strokes and heart attacks; flat feet; varicose veins; and uterine prolapse.[15] Walking, swimming, and low-impact aerobics are safer alternatives.

Herbal and Other Remedies

Although Dr. Walker has found serotonin homeopathic drops to be more effective, among herbal remedies for depression, St. John's wort is the market favorite. A review of twenty-three controlled studies published in the *British Medical Journal* in August 1997 concluded that St. John's wort worked as well as prescription drugs and nearly three times better than a placebo in countering depression, without the unwanted side effects accompanying the drugs. Mild, reversible side effects did occur in some patients, but they were far less frequent or serious than pharmaceutical antidepressants.[16]

DEPRESSION RELIEVED WITH NATURAL SEROTONIN STIMULANT

Joan, age 60, had a good job in a real estate office, to which she dutifully reported every morning. But when she came home in the evening, she locked the door and never left the house. She could barely drag herself out of bed to get to work, and she saw no one except at the office. She was extremely depressed. She had gone on like that for many years when she began taking Serotonin homeopathic drops. She called two weeks later, quite excited, to say she had painted her fingernails. So? She said she would never have done that before; she had started caring for herself. This breakthrough was followed by tap dancing lessons and calling friends to get together to do things. Soon, Joan actually had a life outside the office.

Another effective herbal remedy for depression is Skullcap Oats by Eclectic Institute. Take fifteen to thirty drops in warm water one to five times daily as needed.

Cherry Plum and Rescue Remedy are Bach flower remedies that can help relieve depression and anxiety and are entirely safe. Put four drops in 4 ounces of water and sip throughout the day.

Supplemental estrogen, progesterone, and thyroid hormone can help elevate the mood in women low in those hormones. Natural forms are better than synthetics.

Nutritional supplements can help as well. One is magnesium, a mineral in which people with depression tend to be low. Low magnesium levels heighten the nerve impulses that lead to nervous conditions. A good dose is 400 mg once or twice daily.

B vitamins can also give the spirits a lift. (B Complex 100 is good; take one tablet daily.) For adrenal stress, try Bragg Liquid Aminos, a tasty supplement used as a condiment on food. Inositol (a cousin of glucose) can also help. (IPG by Jarrow is good; take one to six capsules daily on an empty stomach.) Phosphatidylserine may also help.[17] Follow recommendations on the label.

For bipolar disorder, a recent study found that patients who did not respond to treatment with the standard drug lithium responded to treatment with choline.[18]

Homeopathic *Lithium* (something quite different from the drug lithium) is good for depression (ten drops three times daily). *Aurum metallicum* 30C is a homeopathic remedy that is specific for suicidal depression. Take three pellets three times daily or as directed by a practitioner.

For seasonal affective disorder (SAD), full spectrum lights or blue light, customized colored glasses, and homeopathic Melatonin 12X can give relief. Take three pellets as needed.

The Eastern Approach

In Chinese medicine, depression is attributed to liver stagnation. When the liver energy gets sluggish, the body becomes sluggish, not wanting to move; and the emotions become dull, depressed, and irritated. Liver stagnation can result from a bad diet, environmental toxins, and emotional factors such as suppressing anger. The Chinese herbal formula for liver stagnation is called *Xiao Yao Wan* (or *Hsiao Yao Wan*). It stimulates the liver energy to work more actively, relieving the stagnant feeling. Depression typically lifts within a few days.

American-made versions of this formula are Relaxed Wanderer and Bupleurum & Peony. Consult a Chinese medical practitioner for recommendations and dosages.

The liver energy can also be moved with greens. Chlorophyll and milk thistle are good for this purpose. An excellent product called Ultimate Green by Nature's Secret includes chlorella, blue-green algae, barley grass, wheat grass, spinach, alfalfa, kale, and turnip greens. For use, follow label directions. For the Liver Cleanse Diet, see Chapter 4.

If depression is also linked to anxiety, palpitations, nightmares, or panic attacks, Chinese doctors say the heart meridian is likely to be involved. For a heart meridian that is out of balance, appropriate Chinese herbal formulas include *Anmien Pien, Pai Tzu Yang Hsin Wan,* and *Hu Po Yang Xin Dan.* Again, consult a Chinese medical practitioner for recommendations and dosages.

DERMATITIS

See SKIN PROBLEMS.

DIABETES

Diabetes is a chronic condition in which the body does not properly metabolize glucose (blood sugar) due to inadequate production or use of insulin, resulting in too much glucose in the bloodstream. (Insulin is a hormone secreted by the pancreas that helps sugar get into the tissues.) Diabetes is the seventh leading cause of death in the United States. It strikes women more frequently than men, carries greater risks of degenerative disease for women, and can impact on the health of their unborn children. Prolonged hyperglycemia (elevated blood sugar) is a risk factor for the development of heart disease and other chronic complications, including vision loss, kidney failure, high blood pressure, and neurological disorders. Early warning signs include excessive thirst, urination, and hunger; sudden weight loss; fatigue; nausea and vomiting; blurred vision; and numbness in the extremities.

About 90 to 95 percent of women with the disease have type 2 or adult-onset diabetes (non-insulin dependent diabetes mellitus or NIDDM), which usually develops after age 40 and occurs when the body's cells become resistant to insulin. Type 1 diabetes (formerly known as juvenile-onset diabetes), by contrast, occurs because the pancreas actually makes little or no insulin. People with adult-onset diabetes may have normal or even elevated levels of insulin; the hormone just isn't working properly. The chief predisposing risk factors for type 2 are obesity, weight gain, and physical inactivity. Among older women with diabetes, 70.4 percent are 20 percent over their desired weight (compared with 38.2 percent of men), and 25 percent are obese (50 percent over their desired weight). In the 1990s, diabetes rates increased 70 percent for women aged thirty through thirty-nine and increased tenfold in adolescents. The increased prevalence of obesity in these age groups may play a role.

Other risk factors for developing type 2 diabetes include drugs—including birth control pills, steroids, and diuretics—which can induce the disease in otherwise-normal adults. Diabetes or impaired glucose tolerance often develops during antihypertensive therapy with diuretics, and the condition may not go away when treatment is discontinued.[1] Other drugs can either increase blood glucose levels or decrease them, thus increasing the risk of hypoglycemia (low blood sugar) in combination with sugar-lowering drugs. Blood glucose levels are decreased by aspirin and other salicylates, phenylbutazone (a nonsteroidal anti-inflammatory agent), coumarin anticoagulants, ethanol (in alcoholic beverages), sulfonamide antibiotics, and trimethoprim (for urinary tract infections). Blood glucose levels are increased by caffeine (in large quantities), corticosteroids, diazoxide, ephedrine, estrogen, furosemide and thiazide diuretics, lithium, nicotinic acid (in large doses), phenobarbital, phenytoin, rifampin (for the treatment of tuberculosis), sugar-containing medications, and thyroid preparations.[2]

Between 2.5 percent and 4 percent of women in the United States develop gestational diabetes during pregnancy. Increased insulin resistance during pregnancy is caused by hormones produced by the placenta. Gestational diabetes usually ends after the baby's birth, but women who have had it have up to a 45 percent risk of recurrence with the next pregnancy and up to a 63 percent risk of developing type 2 diabetes later in life. Diabetic expectant mothers are also at greater risk for complications such as preeclampsia, cesarean section, and infections. Children of diabetic mothers have as much as a tenfold increase in risk of obesity during childhood and of developing glucose intolerance in puberty—both risk factors for type 2 diabetes.[3]

CONVENTIONAL TREATMENT

Serious cases of diabetes at the beginning of this century inevitably led to severe dehydration, coma, and death. Then it was discovered that the disease could be treated with extracts of the pancreas, the organ that releases insulin. Advances since then have progressively improved the treatment. Type I diabetics still must test their blood-sugar levels and inject themselves with insulin several times a day (usually before meals and before bed), and keep their blood sugar levels stable by eating at regular times and avoiding sugar or sugary foods; however, new single-step devices allow hourly monitoring of blood sugar levels and more accurate insulin dosing, and newer forms of insulin afford better control.[4]

NATURAL REMEDIES

Although insulin injections have improved, correcting the underlying problem is obviously preferable if possible. For type 2 diabetics without symptoms or with only mild disease, nondrug solutions involving diet, nutritional supplements, and exercise are safer and more satisfactory alternatives.[5]

Dietary Solutions

Epidemiological evidence suggests that Type 2 diabetes is a lifestyle disease that is both preventable and reversible. In traditional societies like the Australian Aboriginal and Pacific Island populations, urbanization has resulted in a dramatic increase in type 2 diabetes during this century. Between 10 percent and 35 percent develop the disease when they move to the city (compared to only 3 percent of Caucasians of European descent).

The condition in diabetic Aborigines has shown dramatic improvement when they returned for as few as seven weeks to their traditional diet of legumes and other whole, natural foods.[6]

For many type 2 diabetics, simply shedding 10 to 20 percent of body weight has dropped elevated blood sugar to near-normal levels.[7] Even for type 2 diabetics who need insulin, dietary change can reduce and sometimes even eliminate insulin requirements. This was shown in a study in which the carbohydrate intake of diabetics was nearly doubled by substituting high-fiber complex carbohydrates for animal foods. Type 2 diabetics on low doses of insulin managed to give up the drug altogether, and those on high doses substantially reduced their prescriptions.[8]

The high-carbohydrate, high-fiber diet recommended in that landmark study represented a radical reversal in diabetic theory. Since carbohydrate is what sugar is made of, eating it was formerly assumed to raise blood sugar. Early recommendations therefore involved *reducing* carbohydrate and *increasing* fat and protein. But the high-fat, high-protein diet tended to cause weight gain, and its excess fat contributed to the risk of heart disease. Complex carbohydrates (whole grains and beans) are digested more slowly than simple carbohydrates and actually help regulate blood sugar levels. Fiber also helps regulate glucose metabolism by delaying glucose absorption from the intestines. A high-fiber diet takes longer to be digested, and sugar from the food is absorbed over a longer period. Soluble fibers are particularly effective at regulating blood sugar. They improve glycemic control, reduce fasting plasma glucose levels, reduce insulin requirements, and lower cholesterol and triglyceride levels. Fiber also helps keep your weight down by filling you up with fewer calories and giving you more opportunity to chew.[9]

Beans and other legumes that are slowly digested and absorbed are particularly good foods for diabetics. Studies show that diets based on legumes improve diabetic glucose and insulin profiles, and that slow-release carbohydrate can help relieve the symptoms of the disease. Legumes remain the traditional staples in parts of the world like Africa and India where diabetes is uncommon.

The ideal diabetic diet is also low in fat. Fat not only adds pounds but can also impair insulin activity. Diabetes is most prevalent in beef-eating countries. Two-thirds of the fat in the American diet is derived from animal foods, while all of its fiber comes from plant foods. In one study, the risk of developing diabetes was four times as great for men who ate meat daily as for those who ate it once a week or less. Interestingly, however, no such association was found with the consumption of eggs, milk, or cheese, although those foods are also high in saturated fat.[10]

Regulating Blood Sugar Naturally

Diabetics are known to have low levels of chromium, an essential mineral involved in blood sugar regulation. Supplementing with chromium picolinate helps even out the blood sugar level, preventing dramatic highs and lows.

Anecdotal reports of improvement after chromium supplementation were discounted by the medical mainstream, until a 1996 Department of Agriculture study produced results that were called "spectacular." The difference between it and earlier studies was that chromium picolinate was given in doses of 1,000 mcg—five times the standard dose. The test subjects were 180 type 2 diabetics in China (where nutritional supplements are rarely taken, so effects would be easy to document). High doses restored normal glucose and insulin levels and eliminated the classic signs of diabetes in nearly all of the subjects.

The researcher heading the study advised diabetics who want to try chromium to consult with their doctors first, since insulin intake may have to be reduced. He observed that most diabetics need only 400–600 mcg of chromium daily. He warned that diabetics with long-standing disease or complications won't benefit from chromium.[11]

Chromium is recommended not only for diabetics but for people with hypoglycemia and impaired glucose tolerance, in whom it might help prevent the development of full-blown diabetes. By lowering insulin resistance, blood cholesterol, and blood pressure, it also seems to lower heart disease risk.

Helpful Nutritional Aids

Recent research indicates that alpha lipoic acid, a powerful antioxidant found naturally in spinach and other foods, can lower glucose levels by 20 to 30 percent.[12] Recommended daily dosage is 20–50 mg for nondiabetics and 300–600 mg for diabetics.

Supplementing with 4 grams of evening primrose oil per day for six months has been found to reverse the cause of diabetic nerve damage and relieve nerve pain.[13]

People with low levels of vitamin E have been found to be more likely to develop type 2 diabetes. Diabetics also typically have low levels of vitamin C. They need vitamin B_6 for normal functioning of nerve cells, and carnitine to properly use fat for energy. Also recommended are fish oil, brewer's yeast, magnesium, vanadium, zinc, CoQ_{10}, inositol, taurine, and quercetin. For dosages, you can follow label directions, but everyone is different. It is best to see a practitioner for recommendations specific for your body.

Supplementing with digestive enzymes can also help (two or three tablets with each meal). Besides insulin, the pancreas makes other enzymes, including amylase to break down starches, lipase to break down fat, cellulase to break down vegetable fiber, and protease to break down protein. Diabetics are liable to be low in these enzymes, impairing proper digestion.

Homeopathic and Herbal Remedies

Homeopathic remedies are also available that stimulate the pancreas to make its own enzymes. A good option is Pancreas-Total Endotox M-17 by Apex (ten drops three times daily).

The herb milk thistle, containing the antioxidant silymarin, was shown by Italian researchers to significantly drop and stabilize glucose levels without hypoglycemic episodes.

INSULIN NEEDS REDUCED

After Pat, a hospital receptionist, was diagnosed with type 2 diabetes at age 48, she began taking chromium picolinate (200 mcg with each meal). She was amazed at how much better she felt and at how she could maintain her blood sugar with only half the medication she was taking previously.

INSULIN INJECTIONS AVOIDED

A 36-year-old dietitian sought help after being diagnosed with type 2 diabetes a month earlier. Although she had a family history of diabetes and insulin had been prescribed, she felt that her doctor had been too cavalier about the whole matter. He had not given her an adequate explanation concerning how she had developed diabetes or how she could help herself. On Dr. Walker's recommendation, she started taking 200 mcg of chromium with breakfast and lunch. She also took homeopathic *Syzygum jambolanum* 3X (five drops in water three times daily) and the trace mineral vanadyl sulphate (five drops three times daily). Within two weeks, she was off insulin and controlling her diabetes with her diet. She continues to be very careful about her diet and her doctor visits but is grateful that she no longer has to give herself injections.

The herb also helps with the utilization of insulin, reducing the amount needed.[14] Products vary; follow label directions.

In Chinese medicine, the herb chrysanthemum is used to treat diabetes. *Stevia rebaudiana*, a sweetener, is an herb of the chrysanthemum family. Stevia in its natural form is ten to fifteen times sweeter than common table sugar, and in extract form, it's 100 to 300 times sweeter. Yet it doesn't affect blood sugar metabolism. Studies have verified that stevia aids in reducing plasma glucose levels in normal adults.[15]

Another herb that is growing in popularity with diabetics is one used for centuries in India to support the pancreas and help regulate blood sugar, *Gymnema Sylvestre*. It should be taken with water fifteen minutes before each meal: one capsule with a small or low-sugar meal, two with a larger or high-sugar meal. A homeopathic remedy called *Syzgium jambolanum* can also help.

An excellent combination nutritional and herbal product is Diabetrol by Cardiovascular Research.

Other beneficial herbs available at health food stores include Asian ginseng, bilberry, ginkgo, fenugreek, bitter melon, aloe vera, Siberian ginseng, and Maitake mushroom.

Other Natural Blood Sugar Regulators

Exercise can aid in the control of diabetes, not only by burning up excess calories but by improving glucose utilization and cardiovascular performance. Sunlight is another natural insulin stimulant. When diabetics have been exposed to sunlight treatments, their blood sugar has dropped and the sugar in their urine has decreased or disappeared. Natural sunlight seems to produce the best results.

Warning: Diabetics need to enter sunbathing and exercise programs gradually and to keep in close touch with their doctors. The insulinlike effect of sunlight is so dramatic that it can precipitate a hypoglycemic episode when compounded with insulin injections. Major changes in exercise levels may also require a change in drug dosage to avoid this result.[16]

DIARRHEA

See BOWEL DISORDERS.

DIGESTIVE PROBLEMS

Minor stomach problems, such as indigestion, bloating, cramps, and gas pains, are normally traceable to stress or to bad eating habits (too much or the wrong types of food). They can also be symptoms of menopause. Other stomach complaints can be traced to drugs, including birth control pills, antihistamines, Valium, steroids, and NSAIDs.[1]

More serious digestive ills include gastritis, or inflammation of the stomach lining, which can produce indigestion, diarrhea, and stomach pain; esophageal reflux, a digestive complaint resulting when acid escapes from the stomach into the esophagus; and hiatal hernia, which results when the esophagus becomes herniated, or pushed out, usually from eating something large and hard to swallow. (A common offender is doxycycline, a popular antibiotic that comes in the form of a large pill that can injure the esophagus.) Heartburn is a burning feeling in the chest near the heart, sometimes mistaken for a heart attack. Heartburn actually has nothing to do with the heart but results when stomach acid enters the esophagus.

Warning: A heart attack can also be mistaken for heartburn. Call your doctor if you experience heartburn symptoms along with shortness of breath, problems swallowing, sweating, dizziness, vomiting, diarrhea, fever, bloody stools, or severe abdominal pain.

CONVENTIONAL TREATMENTS

Many women who take Tums or Rolaids for digestive complaints believe they are killing two birds with one stone, since the antacids are promoted commercially as good sources of the calcium needed by women to prevent bone loss after menopause. But these and other antacids actually inhibit calcium absorption by neutralizing stomach acid, raising the pH of the stomach. Calcium can be absorbed only in its soluble ionized form, which requires a low pH.[2] Antacids can also have other unwanted side effects; if taken regularly for long periods, these effects can be quite serious. Different brands contain different principal ingredients, but all of them are subject to negative effects of some kind.

Calcium carbonate, the chief ingredient in Tums, used to be the antacid of choice until prolonged use was found to raise calcium level in the blood, leading to impaired kidney function and kidney stones. The problem is particularly serious for people whose kidneys are already impaired or who drink a lot of milk, since milk is high in calcium. Calcium carbonate can also impair iron absorption, cause constipation, and produce an "acid rebound" in which its use is followed by significant *increases* in stomach acid. That means you can wind up with more acid in your stomach than before you started on the drug.[3]

Sodium bicarbonate, or baking soda, is the major ingredient in Alka-Seltzer and Bromo-Seltzer. While relatively harmless for occasional use, if used repeatedly, it can disturb the body's acid-base balance, especially in people with kidney problems. It can also lead to kidney stones and recurrent urinary tract infections. Sodium bicarbonate is high in sodium, so it's not good for people on low-sodium diets. Also, like calcium carbonate, it can impair iron absorption.

Alka-Seltzer combines sodium bicarbonate with aspirin. If your objective is to relieve a headache, this combination, dissolved in water, can relieve some of the stomach irritation produced by ordinary aspirin tablets. But if you have an upset stomach, the combination is calculated to make it worse, since the aspirin can further irritate your stomach, particularly if your problem is caused by ulcers.

Bromo-Seltzer, which combines sodium bicarbonate with acetaminophen instead of aspirin, is easier on the stomach than Alka-Seltzer. But it's harder on the liver, a hazard especially for alcoholics.

Pepto-Bismol is approved by the FDA both as an antacid and as a diarrhea and hangover remedy. Besides salicylate, which can have the same adverse effects as aspirin, it contains bismuth, a potentially lethal nerve poison. Bismuth hasn't been detected in the blood or urine of people taking recommended doses, but overdose can result in kidney failure and liver damage. In France and Australia, reports of bone and joint disorders and encephalopathy (a degenerative disease of the brain) from the use of bismuth salts even at recommended doses have led to restriction on their use.[4]

Magnesium salts (as in Phillips' Milk of Magnesia) tend to cause diarrhea, which can become severe if the medication is used regularly for more than a week or two. They can also exacerbate kidney problems and cause drowsiness in some people. Aluminum salts (as in Rolaids) have the opposite drawback: they can obstruct the intestines and cause intractable constipation. The industry solution was to combine these two ingredients, as in Maalox, Mylanta, Gelusil, and Di-Gel. The theory was that their opposing side effects would cancel each other out, but in practice, these combination products can cause the side effects of either ingredient. In one case, Gelusil tablets became the subject of a lawsuit when a patient on it died of peritonitis and gangrene resulting from a bowel obstruction.[5]

There is also evidence of a link between aluminum antacid preparations and more serious side effects, including bone disease and Alzheimer's disease.[6] Aluminum displaces calcium from the bones, causing them to be brittle and to break easily. Aluminum-containing drugs are particularly dangerous when taken with orange juice, with any other citrus fruit or juice, or in drugs containing citrate, a combination that increases the absorption of aluminum into the bloodstream by as much as fifty times. Anyone who takes aluminum-containing antacids on a regular basis can end up with both brain damage and thinning of the bones.[7]

The H2-blockers (Tagamet, Zantac, Pepcid, Axid, and others) are drugs that were once reserved for ulcers but are now being promoted for symptomatic relief of gastritis and other less serious stomach complaints. The H2-blockers work by blocking the flow of stomach acid. As with antacids, the problem with using these drugs for gastric distress is that the symptoms are often due to *insufficient* stomach acid. In these cases, the H2-blockers are actually worsening the condition. In any case, the drugs, which need to be taken repeatedly, aren't addressing the underlying problem. H2-blockers are also expensive and can have side effects, including diarrhea, hair thinning, confusion in the elderly, and sexual impotence.

Less obvious than the immediate side effects of H2-blockers are their subtle and long-term effects. Whenever you tamper with the body's natural secreting mechanisms, you risk upsetting beneficial functions. Histamine receptors are found not only in the stomach but also in the heart and blood vessels. Blockage of these receptors has caused fatal heart attacks in patients receiving H2-blockers by injection. Stomach acid has beneficial functions that can also be suppressed by H2-blockers. One is to aid in the absorption of iron from plant foods. H2-blockers used long term have been shown to block this absorption by 28 to 65 percent.[8] Another function of stomach acid is to kill bacteria and keep your stomach from being colonized by undesirables. Without the acid, you run the risk of infection by a number of organisms, including those that cause typhoid, salmonella, cholera, dysentery, and giardia.[9]

NATURAL REMEDIES FOR IMPAIRED DIGESTION

Rather than suppressing digestive juices, an alternative approach to indigestion is to encourage proper digestion with digestive enzymes. A popular choice is chewable papaya enzymes, which contain papain, a natural digestant. Take two tablets after meals.

Digestive enzymes are produced not only in the stomach but in the pancreas, which makes amylase to break down starch, lipase to break down fat, cellulase to break down vegetable fiber, protease to break down protein, and insulin to break down sugars. Without these enzymes, food goes through the intestines undigested, where it ferments and decomposes in the colon, causing gas, bloating, and intestinal upset. If the pancreas is producing insufficient enzymes, taking pancreatic enzymes can help (two to five with each meal). Good brands include those by Tyler and Transformation (available from practitioners and holistic drugstores). Take as directed on the label. It is also good to take apple cider vinegar and honey before meals (two tablespoons apple cider vinegar in water with one teaspoon honey).[10]

Caution: Digestive enzymes should not be taken if the stomach is inflamed due to ulcers or inflammation resulting from the use of nonsteroidal anti-inflammatory drugs, such as aspirin, Advil, and Motrin.

It is better to fix the underlying problem than simply treat the symptoms. A product called Pancreas Total by Apex helps to stimulate the pancreas to produce its own enzymes. Take ten drops three times daily between meals, while continuing to take digestive enzymes after meals. Used over about a three-month period, this remedy can effectively help the digestive system get back on track.

Liver cleansing can also help. The liver clears toxins from the blood. When the liver gets congested, toxins go to the pancreas and prevent it from producing enzymes. Parasites can also stop the pancreas from making digestive enzymes. For remedies, see "Multiple Chemical Sensitivity" on page 185 and "Parasitic Infection" on page 212.

NATURAL REMEDIES FOR SHORT-TERM RELIEF OF UPSET STOMACH

Herbs and herbal teas can help settle the stomach safely and effectively. Good options include licorice, chamomile, St. John's wort, and ginger. Ginger can be taken as ginger tea (simply put a slice of ginger in boiling water and let it steep for 10 to twenty minutes). Peppermint can be taken as peppermint tea or you can add a couple of drops of peppermint oil to warm water and sip it.

The Chinese herbal formula Pill Curing is another effective remedy for settling the stomach or for relieving what the Chinese call "food stagnation"—the feeling after a large meal that the food is stuck in the stomach. This ancient Chinese patent formula is available from different companies and is sold in Chinese pharmacies. Take one or two vials after each meal or as needed.

A homeopathic remedy that is good for simple indigestion with gas and bloating is *Carbo vegetabilis* 6C. The recommended dosage is three tablets every fifteen minutes. For severe upset, take up to six doses. The homeopathic remedies *Nux Vomica* and Carbo Veg (taken together as needed every fifteen minutes after a meal, up to three doses) and Gastrica by CompliMed (taken as directed on the label) are also good. Marco Pharma makes an effective homeopathic remedy for gas, bloating, upset stomach, sluggish bowels, and spastic colon called Frangula.

To stop the morning-after nausea and headache of a hangover, try *Nux vomica* 6C, (three tablets every fifteen minutes, up to six doses). Hangover (a combination homeopathic by Source Natural) and Vitamin B Stress Tabs are also good for hangovers.

For an upset stomach due to food poisoning or morning sickness, see "Nausea and Vomiting" on page 194.

Natural Remedies for Heartburn, Gastritis, and Hiatal Hernia

For heartburn, Boiron and Hylands both make effective homeopathic products called Heartburn. Use according to label directions. Homeopathic *Robinia* 30C can also help relieve heartburn and acid reflux. Take three pills three times daily.

For many people, heartburn is aggravated by carbohydrates and soft drinks. Some people have reported that their heartburn resolved on an Atkins-type diet, high in protein and low in carbohydrates. For women who wear jeans, another useful suggestion is to wear looser ones. Tight pants are thought to contribute to heartburn by forcing acid to back up through the stomach into the esophagus.

For hiatal hernia, several patients have reported that a probiotic remedy called Probioplex Intensive Care by Metagenics healed their hernias in a week or two. Take one to two tablespoons three times a day for one to two weeks.

Dietary Solutions

Chronic stomach complaints may also have dietary causes: overeating in general, eating wrong combinations of foods, or food allergies and intolerances. Common offenders that can upset sensitive stomachs include the lactose (milk sugar) in milk; the gluten in wheat; yeast, sugar, coffee, eggs, and soy products.

The theory of proper food combining lacks scientific evidence, but sensitive people swear by it. Moreover, many women have lost weight on diets based on it. The theory is that different types of food require different digestive enzymes. If you mix your foods im-

---

CHRONIC STOMACH PAIN HEALED WITHOUT DRUGS

Edna reported having severe heartburn and gastritis for more than two years. Rolaids were part of her daily routine. Her symptoms disappeared after she took homeopathic *Robinia* 30C (three pills three times daily) along with Probioplex (according to label directions). The *Robinia* stopped her excess stomach acid, while the Probioplex healed the damage done to her stomach.

Charlene also had chronic stomach and gastrointestinal discomfort. She felt as if the food she ate got stuck in her chest and had trouble getting digested. Her doctor had diagnosed a hiatal hernia but had offered no solution. To her relief, Probioplex also resolved her problem.

properly, some will sit in the stomach and create havoc while others are being processed. If you're prone to indigestion after ordinary-sized meals, try eating fruits, proteins, and carbohydrates in separate meals. Proteins or carbohydrates can be eaten with greens (salads or cooked vegetables), but proteins and carbohydrates should not be eaten together, and fruits should be eaten alone.

DISRHYTHMIA

See IRREGULAR HEATBEAT.

DRY SKIN

See SKIN PROBLEMS.

EAR AND SKIN PIERCING, INFECTION FROM

See SKIN PROBLEMS.

ECZEMA

See SKIN PROBLEMS.

EDEMA

See BLOATING, GAS, AND EDEMA.

EMPTY NEST SYNDROME

Empty nest syndrome—a form of depression in mothers that is associated with their children growing up and leaving home—tends to occur when menopause is approaching, with its added hormonal and emotional stresses. The depression you may feel at this time may make no logical sense to you. Your children have gone on to do what you have worked so hard to prepare them for—college, a career, and perhaps marriage and a family of their own. They have graduated with honors from your care. You should be happy, but your identity has been built around them and their needs. Who are you if not a busy, needed mom? You have been left in an emotional vacuum. Natural remedies can help you see, feel, and capitalize on your own graduated status and freer circumstances.

HOMEOPATHIC REMEDY OPENS HER EYES TO NEW POTENTIAL

Janet was divorced and her children had gone off to college. The nest was empty and she was left without much to do. She was in a romantic relationship that wasn't going well. She had other vague complaints, but mainly she was just depressed and unhappy. The homeopathic remedy *Nat mur* in a strength of 1M lifted the layer of depression left after her children and husband were no longer center stage in her life, allowing her to start seeing things differently. In two months, she had become happy and easygoing. She took a vacation, something she hadn't done in years. She broke up with her boyfriend, realizing he wasn't right for her, and began looking at other men differently, seeing them as real possibilities.

NATURAL REMEDIES

Rescue Remedy and Walnut are Bach flower remedies that are excellent during times of change or transition. Place two to four drops in half a glass of water and sip throughout the day.

Homeopathic remedies can also help, by removing the layers of suppressed grief that keep you from seeing the exciting possibilities presented by your freer circumstances. They can help you find a new focus. Now is the time to do all those things the kids kept you too busy to do. Possibilities include *Ignatia* and *Natrum muriatican* (*Nat mur*) (30 to 200), but the correct remedy depends on symptoms and personality type; see a homeopath for recommendations.

Natural hormones and hormone stimulants can also help, by easing hormonal imbalances. See "Menopause and Perimenopause" on page 174.

ENDOMETRIOSIS

Endometriosis, a puzzling condition affecting 5 million American women, is the second most common gynecological disorder requiring hospital treatment and a leading cause of hysterectomy. Endometriosis involves the abnormal growth of uterine tissue outside the uterus, causing chronic pelvic pain, disabling periods, internal scarring, and infertility. The endometrium, or lining of the womb, bleeds every time menstruation occurs. In women with endometriosis, endometrial-like tissue migrates to other parts of the body (usually the ovaries, fallopian tubes, and peritoneum), where it behaves like the endometrium: it bleeds. But the blood can't escape, so it tends to form adhesions, which become inflamed and scarred and make the organs stick together.

Endometriosis is conventionally considered incurable. Drugs and surgery can help relieve symptoms but have other downsides, and the condition has a high rate of recurrence. Severity of symptoms varies from being asymptomatic to excruciating and disabling. Lighter cases may regress without treatment, so if the condition is discovered accidentally and produces no symptoms, it should not automatically be treated with drugs or surgery.[1]

CONVENTIONAL TREATMENT

Analgesics (painkillers), hormonal drugs (birth control pills), and surgery are the usual conventional treatments, but none is a cure. Analgesics mask discomfort but don't touch its cause. Birth control pills relieve symptoms but may also be responsible for inducing them, through a sort of rebound effect when the drugs are stopped. The drugs have unwanted side effects, and the condition tends to return when pharmaceutical hormones are discontinued.

A drug called Lupron (leuprolide acetate) is sometimes given to induce menopause, since endometriosis tends to improve afterward. But while the drug may successfully eliminate the pain of endometriosis, its cost is premature menopause, and the drug tends to be given to women who are still young. It also induces hot flashes and can cause bone pain, weakness, and numbness in the lower limbs during the first few weeks of treatment.[2] And women who take it seem to age overnight.

The radical surgical alternative is removal of the ovaries, which also brings on premature menopause. The transition can be so sudden, however, that it brings on quite severe symptoms. The patient winds up resorting to hormone replacement therapy, which can then reactivate the endometriosis. Surgery can also lead to adhesions, which further impair function of the female organs.

When appropriate, most doctors recommend getting pregnant, which generally eliminates symptoms, perhaps because progesterone levels are particularly high during pregnancy. But symptoms can recur several years after delivery, and endometriosis victims tend to have trouble getting pregnant. Whether the condition actually causes infertility isn't clear, but the two tend to go together.

NATURAL REMEDIES

Natural Progesterone Therapy

Despite the medical community's contention that the condition is incurable, cases of endometriosis have been cured. One effective treatment is natural progesterone, estrogen's antagonist. Estrogen can stimulate abnormal endometrial growth, and endometriosis is characterized by high levels of estrogen in the blood, indicating a hormone imbalance. Progesterone balances estrogen levels and is a precursor to other hormones, normalizing their activity in the body. *Note: For menstruating women, natural progesterone should be used only from ovulation to the menstrual period.* See "Premenstrual Syndrome (PMS)" on page 215.

ENDOMETRIOSIS CURED WITH NATURAL PROGESTERONE

Sandy was only 19 years old when her gynecologist recommended a hysterectomy. He believed that her endometriosis was so severe that she would never have children anyway. But Sandy's father, Bruce MacFarland, happened to be one of the developers of ProGest natural progesterone cream. He decided to try to correct her hormone imbalance with that newly developed product. The experiment saved her uterus and gave him a grandchild. Although Sandy had had only four periods since she was 16, she had a normal period the next month. At age 29, she delivered a normal, healthy baby.

HOMEOPATHIC RELIEF FROM ENDOMETRIOSIS

Shelley, a 24-year-old hairdresser, had such painful endometriosis that she had considered taking her own life. Every month she dreaded her period. She had to plan for it and take time off work, since she got such severe cramps that she couldn't stand on her feet. The cramps started about two days before her period and continued until its second day.

Shelley had the odd habit of lying naked on the cold bathroom floor to get relief, a symptom that was important in selecting a constitutional homeopathic remedy. With her type of endometriosis, "cold" feels better than "hot" (for example, a heating pad or hot water bottle). The remedies that worked in her case were homeopathic *Lachesis,* along with a homeopathic series therapy for endometriosis, a Chinese herbal formula by Seven Forests, and ProGest cream. Shelley had to work for many years with natural remedies before her cramps were entirely under control, but it took only a few months before she was able to live with them. Her endometriosis has now been under control for many years. She had been told by a number of doctors that her case was so progressed that she could not have children, but after this program of remedies specific for her condition and personality type, she delivered a nine-pound baby boy.

Homeopathic Therapy

Homeopathy can also help by stimulating the body to rebalance disturbed hormone levels. The appropriate remedy depends on the needs of each woman, but a good beginning in most cases is a combination remedy by Boiron called Cyclease. *Mag phos* 6X is another homeopathic remedy that can help stop the pain of cramps. The underlying endometriosis should be treated with constitutional homeopathic remedies specific to the patient. See a practitioner for recommendations and dosages.

Homeopathic remedies can also be used to detoxify the body of the buildup of toxic chemicals. Good options include Dioxin by Hannah's Herb Shop (for dioxin detoxification), Acetaldehyde by Deseret (for formaldehyde detoxification), and Exchem by Apex (for environmental chemical detoxification). Begin slowly with one drop in one ounce of water daily, working up gradually to ten drops three times daily. For a fuller discussion of homeopathic detoxification, see Chapter 5.

Herbal Therapy

According to Chinese medical theory, liver stagnation contributes to endometriosis by causing hormone imbalance. This imbalance can be corrected with a Chinese patent formula called *Xiao Yao Wan,* in combination with the Liver Cleanse Diet (detailed in Chapter 4). *Xiao Yao Wan* is available from practitioners and Chinese drugstores.

Note: Hsia Yao Wan (or Xiao Yao Wan) also increases bleeding, so its use should be stopped three days before the period is expected and resumed after it has ended.

Herbs can also be used to regulate hormones. The Eastern herb *keishi-bukuryo-gan* has been shown to suppress ingrowth of the endometrium in mice.[3] Hormone levels should be checked by a practitioner who is experienced with herbal remedies to determine which levels are out of balance and which herbs are appropriate for balancing them.

Other Natural Therapies

Acupuncture can help balance hormones and relieve endometriosis symptoms. See a practitioner for a treatment protocol for your case.

TRACKING POSSIBLE CAUSES OF ENDOMETRIOSIS

In Chinese medicine, endometriosis is attributed to the body's *qi* (energy) flowing the wrong way, as a result of using tampons or from having sex during menstruation. The tampon theory has recently gained scientific credence, but for another reason: most tampons contain dioxin. The Endometriosis Protection Agency reports a close association between levels of dioxin in the body and the incidence and severity of the disease. Dioxins are airborne byproducts of manufacturing processes involving chlorine, which is used in making plastics, PVCs, solvents like dry cleaning fluid, pesticides, and drugs. Dioxins are also byproducts of the chlorine bleaching process used to whiten paper, rayon, cotton, and other materials, including the fibers used in most feminine hygiene products. Dioxin can remain in the pulp once it is bleached and, like the insecticide DDT, collect in human fatty tissue. Another major source of dioxins for humans is animal fat (meat and dairy), where the chemicals become concentrated after grazing animals ingest them.

A possible link has been found between the amounts of dioxin in tampons and sanitary pads and various ailments, including not only endometriosis but cancers of the cervix, ovaries, and breast.[4]

Sitz baths may also give symptomatic relief. Alternate between sitting in a hot bath for three minutes and sitting in a cold bath for thirty seconds.

Recommended dietary modifications include avoiding foods to which you are allergic, as well as alcohol, sugar, and processed and heavily chemicalized foods, all of which can inhibit immune function.

Recommended nutritional supplements include vitamins A, C, E, and B_6 with vitamin B complex; the minerals calcium, magnesium, zinc, and selenium; and chlorophyll. They are available from a variety of companies; follow label directions.

Evening primrose oil is also helpful, with the proviso that it increases bleeding, which menstruating women with endometriosis already do too much. It should, therefore, not be taken immediately before or during the period.

ENVIRONMENTAL ILLNESS

See MULTIPLE CHEMICAL SENSITIVITY.

ESOPHAGEAL REFUX

See DIGESTIVE PROBLEMS.

FIBRILLATIONS

See IRREGULAR HEARTBEAT.

FIBROIDS

See UTERINE FIBROID TUMORS.

FIBROMYALGIA

Fibromyalgia is a mysterious pain syndrome of the muscles and connective tissue that seems to be reaching epidemic proportions, by some estimates affecting as many as 10 million people.[1] Seven out of eight of them are women, most commonly in their mid-thirties or in menopause. Called by a number of other names including fibrositis, myalgia, and tension rheumatism, fibromyalgia is a form of muscular rheumatism involving inflammation of the white fibrous tissue of the body, especially the muscle sheaths and fascial layers of the locomotor system. The fascia are thin sheets of connective tissue holding muscles, joints, and organs together. The main symptoms are persistent aches and pains, but the condition can also be marked by exhaustion, numbness, feelings of swelling in the joints, constipation or diarrhea, cold intolerance, disturbed sleep, tingling, and headaches. The syndrome also usually involves emotional upsets—anxiety, tension, suppressed anger, and depression.

Symptoms of fibromyalgia resemble rheumatoid arthritis combined with chronic fatigue. It causes considerable pain and stiffness, yet laboratory tests routinely come out normal. For that reason, victims of the disease were once simply dismissed as neurotic. Fibromyalgia is now recognized as a medical syndrome, but the cause and cure remain mysteries. Linked to the delicate balance between mind and body, fibromyalgia typically involves a physical stress of some sort compounded with emotional factors.

Fibromyalgia is an autoimmune disorder. The body seems to be reacting to itself. The process is known, but what triggers it is unknown. For some reason, the muscles start making too much fibrin—protein in the blood that the body forms into fibers, evidently to protect itself against traumatic injury. The fibrin is what makes the muscles painful to the touch. Often a physical trauma that doesn't hurt at the time you sustain it can become quite painful a couple of hours later. The autoimmune reaction responsible for fibromyalgia, as with lupus and other autoimmune diseases, has also been linked to multiple chemical sensitivities, Lyme disease, and parasites. Fibromyalgia may also accompany arthritis and is more likely to strike where arthritis has already struck.[2]

Fibromyalgia usually begins when a person who is under stress undergoes some further injury. For example, it may strike a woman who is already run down with chronic fatigue or stress who then gets into a car accident, has a bad fall, or contracts an infection. She thinks she is coping well, when suddenly she starts to experience aches, pains, and stiffness throughout her body. At first she feels it only when she wakes up. Then it's all day, every day. She gets tingling in her arms and swelling in her hands. Her legs feel like lead, and she's exhausted. Fear that something degenerative and irreversible is happening makes matters worse. She goes to the doctor, but he finds nothing abnormal. In *Are You Sure It's Arthritis?* Paul Davidson, M.D, explains that the pain is indeed in the body, not in the mind even though there is no physical damage to the bones and joints. Pain can occur without injury or tissue damage. Muscle tension alone can cause it.

To illustrate, he describes an exercise in which you hold yourself with your knees bent and your back pressed against a wall. Soon your thighs will be in pain, although no physical injury has occurred. The pain can be released by sitting on a chair and relaxing. The same thing happens in fibromyalgia: the symptoms seemingly result from an abnormal reaction in which the muscles respond to a combination of environmental and psychological stressors by remaining in a state of tension. The brain interprets this as pain, aching, and stiffness. As in the chair exercise, the key to relief is to provide the muscles time for rest and relaxation, allowing a period of repair and rejuvenation.[3]

Caution: The diagnosis of fibromyalgia should not be made without a doctor's help, since it can be confused with some quite serious diseases requiring early medical attention.

CONVENTIONAL TREATMENT

Conventional treatment for fibromyalgia usually addresses symptoms only. It includes analgesics, antidepressants, anesthetics, or corticosteroids that mask or suppress the problem without addressing the underlying cause.

Recently, drug treatment has been developed using glyceryl guaiacolate, the main ingredient in Robitussin cough syrup. Taken in very high doses over a long period of time, the drug dries up the fluids in the body and stops fibrin production. It can, however, have significant side effects at these doses, including diarrhea, nausea, vomiting, and stomach pain, which can be more daunting than the disease. The medication is expensive and has to be used daily long-term. If you skip a day or two, you're back where you started. And worst of all, for a large percentage of fibromyalgia patients, the medication doesn't work.

NATURAL REMEDIES

A study published in *Arthritis Care & Research* in 1999 found that most fibromyalgia patients are now turning to some form of alternative medicine, an indication that traditional drug treatment is inadequate for this baffling condition. The study suggested that these patients could benefit from acupuncture, homeopathy, manual-manipulative therapies, mind-body therapies, and magnetic therapies.[4] (Nikken magnetic mattresses and other magnetic products have gotten enthusiastic endorsements from fibromyalgia sufferers.)

Dr. Davidson's suggestions for relieving fibromyalgia include retraining the muscles and the mind to relax and release stress, beginning with education to understand the condition followed by stretching and relaxation to release the underlying state of chronic tension.[5]

Homeopathic Treatment: Tracking Hidden Causes

The longer fibromyalgia continues, the harder it is to resolve. Beside stress, chronic muscle pain may have other underlying causes that need to be located and cleared. Possibilities include chemical sensitivities, parasites, and Lyme disease. Dr. Walker tests for these conditions and treats them homeopathically when found.

ROOT CAUSE OF FIBROMYALGIA TRACKED AND ELIMINATED

Denise, age 51, had suffered for the past nine years with fibromyalgia, along with chronic diarrhea and stomach pains. Testing indicated that her underlying problems were Lyme disease and parasites. She was treated with homeopathic series therapy for both. (See "Lyme Disease" on page 172 and "Parasitic Infection" on page 212.) Her symptoms got worse before they got better, a normal homeopathic "aggravation"; however, after three weeks of treatment, she called to say she was much improved. Four months later, she could hardly believe the transformation in her health. She was energetic and had almost no pain, except for some mild stiffness when she overdid her activities. Her parasite-induced diarrhea was also gone. She said she felt twenty years younger.

Debbie also came to Dr. Walker complaining of fibromyalgia, with severe pain all over her body. Testing indicated she was extremely sensitive to petroleum products. When asked about her cosmetic usage, she acknowledged lathering her body nightly with Vaseline Intensive Care Lotion. Dr. Walker suggested she stop using it and take homeopathic Petroleum by Apex to eliminate its residues from her system (beginning with a single drop in half a glass of water, increasing slowly to ten drops daily). With this simple protocol, Debbie's symptoms were dramatically reduced in less than two months.

Nutritional Supplements

Antioxidants have been shown to benefit fibromyalgia sufferers, sometimes dramatically. Vitamin E is one. Take 400–800 IU daily.

Another antioxidant found to help in cases of both fibromyalgia and arthritis is Pycnogenol, a natural compound extracted from the bark of the French maritime pine tree and from grape seeds.[6] Pycnogenol reactivates damaged collagen by binding to collagen fibers and realigning them to a more youthful undamaged form, quenches free radicals, reduces inflammation, and boosts the immune system. Take 100 mg up to three times daily.

Other beneficial antioxidants include grapeseed extract (high in oligomeric proanthocyanins [OPCs]), green tea extract, and CoQ_{10}. Combination antioxidant formulas are marketed by several companies. For all of these products, follow label directions.

DHA, an essential fatty acid, can also help. DHA Max by Jarrow is particularly good. Take two capsules three to four times daily.

A relatively new addition to the nutritional supplements available for relieving the pain of fibromyalgia is S-adenosyl-methionine (SAMe). Sold in Europe as an antidepressant drug, SAMe is the activated form of methionine, an amino acid. In a crossover study reported in the *The American Journal of Medicine* comparing SAMe and a placebo in the treatment of fibromyalgia, the number of trigger points and painful anatomic sites decreased in fibromyalgia sufferers after administration of SAMe but not the placebo. Scores for depression also significantly improved on SAMe but did not change on the placebo. The researchers concluded that SAMe is a safe and effective therapy in the management of fibromyalgia.[7] SAMe is made by many supplements companies and is widely available in health food stores; follow label directions.

Fibromyalgia symptoms have also been relieved by a combination of malic acid (magnesium maleate) and boswellia, an herb used traditionally in India. Although malic acid alone can help fibromyalgia pain, the combination is more effective. Malic Acid Plus includes boswellia. One downside is that two capsules need to be taken every morning and evening. If they are stopped, the pain returns, indicating they are still only masking pain.

But they do avoid the side effects of conventional drugs and are more effective than ordinary analgesics and antidepressants.

Manual Manipulation Techniques

Massage, chiropractic adjustment, and other forms of manual manipulation of the joints, fascia, and connective tissue can also help fibromyalgia sufferers.

Craniosacral therapy is a painless form of manual manipulation that is particularly good for relieving fibromyalgia and other rheumatic pain. Emphasizing the importance of maintaining normal blood and nerve flow and the release of blockages in the energy patterns of the body, it improves the flow of nutrients to tissues and organs, boosts the immune system, and assists the elimination of waste products through the lymphatic system. Craniosacral therapy is a technique taught by the International Association of Health Care Practitioners in Palm Beach Gardens, Florida, headed by John Upledger, D.O.

Oram Miller, D.O., a San Diego chiropractor proficient in the technique, explains that the cranial motion of the skull bones needs to be as free, balanced, and symmetrical as possible for optimum health. Whenever there is a traumatic blow, such as a fall, this cranial motion becomes jammed and compressed in the head or body. This can cause a host of medical problems, including chronic pain syndromes, arthritis, jaw pain, middle ear infection, depression, and fibromyalgia. These strain patterns not only stay with the person for decades afterward, but one injury strain pattern winds up layered upon another, weaving into a latticework within the connective tissue structures of the body—the muscles, joints, ligaments, and tendons. Much of the energy of a car accident goes through the body and out the other side, but some of it gets locked in the tissues as "energy cysts." Cranial manipulation breaks up these energy cysts in a very gentle way.

Anyone who ends up with a diagnosis of fibromyalgia, states Dr. Miller, has had injuries in the past that resulted in whole-body strain patterns that were never fully released. There are also sleep deprivation, stress, and emotional components to fibromyalgia. These are the triggers, which cause the body to lose its previous ability to compensate for the strain patterns that never fully went away at the time of injury. Unless the person gets evaluated and treated by a practitioner of cranial technique within days or weeks of an accident to get these subliminal patterns out, they will be carried around for years.

For a craniosacral therapist in your area, call the Cranial Academy in Indianapolis (telephone [317] 594-0411), or check the Web site of the Upledger Institute, www.upledger.com.

FUNGAL INFECTIONS

There are many types of fungal infections, but the conditions in which they thrive are similar, and so are the natural methods of reversing them. Fungi thrive on sugar and dead matter, including hair, nails, and superficial layers of skin, and in moist areas, particularly the vagina.

Fungal invasion of any sort usually indicates candidiasis, a toxic overgrowth of the fungal yeast *Candida albicans*. Although it is particularly noticeable in the vaginal area, candidiasis is typically a symptom of an underlying imbalance affecting the whole body. When this ubiquitous yeast is growing out of control in the body and the blood, the body becomes more susceptible to invasion by other fungi. Anyone with nail or skin fungus is likely to have an overgrowth of *Candida* as well. Common fungal infections of the external layers of the body include athlete's foot, showing as a rash or patch of cracked, scaly, very itchy skin on the feet; and tinea, or ringworm, a fungal infection of the scalp, hair, skin, and nails. Onychomycosis, or tinea of the toenails and fingernails, particularly affects the elderly and has increased by a factor of four in the last twenty years. In one survey, it struck nearly half of patients over 70.[1] Yellowed toenails are typically a sign of this fungus.

Candidiasis can manifest as vague symptoms including depression, anxiety attacks, mood swings, lack of concentration, drowsiness, poor memory, headaches, insomnia, fatigue, bloating, constipation, bladder infections, menstrual cramps, vaginal itching, muscle and joint swelling, pain, hypothyroidism, and skin problems. *Candida* has been found to produce seventy-nine different toxins that can wreak havoc with the immune system. Thought to affect as many as one in three American women, *Candida* infection has been linked to drug use, including antibiotics, birth control pills, cortisone, and estrogen (on which *Candida* feeds).[2] *Candida* yeast is a natural resident of the body, normally found in harmless proportions. The body's natural defense against fungal overgrowth is its resident population of normal bacterial flora. But yeasts are impervious to the antibiotics that wipe out bacteria. When friendly bacteria are wiped out along with unfriendly ones by antibiotics, the field is left wide open for the yeasts to move in. Steroids and other drugs that suppress the immune system can also allow yeasts to grow.

CONVENTIONAL TREATMENT

To treat fungal invasions resulting from antibiotic "overkill," the conventional approach is to prescribe another drug. For vaginal yeast infections, there is clotrimazole (Lotrimin, Gyne-Lotrimin, and Lotrisone). For strictly local infections, nystatin (Mycostatin), used topically or as a "swish" in the mouth, is relatively safe although it can produce nausea, vomiting, and diarrhea. Antifungal creams like Tinactin or Lotrimin are the conventional remedies for athlete's foot. These drugs can work temporarily but the fact that the infection tends to recur suggests that they don't reach the underlying problem, which is systemic.

For systemic fungal invasion and for nail fungus, the drugs used until recently were griseofulvin and ketoconazole, but side effects ranging from annoying to serious, along with a high relapse rate, made doctors reluctant to prescribe them. A new line of broad-spectrum oral antifungal agents are promoted as working quickly and safely on systemic fungal conditions, including itraconazole (Sporanox), terbinafine (Lamisil), and fluconazole (Diflucan).[3] Research indicates, however, that these drugs too can be hazardous. All three have been linked to liver damage or liver failure leading to death or liver transplants, and Sporanox has been linked to congestive heart failure.[4] The drugs are also very expensive and need to be taken for months, and still the fungus tends to recur. Women wind up taking multiple courses of the drugs, at several dollars a tablet.

New topical medications are available for nail fungus, including Tineacide, Fungoid Tincture, and Mycocide NS, but they need to be applied daily for at least a year, and they don't work well unless the problem is caught early. When the topical drugs fail, the broad-spectrum oral antifungals (Sporanox or Lamisil) are typically recommended, with their concomitant risks.[5]

NATURAL REMEDIES

The Homeopathic Approach

Drugs aimed at killing the fungus are an imperfect solution because the fungus tends to return when the drug is stopped. Homeopaths feel that the underlying candidiasis is a symptom that the immune system is not working properly. Once this infection invades the body, it can further suppress the immune system and cause a variety of problems including depression, fatigue, foggy thinking, and poor digestion. Reversing the damage done to the intestinal flora by years of taking antibiotics, steroids, and other drugs, eating antibiotic-containing meats, and using antibacterial soaps is a long and difficult process. The problem won't go away in a month.

Some practitioners recommend special diets to control *Candida*, involving the elimination of the foods on which *Candida* feeds. But these diets too are imperfect solutions, since *Candida* returns when sugar or fermented foods are again eaten. Rebalancing the flora with acidophilus helps, but for most women fungal infection is a very deep, long-term problem needing deep-acting solutions. Homeopathic remedies work, but a year or more of treatment may be needed to eliminate the condition, along with dietary and lifestyle changes. Women who live in houses with moldy basements or ceilings that leak, or who get through the day on an adrenaline rush fed by sugar and coffee, or who are heavy wine drinkers, will have a hard time overcoming the condition.

With these provisos, homeopathic remedies can work quite well to boost the immune system, preventing the fungus from multiplying out of control. An effective protocol for eliminating yeast of every sort involves the following remedies by Deseret Biologicals: Candida 1M (two or three drops daily for four months), followed by Candida 200 (ten drops daily for four months), followed by Candida Plus (ten drops three times daily). Other options are Mycocan Combo by PHP, FNG by Deseret, and Fungisode and Molds/Yeast/Dust by CompliMed (for all, take ten drops three times daily).

ELUSIVE FUNGAL INFECTIONS CURED HOMEOPATHICALLY

Lynette had a distressing fungul infection under her arms. Colloidal silver spray eliminated her symptoms, but the infection kept coming back. The problem went away permanently after she took homeopathic FNG (ten drops three times daily until the bottle was empty).

Sherry's high-stress job in the garment district kept her at work ten to fourteen hours a day, where she was constantly breathing in the fabric's formaldehydes. She had chronic recurring vaginal yeast infections, craved sugar, and had trouble sleeping at night. She had been diagnosed with and treated for *Candida* on several occasions, but the infection kept coming back. While on a *Candida* diet (described under "Helpful Tips"), she was fine, but if she ate a piece of cake or drank a beer, the next day her yeast infection would return. The "maintaining cause" was evidently her job, which kept her body run down and exposed her to toxic fumes. For her extreme case, Sherry was given homeopathic series therapy for *Candida* called Monilia Albicans. She also went on a Liver Cleanse Diet (detailed in Chapter 4) and formaldehyde detox program (detailed in Chapter 5). At the end of two months, her yeast infections were gone, and they have not returned.

Herbal and Nutritional Remedies

A variety of herbs and nutrients also have antifungal properties. Garlic is one. In laboratory experiments, its antifungal activity has been shown to be greater than that of either nystatin or amphotericin B.[6] Health food stores now sell deodorized garlic tablets that make this age-old remedy both easy to take and socially acceptable. Other useful herbal and nutritional antimicrobials include grapefruit seed extract (Nutribiotic or Proseed), olive leaf extract, barberry, pau d'arco (a South American anti-infective herb), caprylic acid (a medium-chain fatty acid found naturally in the body that counters microorganism growth), undecylenic acid (another fat found naturally in the body, produced commercially from castor bean oil), and oregano. There are many brands of these products available at health food stores. A combination product that is convenient and easy to use is Candistroy by Nature's Secret. It contains a variety of herbs that fight *Candida* and boost the immune system, along with acidophilus. Follow label directions.

For fungal infections of the skin, a popular topical anti-infective that is more natural and less toxic than drugs is colloidal silver (silver suspended in a liquid medium). It can be used topically as a spray or taken orally if the spray is insufficient to eliminate symptoms. It works in difficult cases, but like antifungal drugs, it doesn't necessarily cure the problem for good. And although it doesn't have serious reported side effects like the drugs, silver is still a heavy metal, with unknown long-term effects.

Other natural topical agents that are effective and have no side effects are tea tree oil and a combination Chinese remedy called Wo oil. Wo oil may also be used for cleaning under the nails with a scrub brush to help eliminate parasites.

Lactobacillus acidophilus, Bifidobacterium bifidum, and *Lactobacillus bulgaricus* are "good" bacteria that protect the digestive tract from invasion by unwanted microorganisms.[7] If you have taken antibiotics, lost beneficial bacteria should be replaced with these cultures. Some experts recommend yogurt, but not all yogurts contain live acidophilus cultures, and yogurt itself is a fermented food. Acidophilus supplements in liquid or capsule form are better choices than yogurt. Jarrow and Natren are good brands, but there are many others; follow label directions.

For additional natural remedies for vaginal yeast infections, see "Vaginitis and Vaginal Infections" on page 240.

Helpful Tips

To help control *Candida,* try these measures:

◆ Avoid antibiotics unless critically necessary. If you must use them, replace friendly flora by taking acidophilus and bifido supplements after completing the course of drugs.

◆ Avoid foods on which yeast thrive—that is, foods containing sugar, molds, or yeasts; mushrooms and aged or fermented foods, including breads made with yeast; aged cheeses; vinegar; and beer. Eat pure, sugar-free foods.

◆ Avoid toxic chemicals, tap water, fabric softeners on underwear, and scented detergent.

◆ Don't wear damp socks or wet clothing after perspiring.

◆ Practice safe sex. If using oral contraceptives or a spermicide with nonoxynol-9, supplement with beneficial flora (acidophilus or bifido products).

◆ Get enough sunshine and exercise.

◆ Avoid stress.

To prevent fungal infection of the toes or to keep an infection from spreading, try these measures:

◆ Wear cotton or wool socks and change them frequently.

◆ Air out your shoes after use.

◆ Dry your feet well after washing and use foot powder, if needed, between the toes.

◆ Avoid walking barefoot in public bathrooms or shower areas. Try waterproof sandals.[8]

AN ANTI-*CANDIDA* pH BALANCE DIET THAT DELIVERS

The problem with anti-*Candida* diets is that as soon as you go off them, the candidiasis tends to return. But Ellen (one of this book's coauthors) found one that made her feel so much better that she was actually motivated to stay on it. In their 2002 book *The pH Miracle,* Dr. Robert Young and his wife, Shelley, present a program promoted as reversing a broad range of symptoms including fatigue, joint pain, poor digestion, and overweight. Ellen found that their claims were true. The program involves avoiding anything that turns the body pH acidic, a medium in which pathogens flourish, and concentrating instead on foods that promote alkalinity. The key to quick results are copious daily green drinks composed of a broad variety of vegetables and grasses, laced with chlorine dioxide or hydrogen peroxide drops (which wipe out pathogens). A mere three days on these drinks, without substantial dietary change, made Ellen feel so rejuvenated that she actually looked forward to modifying her diet to experience more.

Foods stressed include vegetables, grasses, raw fresh organic foods, nonanimal protein, soy, fresh fish (occasionally), essential fats, sprouts, herbs and spices, lemons, limes, grapefruit, tomato, avocado, and water. Foods to avoid include sugar in all forms, simple carbohydrates, refined and processed foods, sweet fruit, dairy products, salt, saturated and other unhealthy fats, meat and eggs, stored grains (meaning last year's crop), yeast, edible fungus, spirulina and algae (which thrive in acid conditions—other forms of chlorophyll are recommended instead), fermented and malted products, alcohol, caffeine, corn products, peanut products, heated oils, microwaved food, and artificial sweeteners. Although it sounds hopelessly spartan, Ellen found that cutting back on sugar and eating in this way actually modified her taste buds so that simple vegetable-based meals tasted delicious.[9]

GALLBLADDER DISEASE AND GALLSTONES

Ninety percent of gallbladder problems are due to gallstones. The most common and costly digestive disease in the United States, gallstones affect approximately one in ten Americans, and two out of three of them are women. The greater prevalence in women is thought to be due to multiple pregnancies, obesity, and cycles of rapid weight loss.[1]

The gallbladder, located on the upper right side of the abdomen under the liver, is a small organ that stores the bile excreted by the liver to break down fats in the digestive tract. It also stores cholesterol, toxins, and metabolized drugs. These substances can all coalesce to become gallstones when the bile gets oversaturated with cholesterol. The cholesterol precipitates out and forms crystals. Then minerals, bile pigments, and calcium are deposited around these crystals.

Increased gallstone formation is also associated with increased estrogen levels from estrogen replacement therapy (ERT), oral contraceptive use, and pregnancy. Estrogen increases the amount of cholesterol relative to bile salts and lecithin in bile. This increases the saturation of bile with cholesterol, leading to crystal formation. Estrogen also alters bile acid composition, increasing the chance of gallstone formation.[2]

Gallstones are not harmful in themselves, and many women have them for years without being bothered by them. Problems arise when stones are driven out of the gallbladder and into the bile duct, blocking it. This typically happens after eating a large fatty meal. The gallbladder tries to expel its fat-digesting substances and winds up expelling a gallstone as well. The victim then feels acute symptoms, including a severe steady pain and tenderness in the gallbladder area, nausea and vomiting, jaundice, and fever. An acute attack is typically described as a sudden, severe pain in the gallbladder area that radiates to the back between the shoulder blades.

Epidemiological studies suggest that gallstones are largely a disease of civilization, related to the high-fat, low-fiber Western diet. Gallstones are very rare in wild animals and are almost as rare in people living in nonindustrialized countries. They're common, however, in Westerners—including African-American Westerners, although rare among their West African relatives. North Americans, with a high incidence of stones, have bile that is nearly saturated or supersaturated with cholesterol. Rural Africans, with a very low incidence of stones, have bile that is almost always highly unsaturated.[3]

CONVENTIONAL TREATMENT

Gallstones are so common in the United States that at one time doctors were known to remove the gallbladders of symptom-free patients as a preventive measure. Enthusiasm for gallstone surgery was tempered when a landmark 1982 study found that most people with gallstones never developed symptoms. In the 1980s, alternatives to surgery were developed that destroy gallstones with strong drugs or shock waves. But unless the gallbladder itself is removed, the gallstones will often return. Stones cause pain when they get stuck in the bile duct. This can't happen when the gallbladder has been removed, because the bile is then secreted directly into the intestines.

Gallbladder surgeries jumped by 20 percent after 1988, becoming the third most popular major operation in the country after cesarean section and hysterectomy. This was not because gallbladder disease had suddenly increased but because 1988 was the year laparoscopic cholecystectomy was introduced. This "Band-Aid" surgery involves only a tiny cut instead of the six-inch abdominal incision required for standard gallbladder surgery, substantially reducing pain and recovery time.[4] But enthusiasm for this surgery was tempered when the complication rate suddenly skyrocketed. Laparoscopic surgery, it seems, is much more sophisticated than the old operation, since the internal organs are no longer exposed to plain view. Because the surgeon has to "see" through a laparoscope, errors can go undetected. The patient may be sewn back up while potentially fatal bleeding continues inside.[5]

A review published in *The New England Journal of Medicine* found that few gallbladder problems require surgery. Even recurrent gallstone pain may resolve spontaneously without surgery after several months. Intolerance to fatty foods, bloating, and flatulence are often attributed to gallstones, but the only symptoms for which surgery is now considered medically necessary is a specific type of abdominal pain called biliary colic (a steady pain in the upper right side of the abdomen) and jaundice.[6]

NATURAL REMEDIES

The Eastern Approach

Doctors who practice in the tradition of the Far East maintain that gallbladder surgery merely compounds the patient's problems and worsens her symptoms by throwing the gallbladder meridian further out of balance. Western medicine diagnoses gallbladder disease only when the condition is so acute that surgery is already necessitated. In Chinese medical practice, diagnosis is made long before the gallbladder is in such serious condition that it needs to be removed. Early warning signs include belching, burping, nausea, and problems digesting fat or fried foods.

Li Dan is a classic Chinese formula that dissolves stones without surgery. The remedy is appropriate for people who have problems digesting fat, and who feel worse after a fatty meal. It should be used for approximately three weeks, and may be followed by the Gallbladder Flush (described on page 124). *Li Dan* is available from Chinese pharmacies or licensed acupuncturists. K'an Herbs makes a good *Li Dan* product.

A variation of this herbal formula that has been used by the Chinese for thousands of years to dissolve gallstones is *Li Dan Paishi*. Composed of pig bile, the formula is anecdotally reported to be as effective as the prescription gallstone drug derived from ox bile and is much cheaper (about $4 per week).

Homeopathic Remedies

Homeopathic remedies can also reverse gallbladder disease before it becomes so acute as to require surgery. An excellent combination product is CompliMed's Liver and Gallbladder Homeopathic Formula. It can help even people who have had their gallbladders removed, since the problem is not with that organ alone but results when the gallbladder is deprived of energy from some other source, causing the organ to no longer work properly. The homeopathic formula rebalances the body, clearing the energy field around the gallbladder area. The recommended dose is ten drops three times per day.

GALLBLADDER SURGERY AVOIDED WITH CHINESE REMEDY

Amy became distraught and sought a remedy after a sonogram indicated that she had gallstones. Her physician scheduled gallbladder surgery for her, but Amy said she would do anything to avoid it. She postponed the surgery and took *Li Dan* herbal liquid faithfully for four weeks. Then, she had another sonogram. The result so surprised her doctor that Amy asked for a copy of the report. It indicated that her gallstones had completely disappeared.

STOMACH AILMENTS RELIEVED WITH SIMPLE REMEDIES

Maria had been suffering for weeks from burping, bloating, stomach pains, low energy, heartburn, and nausea. Nearly every night between 2 A.M. and 4 A.M., she'd wake up feeling anxious and unable to sleep. She said her first attack had begun after a lunch consisting of a large helping of French fries, the only thing she had eaten that day. On questioning, however, she recalled having had "stomach problems" off and on for years. She had never been able to eat a fatty meal without being uncomfortable for days afterward. Maria had seen a medical doctor, who had run tests. He had found that her gallbladder, while inflamed, had no stones. He had, therefore, ruled it out as the source of her stomach problems. Instead, he had put her on a stomach acid-blocking drug called Prilosec. The drug had eased her symptoms somewhat, but it masked rather than addressed her underlying condition. In the ordinary course, her inflamed gallbladder would have continued to deteriorate until it needed to be removed.

To Chinese doctors, Maria's symptoms were classic signs of first-stage gallbladder disease. The liver and gallbladder are said to share energy. When the liver is in a state of excess (for example, in women with PMS), the gallbladder is in a state of deficiency. The "time of the liver" is from 2 A.M. to 4 A.M., a factor reflected in Maria's inability to sleep at that time. She was given the Chinese herbal formula *Li Dan* and CompliMed's Liver and Gallbladder Homeopathic Formula. Several days later, she reported that she was finally sleeping through the night, and that her stomach symptoms and belching were gone.

Dietary Approaches

Also important for avoiding gallbladder problems is dietary regulation. Bingeing and dieting can throw off the gallbladder, which functions to release bile for incoming fat. If no fat comes in, the fluid thickens and can cause painful stones. Fat should be processed at a steady rate. Don't go for long periods without eating and then eat a huge meal. Periodic onslaughts can overload the gallbladder. Fat should be eaten in moderate amounts spread throughout the day in order to flush the bile and the gallbladder.

Another important dietary factor is fiber. Denis Burkitt, M.D., attributed the low incidence of gallbladder disease among rural Africans to the fact that their diets include enormous amounts of fiber. Americans on refined-foods diets, by contrast, eat unnaturally little of it. Fiber binds bile acids in the intestines so they can be eliminated in the stools rather than reabsorbed and returned to the liver. Since bile acids are made from cholesterol, more cholesterol must be used to replace its loss in the bile, leaving less cholesterol available for forming stones.

Wheat bran is a popular source of fiber, but it can irritate the delicate lining of the intestines and inhibit mineral absorption. Safer and more digestible alternatives are raw vegetables, raw and dried fruits, and most beans and whole grains. Dr. Burkitt's dietary suggestions for avoiding gallstones (as well as diverticulosis, kidney stones, and many other "Western" diseases) included substituting complex carbohydrates for fiber-depleted carbohydrates (white sugar and white flour). Complex carbohydrates include whole-grain breads (wheat, rye, oats, corn, and millet), whole-grain cereals (wheat bran, oat bran, and corn bran), and high-fiber vegetables (potatoes, carrots, beans, Brussels sprouts, and onions).[7]

Certain specific foods are also beneficial for preventing and treating gallstones. One is soy. There is evidence that soybean products not only guard against stones but also dissolve those that have already formed.[8] In *Healing with Whole Foods*, Paul Pitchford recommends apples (particularly green apples) to help soften stones; radishes to help remove

FULL RECOVERY FROM PAIN

Debbie had recurring gallbladder attacks, which were particularly severe at night. She suffered from belching, bloating, pain that radiated to the back between the shoulder blades, and continual abdominal discomfort that was worse after eating. Her treatment consisted of *Li Dan Paishi* tablets for four weeks (six pills two to three times daily), followed by three days of eating only apples or drinking apple juice, and then the gallbladder flush. She got quite sick the night of the gallbladder flush but was dramatically better the next morning. The flush was followed by Liver and Gallbladder Homeopathic Formula by CompliMed (ten drops three times daily) to rebalance her meridians. Debbie has had no more gallbladder problems since.

stones and deposits from the gallbladder; and pears, parsnips, seaweed, lemon, limes, and turmeric to hasten gallstone removal. In addition, he suggests a two-month course of 3 to 5 cups of chamomile tea daily, along with 5 teaspoons of fresh flaxseed oil added to food.[9]

Recent research indicates that vitamin C can help women avoid gallbladder disease, and that a lack of it may be a risk factor for the disease. Increasing vitamin C intake can be done with supplementation (250–500 mg daily), a large orange per day, or an increased intake of other fruits and vegetables.[10]

The Gallbladder Flush

Gallstones have been released naturally with a protocol called the "gallbladder flush." The procedure, however, is controversial. The *Encyclopedia of Natural Medicine* maintains that "stones" passed in this way are actually a complex of minerals, olive oil, and lemon formed within the gastrointestinal tract, and that large amounts of olive oil will contract the gallbladder and increase the likelihood of a stone blocking the bile duct.[11] But good results have been obtained with the procedure when it has been preceded by a three-week course of *Li Dan* to break up the stones. Paul Pitchford's version of this treatment consists of sipping a mixture of ⅔ cup warm olive oil and ⅓ cup fresh lemon juice at bedtime, then sleeping on the right side. In the morning, the stones usually pass in the stool.

Naturopathic doctors have long used coffee enemas to help flush out the gallbladder and stimulate it to release bile. Although not recommended for long-term use, used short term, coffee enemas can be quite beneficial. For protocols, see Paul Pitchford's *Healing with Whole Foods* or Bernard Jensen's *Dr. Jensen's Guide to Better Bowel Care.*[12]

GAS

See BLOATING, GAS, AND EDEMA.

GASTRITIS

See DIGESTIVE PROBLEMS.

GENITAL WARTS

As many as a million cases of genital warts are diagnosed each year.[1] Among other places, they can occur on a woman's anus, urethra, vulva, vagina, or cervix. Genital warts are caused by infection with the human papilloma virus (HPV), which is linked to cervical cancer. HPV is sexually transmitted, but the source is sometimes hard to trace, since the warts may not show up for two to eighteen months after exposure and Pap smears don't necessarily catch them. In one study of women age 15 to 50, HPV was found in 10 percent of those with normal Pap results, as well as in 35 to 40 percent of those with abnormal smears.

CONVENTIONAL TREATMENT

Genital warts are easily removed with topical drugs, laser surgery, or freezing, but the recurrence rate is high. Removing the warts doesn't eliminate the virus, which can remain latent in the skin. Repeated treatments may be necessary.[2]

Recommended preventive measures include abstaining from sex, regular checkups, and the use of condoms. There is some concern, however, that HPV is so small that it may be able to penetrate a condom. Moreover, it can be transmitted from skin to skin in areas not covered by a condom.

NATURAL REMEDIES

Homeopathic series therapy can clear not only the warts themselves but also the underlying infection. Homeopaths maintain that clearing the system of HPV homeopathically also substantially reduces the risk of contracting cervical cancer. Particularly effective is Human Herpes 6 Virus series therapy by the German company Staufen, taken along with the vibrational remedy Warts by Kroeger Herbs. Also good is Condylomata series therapy by Staufen, taken along with the constitutional homeopathic remedy *Thuja*. Series therapy consists of a box of ampules of the remedy in different potencies to be taken in a particular order. The remedies should be taken at the rate of one ampule every three days for a month. Any warts that have been burned off are liable to reappear, but don't panic; that's how the remedy clears the virus from the body. Sex should be avoided during this process, since infections that have reached the surface of the skin can be contagious.

ALARMING INFESTATION OF GENITAL WARTS CLEARED

Sarah confided to Dr. Walker that her vagina was covered with hundreds of warts. Her gynecologist had said it was the most rampant case he had ever seen. Sarah had suffered for years with chronic fatigue syndrome, and her system was so run down that she had no immune reserves to fight off the virus. She had previously undergone a series of extremely painful laser treatments to burn off the warts, but they had returned. She tried a homeopathic series therapy, but complained that it was aggravating the infection. Dr. Walker assured her that it was merely a healing crisis and that the warts would go away. To her relief, in about two months they did; and they have not returned. Since then, Dr. Walker has helped a number of women reverse a diagnosis of HPV using Condylomata series therapy, lymph drainers, and vitamin A.

GONORRHEA

Each year, approximately 650,000 people in the United States are infected with gonorrhea,[1] making it the nation's second most common sexually transmitted disease after chlamydia. Gonorrhea can lead to infertility or to pelvic inflammatory disease. Another potential complication is gonococcal arthritis, the most common form of arthritis caused by an infectious agent. The first symptoms are fever, chills, and body aches. If left untreated, the condition can develop into full-blown arthritis, with rapid destruction of cartilage and bone.

Gonorrhea may produce no symptoms. If there are symptoms, however, they usually develop within one to three weeks after exposure. Symptoms include difficult or painful urination; penile discharge in men; and a yellowish vaginal discharge, bleeding between periods or after intercourse, and pain in the pelvic area during intercourse in women. Gonorrhea isn't detectable by Pap smear and requires other specialized tests.

CONVENTIONAL TREATMENT

Gonorrhea was once easily treated with penicillin, but antibiotic-resistant strains have increasingly frustrated standard treatment. In the 1980s, the germs became resistant not only to penicillin but to tetracycline. In September 2000, the Centers for Disease Control and Prevention reported that gonorrhea is now developing resistance to two newer antibiotics, seriously limiting drug options.[2]

Condoms, diaphragms, and spermicides containing nonoxynol-9 may help reduce the spread of the disease, but nonoxynol-9 is a synthetic estrogen mimic that can have other side effects. See "Uterine Prolapse" on page 237 and "Bladder Infection, Irritation, and Inflammation (Cystitis)" on page 63. The safest course remains abstinence or careful selection of sexual partners.

NATURAL REMEDIES

Gonorrhea victims are required by law to see a medical doctor, who must report each case to the health department; therefore, patients diagnosed with the disease generally wind up on antibiotics. But homeopaths feel that it is still important to seek homeopathic treatment from a qualified practitioner. Even when treated with antibiotics, gonorrhea can cause deep, lingering physical and emotional imbalances, and these can be cleared by an experienced homeopath. The appropriate constitutional remedies are chosen on a case by case basis after taking a detailed patient history.

GRAVES' DISEASE

See HYPERTHYROIDISM.

HAIR LOSS

Female pattern baldness is related to declining levels of female hormones and a relative increase in testosterone. Hair loss can also be caused by drugs (particularly chemotherapeutic agents), scarring from radiation, poor thyroid function, skin disease, stress, poor nutrition, parasites, and high doses of vitamin A. Other suspects are certain hair styles and products, including tight ponytails or buns, curling irons and blow dryers, and harsh chemicals in dyes and sprays.

Chronic dandruff can also result in hair loss. Dandruff is a condition of the scalp involving the shedding of white flakes of dead skin, commonly caused by a disorder of the sebaceous glands. Other causes of dandruff are trauma, hormone imbalance, poor diet, and excess sugar.[1]

CONVENTIONAL TREATMENT

The most popular pharmaceutical answer to hair loss is a drug called minoxidol (Rogaine) used topically to restore hair growth. Rogaine was approved for over-the-counter sale for hair loss in March 1996. Despite quite a bit of media hype, it has not proven itself a miracle cure for reversing time's ravages to the scalp. In controlled trials, it has produced "dense" hair growth in only 8 percent of users after a year's application, and only 16 percent found regrowth sufficient to continue the treatment. Some experienced severe itching, and the long-term effects of the drug are unknown. Up to eight months may be required before effects are noticeable enough to know if the drug will work in a particular case. Also, it has to be applied daily for life to maintain its effects, at an investment of $45 to $55 per month.[2]

NATURAL REMEDIES

A natural alternative that has been reported to be quite effective at early stages of hair loss is a Chinese product called Avacor. Its only downside is that it can upset your stomach if taken with food. The phone number for ordering is (877) 805-9743. Another alternative available at Chinese drugstores is the Chinese patent formula *Sheng Fa*. Eastern doctors say it works by strengthening the kidney energy. Weak kidney energy results in hair loss. The recommended course of treatment is four pills twice daily over a four-month period.

Natural hormones can also stimulate hair growth. Women who are losing their hair report that applying ¼ teaspoon of natural progesterone cream (ProGest) to their scalps each night has resulted in hair that is thick and lustrous.

Nioxin is an herbal hair product that has produced dramatic results. It is sold by beauty supply companies and comes in the form of a shampoo, conditioner, and scalp treatment. Directions are on the labels. For dandruff, tea tree oil shampoos are very effective. Many brands are available at health food stores.

Vitamin products are available that are specially formulated for the hair. Nature's Plus makes Ultra Hair capsules. For people who dont like taking pills, the product also comes in the form of a tasty morning drink. Use according to label directions.

The amino acid cysteine can promote both hair growth and hair curl. Take 500 mg one to three times daily.

To detoxify the body of harsh chemicals in hair products and cosmetics, an effective homeopathic remedy is Beautex by Mediral. To help avoid cleansing reactions (achy, flu-like symptoms), start slowly with one drop in water daily, increasing gradually to ten drops three times daily.

HEADACHES

Eighteen million American women suffer from headaches of various sorts. Until puberty, boys and girls are equally likely to get them. After puberty, however, female headache sufferers outnumber males in all age groups. Women's headaches also tend to be more frequent and more severe.[1]

More than 90 percent of headaches are caused by tension, which constricts blood vessels in the head. Tension headaches can be a symptom of anxiety, stress, or physical tension; lack of sleep; overconsumption of caffeine; food allergy; eyestrain; fever; hypoglycemia; drug side effects; PMS; dehydration; or trauma. Tension headaches are typically dull and persistent, affecting both sides of the head.

Migraine headaches, which trouble about 17 percent of American women and 6 percent of American men, are more serious than tension headaches. They are severe, recurrent headaches typically accompanied by nausea, vomiting, "auras" (visual disturbances), lightheadedness, intolerance to light, and numbness or tingling in the head or arms. Attacks last from four to seventy-two hours and strike on average one to four times a month. While migraine headaches are more common in women, cluster headaches are more common in men. Cluster headaches usually occur in clusters (from three to six attacks per day) over a period of weeks or months. Both cluster and migraine headaches usually affect one side of the head, but migraines tend to last longer.[2]

Heredity is a factor in migraine headaches; one or both parents of most migraine sufferers suffered with them as well. Hormones also play a role. The hormonal changes that occur during puberty, the monthly menstrual cycle, pregnancy, childbirth, breast-feeding, and menopause all affect migraine incidence. About 15 percent of women who have migraines only get them two or three days before or after the start of their menstrual period, and more than 60 percent say migraines worsen at this time. Others report that they have a predictable headache at some part of their cycle, perhaps at ovulation.

Some women report improvement of migraines while taking oral contraceptives, but more commonly, migraine headaches will worsen with hormonal drugs. In fact, birth control pills have been known to bring on migraines in women who never had headaches previously. Discontinuation of the drugs may not result in improvement for many months. Non-estrogen hormonal methods of birth control such as Depo-Provera injection can also aggravate headaches in some women.[3]

Migraines peak for women during their childbearing years. A preexisting migraine condition can become worse during the first trimester of pregnancy and then disappear for the last two. Migraines can also appear for the first time during pregnancy or soon after giving birth, but many women who suffer from migraines notice an improvement during pregnancy. This is probably due to the sustained high levels of hormones. Managing migraines with drugs during pregnancy and breast-feeding can be a problem; babies should not be exposed to drugs they don't need. Avoidance of headache triggers, exercise, biofeedback, and other relaxation techniques are better options.

At menopause, headaches may reappear after years of absence or become more severe or frequent. Following natural menopause, however, there is a reported 60 percent decrease in headache incidence and severity. Women whose migraines were mainly menstrual related seem to benefit most in this way from menopause. As with birth control pills, some menopausal women with migraines improve on hormone replacement therapy, while others find that their headaches get worse.[4]

Note: Sudden severe headaches can indicate a condition that is more serious than tension or hormonal changes—possibly hemorrhage or bleeding inside the brain. A severe headache with stiff neck and fever could indicate meningitis or meningoencephalitis. Other danger signals are headaches that begin after exertion, straining, coughing, or sexual activity; or headaches that are accompanied by changes in mental state, drowsiness, confusion, or memory loss. If these symptoms accompany a headache, seek professional medical help.

CONVENTIONAL TREATMENT

Most tension headaches are treated with over-the-counter analgesics (aspirin, acetaminophen, and ibuprofen). For habitual users, however, these drugs can become progressively less effective and can precipitate a syndrome of "rebound headaches." The sufferer pops more analgesics, but the headache never really goes away. The result is a constant dull headache perpetuated by the very drugs intended to relieve it.

To treat migraines and cluster headaches, prescription drugs are often used. For migraines, sumatriptan (Imitrex), ergotamine tartrate, or dihydroergotamine (DHE) may be prescribed. Imitrex, which is particularly popular, changes serotonin levels in the brain. By 1995, Imitrex was being used by more than 2 million people worldwide. However, the FDA had received 3,526 voluntary reports by then of suspected side effects, including 83 deaths and at least 273 life-threatening complications. Lawsuits followed. Safety concerns eventually prompted the manufacturer to change its labeling to emphasize that Imitrex should be used only when a doctor has clearly established that a patient is suffering from migraine, and that it should "not be given to patients in whom unrecognized coronary artery disease is likely without a prior evaluation for underlying cardiovascular disease." The question is, how do you recognize patients likely to have "unrecognized" coronary artery disease? Deaths of people who were apparently healthy and had no heart disease detectable even at autopsy have been blamed on the drug. Research also suggests that Imitrex can gradually damage heart vessels in otherwise healthy people.[5]

Other drugs may be prescribed to prevent migraines, including beta-blockers, calcium channel blockers, and certain antidepressants and anticonvulsant drugs; however, none of these drugs is very effective for this purpose.

NATURAL REMEDIES

For simple headaches, relaxation can be effective. Muscle contraction headaches, including common migraines, may respond to easy neck stretches. Move the head to one side and then to the other, resisting with the head against the palm of the hand.[6] Tension headaches caused by the neck muscles pulling on the scalp may be helped by chiropractic or craniosacral manipulation.

Aromatherapy is another option. Try rubbing peppermint oil directly on the forehead. Peppermint oil is a natural antispasmodic and diuretic that has been shown in German research to be as effective as Extra Strength Tylenol in easing tension headaches.[7]

The old-fashioned ice pack to the forehead also works. In fact, it has been found to work in about the same amount of time as an analgesic takes to kick in. The ice constricts the swollen blood vessels that cause the head to ache.[8] If an ice pack isn't enough, emersing the arms up to the elbows in ice water is also helpful.

For sinus headaches, hot compresses on the sinuses can relieve pain.

For headaches brought on by stress or tension, a gemmotherapy called Black Currant by Dolisos can help. Liquid tinctures derived from the immature shoots of plants, gemmotherapies are available in health food stores. Follow label directions.

Magnesium supplements have been found to reduce nerve excitability and migraine susceptibility. Low levels of magnesium increase nerve cell excitability and pain.[9] Magnesium and calcium levels should be in balance; for example, 500 mg daily of each.

For migraines, the herb feverfew has been touted as a miracle cure that can eliminate the need for drugs. British researchers have found that the herb not only cuts the number and severity of headaches but also reduces the nausea that goes with them. Feverfew suppresses the release of prostaglandins and histamines that produce inflammation. In one study, migraine victims who took feverfew capsules for six months were relatively free of migraines, while those taking a placebo had three times the normal incidence of them. In another study, the herb reduced the incidence of migraines by 25 percent and lessened their severity dramatically.[10] Feverfew is readily available in health food stores; again, follow label directions.

The herbal form of aspirin is willow bark. Used by Chinese physicians 2,500 years ago, it contains salicin, a pain reliever that is very similar to that found in aspirin. Another herbal analgesic is meadowsweet tea. These herbal options, also available at health food stores, can be just as effective as aspirin at much lower risk.[11]

Acupuncture and EMG (electromyographic) biofeedback have been used successfully in the treatment of both tension and migraine headaches.[12] Physical therapy, self-hypnosis, and relaxation can also offer relief.[13]

Homeopathic Solutions

Homeopathic remedies get to the root of the problem. For migraines, the easiest homeopathic option is a combination remedy by CompliMed called Migramed. The dosage is ten drops three times a day. BHI also makes a combination remedy called Headaches that helps in cases of migraine. Hyland's makes a headache formula that is good for occasional headaches. Follow label directions.

Finding the right constitutional homeopathic remedy usually requires consulting a homeopathic physician, who will take a detailed patient history. However, you may be able

TRACKING THE CAUSE OF HEADACHES

The ideal solution to intractable headaches is to find and eliminate the cause. Beside fluctuations in the menstrual cycle, headaches can start with particular triggers, which can often be tracked by keeping a log of your headaches and correlating them with your habits. Stress is by far the most common trigger. Women who juggle many different roles—mother, wife, working woman, caretaker of the home, and caregiver for small children, aging parents, or ill family members—are prone to headaches. Environmental and behavioral triggers of headaches include heat, humidity, sudden changes in barometric pressure, dust, smoke, glare, and strong odors. Eyestrain, physical exertion, chronically tensing muscles, irregular sleep schedules, insomnia, and oversleeping can also bring on headaches.

Common dietary triggers of headaches include alcohol, aged cheeses, nuts, dairy products, shellfish, chocolate, and food additives and preservatives such as MSG, aspartame, and nitrates. Headaches have also been blamed on "reactive hypoglycemia"—the plunge in serum insulin levels that follows a sharp rise after you overdose on sugar.

Other headaches have been traced to a misaligned bite. Temporomandibular joint dysfunction (TMJ) is a dental condition that results from irritation of the disk connecting the jaw to the skull. If this is your problem, before you succumb to expensive mouth reconstruction, try making a studied effort to relax your jaw. Tension can throw your bite off, resulting in headaches. Your dentist can also fit you with a mouthpiece to wear at night to relieve jaw tension.[14]

to recognize your symptoms from the following list. If no relief results, a different remedy is needed. Use 30X concentrations. The dosage of each remedy is three pills every fifteen minutes for a total of eight doses.

Homeopathic Options for Treating Migraines

◆ *Iris versicolor*—for classic migraine, usually on the right side of the head; pain typically centered in the temple, above or below the eye; vomiting that gives no pain relief; blurred vision preceding headaches; a tight feeling in the scalp.

◆ *Lac caninum*—for headache on alternating sides, either during one attack or from one headache to the next; headache of the occiput (back part of the head) radiating to the forehead.

◆ *Lac defloratum*—for migraine preceded by an aura or dim vision; worse with noise, light, and menses; nausea and vomiting present with headache; frontal headache with nausea, vomiting, and chills; headache better with cold applications, lying down, or in the dark.

◆ *Natrum muriaticum*—for the throbbing, blinding headache or migraine that can be felt in any location; often on the right side of the head; "feels like a hammer beating the head"; headache from grief; numbness in face or lips; worse with light, in the sun, when reading, before or after menses, with noise, with head injury, between 10 A.M. and 3 P.M.; better lying in a dark, quiet room; better with perspiration and cold applications.

◆ *Sanguinaria*—for the migraine headache that is better after vomiting, with sleep, or after passing gas; migraine on the right side, typically beginning in the neck on the right side and extending to the forehead and eye.

Homeopathic Options for Cluster Headaches

◆ *Glonoinum*—for the pulsating, bursting headache; headache with flushed face and pounding pulses/carotids (arteries in the neck); headache worse from the sun, or that comes and goes with the sun, even without direct exposure; worse from alcoholic drinks, motion, heat, jarring, tight collars; better with external pressure or when lying in the dark.

◆ *Belladonna*—for cluster or migraine headache that begins in the occiput and radiates to the right temple or forehead, settling around the right eye; headache worse after a hair cut; head sensitive to cold, drafts, washing hair.

◆ *Lachesis*—for pulsating, bursting headache; left-sided headache that can be migraine; headache that begins on the left and moves to the right; headache that comes before the menstrual period and is better after the flow begins; headache with flushed feeling.

Homeopathic Options for Tension Headaches

◆ *Aconite*—for the headache that comes on suddenly; headache after shock or fear, exposure to wind or cold; severe headache during fever.

◆ *Apis*—for head pain behind the left ear, extending to the left eye or temple; the brain feels tired or the head feels swollen; feeling of heat; throbbing pains; better with pressure; worse with motion.

◆ *Bryonia*—left-sided headache; headache over the left eye extending to the occiput, then to the whole head; worse from coughing, in the morning, when constipated, when ironing; better with pressure or with eyes closed.

◆ *Gelsemium*—for the headache beginning at the occiput or neck and radiating to the forehead; worse at 10 A.M.; better with urination; head feels very heavy.

◆ *Ignatia*—for the headache that is worse after sweets; headache pain like a nail driven into the head; headache after grief, characterized by sighing.

◆ *Coffea*—for headache resulting from coffee withdrawal, strong stimulation, or strong emotions; headache worse with music, noise, footsteps; headache or migraine pain like a nail driven into the head.

◆ *Chamomilla*—for headache from tooth pain, teething, or earache.

◆ *Lycopodium*—for headache that's worse on the right side, worse from 4 P.M. to 8 P.M. or when trying to concentrate; pain as if temples are being screwed together.

◆ *Pulsatilla*—for tension or migraine headache that occurs at the end of the menstrual flow; headache that's worse with menopause, heat, sun; worse on exertion or after emotional stress; better with open air, cold applications, pressure; headache pulsates or feels as if it's pressing outward.

HOMEOPATHIC REMEDIES GET TO THE ROOT OF HEADACHES

Mary had been married for twenty-four years, and for twenty-four years she had suffered with severe weekly migraines, involving nausea and vomiting for two or three days at a time. She had taken every conceivable drug for them, including Prozac and Imitrex. The Prozac did nothing. The Imitrex was effective at first but she had to keep increasing the dose, until she was up to ten or twelve injections per headache. At $40 per injection, this was a prohibitively expensive proposition.

Mary's problem appeared to be emotional. She wasn't getting along well with her husband. Homeopathic remedies were recommended based on her particular symptoms: *Ignatia,* then *Chelidonium,* then *Staphysagria,* then *Lac caninum.* At first, the remedies aggravated Mary's emotional state. She cried more. She saw what a disaster her marriage was, a fact she hadn't really faced before. She realized that her husband was treating her unfairly. Eventually, the homeopathic remedies helped her rebalance her life and her outlook. She began expressing her feelings more openly to her husband. Not only has her marriage improved, but she has had no migraine headaches in more than four years. She is still working out her problems, but homeopathic remedies are helping her move past an emotional trap in which she had become "stuck."

◆ *Silicea*—for headache or migraine that begins in occiput and radiates to the forehead or right side of the head; worse from cold, drafts, mental exertion, menstruation, uncovering the head; better when lying with eyes closed or in the dark, or from warming or wrapping the body.

◆ *Arnica*—for headache from trauma or concussion; the head that feels bruised or has an aching, sharp pain; worse when stooping.

◆ *Hypericum*—for the bursting, aching headache; worse in damp and fog; headache from contusions or dental work.

◆ *Nux vomica*—for the headache of a hangover; worse with noise, light, mental activity, before menses; head highly sensitive to stimulation; allergy headache.

HEART ATTACK

See HEART DISEASE.

HEART DISEASE

Although women have a significantly lower risk of heart disease than men before menopause, they catch up after menopause. Heart disease remains the number one cause of death among American women, killing more than 226,000 each year. Underlying heart disease is atherosclerosis, or hardening of the arteries, which results from an accumulation of calcified fatty plaque in the blood vessels. Atherosclerosis is the chief cause of coronary heart disease (CHD) and strokes, is a major cause of high blood pressure, and contributes to circulatory disorders including Raynaud's syndrome. When the heart is too weak to pump as hard as it should, blood backs up into the lungs and veins, causing congestive heart failure. When the blood can no longer get through the vessels, a heart attack may result. Angina, or chest pain on exertion, can warn of an impending heart attack.

Cardiac arrhythmias, or irregular or racing heartbeats, are other warning signs. In women, however, they are also common symptoms of menopause and are not necessarily cause for alarm. (See "Irregular Heartbeat" on page 165.)

Though heart disease manifests in different ways, a common dysfunction runs through them all. Chinese doctors believe the underlying problem is an imbalance in the heart meridian. Supporting it with vitamins, minerals, homeopathic remedies, and herbs can help.

Whether taking hormones can also help is controversial. As recently as 1995, the American Heart Association (AHA) advised that all women with heart disease should consider taking estrogen, since premenopausal women with higher estrogen levels have a significantly lower risk of heart disease than either men or postmenopausal women do. But in July 2001, the AHA came out with new guidelines that represent a drastic reversal in its approach. The AHA said healthy women should *not* take hormones after menopause to prevent heart disease, and those who already have heart disease should not start on hormones. The advisory was based on the results of several studies of hormone replacement therapy (HRT) and heart disease, including the Heart and Estrogen/Progestin Replacement Study (HERS). It found that for women with heart disease, taking oral estrogen plus progestin actually raised the risk of recurrent heart attack and death during the first year of use, and lowered it only slightly thereafter.[1] Worse, estrogen is linked to an increased risk of breast cancer, another growing epidemic, as discussed in Chapter 2.

An alternative theory explaining the lower risk of heart disease in premenopausal women relates to the iron lost in menstruation. Excess iron stores have been associated with an increased risk of heart attacks in men, who have no mechanism like menstruation for cleansing the body of excess iron buildup.[2] Menopausal women also have no such mechanism, so their heart disease rates go up.

CONVENTIONAL TREATMENT

The conventional approach to preventing heart disease is to use drugs to reduce its major risk factors—high blood pressure and high cholesterol levels. This approach grew out of the Framingham Heart Study, in which 5,209 adults living in Framingham, Massachusetts, were followed for eighteen years beginning in 1949. People with lower blood pressure and serum cholesterol levels were found to live significantly longer than people with higher levels.[3] Long-term studies of people on low-fat, high-fiber vegetarian diets have also consistently shown a reduction in serum cholesterol and blood pressure levels, as well as an actual increase in life expectancy.[4]

The wrinkle in those studies is that the long-lived people in them did not achieve low blood pressure and cholesterol levels by using drugs. Their low risk factors came either from their lifestyles or their genes. In most studies that have looked at lowering cardiac risk factors with drugs, long-term benefits have been disappointing. In some studies, the drugs have actually been linked to an *increased* risk of death from heart disease. For a detailed discussion, see "Cholesterol, High" on page 83 and "High Blood Pressure (Hypertension)" on page 142.[5]

Julian Whitaker, M.D., suggests that the increased use of beta-blockers to lower blood pressure may actually be responsible for the modern epidemic of congestive heart failure. Ten to 20 million people are on beta blockers, which act by slowing the heart's pumping.

TRACKING THE CAUSE

Tracing the history of modern heart attack treatment in the January 1998 *Townsend Letter for Doctors and Patients,* Wayne Martin observed that before 1925, heart attacks were practically unknown. Seventy years ago they were blamed on blood clots in the arteries and were called "coronary thrombosis." But when warfarin, an anticoagulant that breaks up clots, didn't do much to prevent a second heart attack in people who had already had one, attention was switched to cholesterol and the disease was renamed "myocardial infarction." Butter was abandoned en masse for margarine, and polyunsaturated liquid vegetable fats like corn oil were recommended. Yet heart disease and heart attacks steadily increased.[6]

Ironically, researchers are now blaming the epidemic of heart attacks in part on the widespread use of polyunsaturated vegetable fats once thought to prevent them. Heart attack deaths have increased by a factor of eighty in the same time that polyunsaturated fat use has tripled. The problem with this fat is that the protective antioxidants have been removed during processing. Antioxidants are substances that keep your internal tissue from reacting with oxygen and breaking down into harmful, free-floating pieces called free radicals. Antioxidants are lost in the modern diet not only in commercial fats but also in bleached flour and other processed foods. Homogenization and pasteurization of milk have also been linked to an increased risk of heart disease.

In 1980, cardiologists returned to their first theory and decided that sticky platelets and blood clots were the problem. Everyone over age 40 was advised to take aspirin, an anticoagulant, to avoid a heart attack. But doctors began to reconsider that advice too, when several trials with aspirin merely produced a run of ulcers without preventing heart attacks. Aspirin taken habitually can eat holes in the stomach and can lead to other unwanted side effects. (See "Pain and Inflammation" on page 209.)

Then, a large American trial showed that regular aspirin use reduced heart attack incidence by 40 percent in male doctors. A daily aspirin again became the rage. But critics pointed to a subtle discrepancy in the study: unlike the studies in which aspirin was ineffective, it used Bufferin, which contains magnesium. Magnesium is a natural vasodilator that reduces platelet adhesion independently of the effects of aspirin.[7]

There is another discrepancy in the data: while a reduction in heart attack incidence has been shown in middle-aged men regularly using Bufferin, an increase in overall survival from a daily aspirin habit in that population has not been shown. One reason seems to be that while the drug reduces heart attacks, it also increases a certain type of stroke. When blood clotting is prevented, bleeding times are extended, sometimes to dangerous lengths. The risk of stroke from cerebral hemorrhage, or bleeding, then goes up.[8]

This is exactly what happens in congestive heart failure: the heart pumps too slowly to move the blood sufficiently to nourish the body.[9]

NATURAL REMEDIES

The Dietary Approach

In 1988, Dr. Dean Ornish, a San Francisco cardiologist, proved that the fatty plaque deposits blocking the coronary arteries of advanced heart patients could be made to shrink using natural therapies alone. The therapies used in his study were a strict low-cholesterol diet, meditation, and yoga. The official position of conventional medicine before that was that heart disease progressed inexorably to the patient's death, no matter what he ate, did, or believed.[10]

Half the patients in Dr. Ornish's study were counseled (but not required) to lower cholesterol and blood pressure and to quit smoking. The other half were required to quit smoking, to walk one hour three times a week, to reduce stress by daily yoga and meditation, and to eat a low-fat vegetarian diet. The only animal products allowed were nonfat milk and yogurt. Only 8 to 10 percent of their total calories came from fat—about a quarter of the usual American intake. After a year, arterial blockage was significantly reduced in ten of twelve patients in the vegetarian group. By comparison, eleven of seventeen patients in the control group got worse. Cholesterol levels also dropped markedly in the vegetarian group, while decreasing only modestly in the other group.[11]

In another study, sponsored by the National Heart, Lung and Blood Institute, the formation of *new* lesions was prevented simply by cutting fat to about 27 percent of total calories (compared to 36 to 37 percent in the normal diet).[12]

While dietary cholesterol in excess or of the wrong type can be dangerous, insufficient fat can also be dangerous. Cholesterol is produced by the body itself and is necessary to repair injuries and protect against irritation to the arterial wall. It is also the substance of which hormones are made. Without enough healthy fats to make cholesterol, your body will be hormone-deficient.

Research has shown that the dangerous form of dietary cholesterol is the form that has been oxidized by high temperatures and exposure to air.[13] Antioxidants can help protect against this damage. Antioxidants can be obtained from foods, but you need to eat the whole food, not the processed version. Eat whole-grain bread, whole oatmeal, whole buckwheat, and the like, along with raw or lightly cooked vegetables and fruits.

Antioxidants

A number of antioxidants have been found to help lower the risk of heart disease. One is vitamin E. In two studies reported in 1992 involving more than 130,000 people, women who took at least 100 IU per day of vitamin E for two or more years reduced their risk of heart disease by 26 percent, and men on the same regimen reduced their risk by 46 percent. Interestingly, people who took megadoses of vitamin E had no greater reduction in risk than those who took 100 IU daily.[14] Vitamin E evidently reduces the oxidation of cholesterol, preventing damage to the heart and arteries.

Matthias Rath, M.D., a German researcher, attributes heart disease to a deficiency of vitamin C, also an antioxidant. The simple cure, he says, is to take more of this vitamin. Though the studies go both ways, most studies have found that high-dose vitamin C (more than 2,000 mg per day) is protective against carotid artery disease.[15]

Another strong antioxidant now available in pill form from various manufacturers is alpha lipoic acid (ALA). ALA prevents cell damage, slows aging, regulates blood sugar, and removes toxic metals from the blood. It has the advantage that it is both water and fat soluble, so it can permeate all the body's cells. A dose of 100–200 mg daily is good. ALA is also found in foods, including spinach, kidney, heart, skeletal muscle (beef), and broccoli.[16]

Among other potent antioxidants are oligomeric proanthocyanins (OPCs). Red wine, which is thought to be responsible for the "French paradox" (low blood cholesterol despite a high-cholesterol diet), contains OPCs. Other sources of OPCs are grapeseed extract and Pycnogenol. Quercetin, a flavonoid antioxidant found not only in red wine but also in black tea and onions, has been shown to reduce heart attack deaths.

The herb hawthorn berry (*Crataegus oxyacantha*) also contains OPCs. Hawthorn berry has been shown in clinical studies to have cardiovascular benefits in the treatment of coronary artery disease, high blood pressure, mild congestive heart failure, angina, and abnormal heart rhythms (arrhythmias).[17]

A placebo-controlled, randomized, double-blind study demonstrated that in patients with cardiac insufficiency (a backflow of blood from the heart), hawthorn berry significantly improves heart rate and endurance and reduces symptoms without side effects.

Other researchers who found significant improvement in heart function from this herb suggested it was appropriate for use instead of digitalis for patients who did not yet need that powerful but toxic drug.[18] Jarrow's hawthorn berry is particularly good. Take one 500-mg capsule one to three times daily.

Coenzyme Q_{10} (CoQ_{10}) is another antioxidant with documented effectiveness in strengthening the heart in patients with congestive heart failure.[19] There are many brands, but NOW Foods makes an inexpensive high-quality product. Take 1 mg per pound of body weight daily.

Other Nutritional Remedies

Beside vitamin E, other natural substances shown to help blood flow without the side effects of aspirin include vitamin B_6 (more than 40 mg a day), purple grape juice (10 ounces a day), gamma-linolenic acid (GLA), ground ginger, and the oils of onion and garlic. Garlic has natural blood-thinning, cholesterol-reducing, and blood pressure–lowering properties. Ginger, like aspirin, reduces pain and is highly anti-inflammatory.

GLA is found in evening primrose oil. GLA is converted in the body to a prostaglandin (a fatty acid that behaves like a hormone) called PGE1. PGE1 prevents the clumping together of blood platelets, a cause heart attacks and strokes; opens up blood vessels and improves circulation; helps the kidneys remove fluid from the body; and slows down cholesterol production. PGE1 also controls arthritis, improves nerve function, gives a sense of well-being, regulates calcium metabolism, aids the immune system, and seems to inhibit cancer development. Recommended dosage is two 1,300-mg capsules of evening primrose oil nightly.

Scientists at London's National Heart and Lung Institute have concluded that natural progesterone has a direct impact on reducing platelet clumping.[20] In 1997, researchers at Oregon Regional Primate Research Center showed that natural—but not synthetic—progesterone may help prevent heart attacks.[21]

Fish or fish oil capsules can also protect the heart. Taking their cue from the heart-hardy Inuit, British researchers found a 29 percent lower death rate from heart attacks in men who ate omega-3 fatty acids (especially EPA, or eicosapentaenoic acid) in the form of fatty fish or fish oil capsules. Omega-3s thin the blood, reducing the risk of blood clots. Omega-3s also reduce blood triglycerides, and they may lower blood pressure and reduce cardiac arrhythmias. Jarrow makes a good fish oil product called DHA Max. Take two capsules three or four times daily.

The mineral magnesium, when given intravenously to patients with suspected heart attacks, has reduced cardiovascular mortality by a remarkable 25 percent.[22]

Arginine, an amino acid, has been shown to decrease blood platelet stickiness in people with very high cholesterol levels. Platelet stickiness is associated with heart failure and stroke. Arginine at a dosage of 8.4 grams a day taken for two weeks decreased blood platelet stickiness for sixteen weeks, and it was well tolerated and without side effects.[23]

Tufts University researchers reported in 1997 that foods rich in B vitamins, particularly folic acid, are essential to a healthy heart. The reason, however, involved a culprit other than cholesterol: homocysteine. This essential amino acid was linked to an increased risk of heart attack and stroke when it accumulated in the blood, perhaps because it damaged the lining of the blood vessels. Folic acid helps keep blood homocysteine levels from going too high. Leafy greens like spinach, fruits, and beans are good food sources of folic acid.[24]

ANGINA SYMPTOMS RELIEVED

Mrs. Hicks had severe angina (chest pain), accompanying heart disease so advanced that her doctor did not expect her to survive. She was extremely weak and barely able to walk. But her husband, Irl, an old-time Idaho farmer, was a firm believer in alternative medicine. He owned a book on homeopathy and had read it through many times. When he sought help in choosing a homeopathic remedy, Dr. Walker recommended a homeopathic *Cactus* combination. In a matter of weeks, his wife was out of bed, walking around, and full of life. Her doctor couldn't believe it. At last report, six years later, she remained alive and well.

Homeopathic Remedies

Homeopathic remedies can also help. Irregular Pulse and Heart Drops by Professional Complementary Health are effective products available from practitioners or at homeopathic drugstores. Consult a licensed homeopath for recommendations and usage.

Herbal Remedies

Artery walls can be injured not only by oxidized fats but also by toxic chemicals, pesticides, and heavy metals. Chelation to eliminate heavy metals from the arteries has effected some remarkable recoveries from heart disease. (See Chapter 5.) The herb mistletoe, which has demonstrated heart benefits, is thought to work like oral chelation in removing plaque from the arteries. Viscum by Marco Pharma is a good brand. Use according to label directions.

Besides congested or toxic arteries, there can be an emotional element to a heart attack. The stereotypical victim grips the chest after suffering some great shock or fright. Natural remedies can help alleviate this emotional factor. Bach flowers are vibrational remedies that are particularly good for treating emotional conditions. Rescue Remedy is excellent. For an appropriate Bach flower remedy for your particular condition, consult an experienced practitioner.

Herbal tinctures that are good for circulatory disorders include Aesculus, Polygonum, and Solidago by Nestmann. Other helpful herbs are butcher's broom, cayenne, and capsicum. Follow label directions.

Chinese herbalists also use acupuncture, which is particularly helpful in circulatory disorders like Raynaud's syndrome.[25]

For other natural remedies, see "High Blood Pressure (Hypertension)" on page 142 and "Cholesterol, High" on page 83.

HEART PALPITATIONS

See IRREGULAR HEARTBEAT.

HEARTBEAT IRREGULARITIES

See IRREGULAR HEARTBEAT.

HEARTBURN

See DIGESTIVE PROBLEMS.

HEMORRHOIDS

Hemorrhoids are swollen blood vessels, or varicose veins, that form in the lower rectum or anus. Most adults get hemorrhoids at some time in their lives. They usually aren't painful, but they can bleed, itch, or protrude. They are aggravated by pregnancy, childbirth, and straining at stool. The typical American diet of refined foods, which lacks the fiber and bulk necessary for forming soft stools, contributes to both hemorrhoids and varicose veins by causing constipation.[1]

CONVENTIONAL TREATMENT

Preparation H has the $100-million-plus hemorrhoid market cornered, but both the FDA and *The Medical Letter* question its advertising claims. These authorities assert that there is no acceptable evidence that Preparation H can shrink hemorrhoids, reduce inflammation, or heal injured tissue.[2] Unfortunately, no other drugs seem to accomplish these feats any better. Not only do topical drugs not cure the condition, but also ointments and suppositories can make it worse by sensitizing the skin.

The vasoconstrictors touted as shrinking hemorrhoids do constrict blood vessels, but the effect is only temporary. After a few days, the drugs may produce a rebound effect, causing the blood vessels to become more dilated than before. Since these stimulant drugs are rapidly absorbed from the lining of the rectum, they can also cause significant side effects, including heart palpitations, sleeplessness, and paranoia.

Benzocaine, a local anesthetic found in products like Americaine and Lanacane, can deaden feeling in the sensitive area. But again the relief is only temporary, and the drugs don't promote healing. In fact, benzocaine, which tends to be irritating, can prolong the healing process. It can also cause sensitization, rendering you allergic not only to benzocaine but also to related anesthetics, including the novocaine used by dentists.[3]

Hemorrhoidal preparations often include agents for wound healing, but these too lack evidence of effectiveness; so do the hydrocortisone products widely marketed for rectal itch. The latter have a further drawback: if used long term, they can cause skin disorders.[4]

The best pharmaceutical product is zinc oxide. It doesn't treat the underlying problem, but it can ease anorectal pain and itch without significant side effects, and it can serve as a protective coating over the skin to prevent further irritation.

NATURAL REMEDIES CAUSE HEMORRHOIDS TO DISAPPEAR

A woman sought help for a severe case of bleeding hemorrhoids. She had had them off and on for several years and they were quite uncomfortable. Asked about her dietary habits, she said she craved hot spicy food and coffee, of which she drank substantial quantities. Dr. Walker advised reducing the coffee and spicy food and taking the Chinese patent formula Fargelin, along with homeopathic *Nux vomica* 30C to correct the imbalance in her system indicated by the craving for spicy food and coffee. The dosage was three pills three times a day for both. The next week, the woman called to say she couldn't believe how much better she was. The bleeding had stopped and the pain was gone. A few weeks later, she reported that the hemorrhoids had cleared up completely.

Fortunately, uncomplicated external hemorrhoids usually go away by themselves in a couple of weeks without treatment. *If the problem persists—and particularly if you are bleeding from the rectum—see a doctor. Blood that is dark rather than bright red may be a symptom of a serious medical condition.*[5]

NATURAL REMEDIES

Chinese doctors explain hemorrhoids as occurring when the *qi*, or life force that holds the abdominal organs in place, is weak so that everything falls, creating hemorrhoids. Fargelin for Piles, a Chinese patent remedy for hemorrhoids, increases the life force and pulls hemorrhoids back up. The dosage is three pills three times a day. Users often report that their pain and swelling are relieved in a day and hemorrhoids and symptoms are gone in three days.

Homeopathy can also help. Possible options include *Aloe, Aesculus, Lycopodium,* and *Nux vomica,* but consulting a homeopath is best for individualized constitutional treatment.

Additional suggestions for easing hemorrhoidal discomfort include wearing porous underwear that won't trap moisture, taking sitz baths, using moist heat, getting enough rest, and keeping the anal area clean (though not with a harsh soap or antiseptic, which can be irritating). It is most important to correct the underlying problem, which is usually constipation. See "Constipation" on page 91.

HERPES, GENITAL

The herpes simplex virus belongs to the group of large DNA viruses that includes varicella-zoster virus, Epstein-Barr virus, and cytomegalovirus. Herpes lesions are painful recurring blisters that break and form crusty sores, shedding millions of viruses that are extremely contagious. Genital herpes is caused by the herpes simplex virus-2 (HSV-2). However, it is also increasingly being traced to the virus that causes cold sores, HSV-1. HSV-2, in turn, can be responsible for cold sores.

To prevent spreading genital herpes, infected people need to be able to recognize a recurrence when it hits, and to studiously avoid sexual contact while the lesions are present. The viruses may emerge before the blisters do, but there is often a feeling of tingling, itching, or general ill health that warns of an impending outbreak.

Genital herpes can kill infants who contract it from their mothers at birth. Because of this risk, delivery by cesarean is recommended for pregnant women with active genital lesions.[1]

CONVENTIONAL TREATMENT

There is no effective conventional cure for genital herpes, but symptoms can be reduced by an expensive drug called acyclovir (Zovirax), at least on the first attack. For patients with frequent recurrences, acyclovir is sometimes given orally three to five times a day and topically up to every three hours. This regimen can reduce the frequency of recurrences by as much as 75 percent, but it doesn't prevent them, and its long-term safety and effectiveness are unknown. *Caution in the use of acyclovir is advised particularly for women who are pregnant or who might become pregnant.*

Anesthetics aren't recommended for herpes, even though the lesions can be very painful. The lesions need to be kept clean and dry, and anesthetics can counteract the desired drying effect.[2]

NATURAL REMEDIES

Homeopathic Treatment

The most popular natural treatment for herpes is the amino acid L-lysine (500–1,500 mg two or three times a day). This treatment works and is safer than Zovirax, but it still addresses only the symptoms.

Homeopathic series therapy called Herpes Simplex (by Staufen or Deseret) actually clears the disease in patients with frequent, recurring herpes outbreaks. Series therapy involves a series of ampules of different potencies to be taken in a particular order. For use, see a qualified practitioner.

If that remedy doesn't work, the problem is likely to be due to a staph/strep infection inside the herpes lesions. The bacteria are taking over after a breakout. For these cases, a remedy called Staph/Strep by Deseret or CM418 by CompliMed needs to be taken in combination with the Herpes Simplex series therapy. Treatment with these homeopathic remedies is generally followed by a particularly bad outbreak, but this is actually a good sign. The virus, which sits on the nerve endings, is being cleared from the body. This healing crisis is liable to occur any time from a week after treatment is started to a week or two after it is completed. The longer the disease has been suppressed with drugs, the worse the outbreak is likely to be; after that, however, outbreaks generally cease or are limited to a few manageable incidents when under unusual stress.

People with occasional minor outbreaks report that Cliniskin-H by CompliMed is also effective, taken at onset at a dosage of ten drops every fifteen minutes for one or two hours. If the remedy is taken before the lesions actually manifest, they often won't break out at all. If taken after the outbreak, the remedy should be continued four times daily until lesions are gone.

Other remedies reported to help include Erpace by Dolisos and calendula and hypericum ointment. Boiron or Nelson are good brands. These remedies are available at health food stores; follow label directions.

HERPES CLEARED WITH HOMEOPATHIC REMEDY

Doris complained of the occurrence of severe herpes outbreaks every two weeks. She had tried everything, including L-lysine and ample doses of Zovirax, but nothing seemed to help. She was given homeopathic series therapy for herpes. Within two weeks, Doris had an unusually bad outbreak (the homeopathic clearing), but she never got another outbreak.

Judy had a similar experience. Her only outbreak after the homeopathic clearing was during an unusually stressful time. She said that this incident, which formerly would have been incapacitating, was minor and manageable.

Relaxation Techniques

Studies have confirmed anecdotal evidence linking herpes outbreaks to psychological stress. In one study, the stress of taking a medical school exam was found to activate latent herpes. Another study found that people who were anxious, depressed, or lonely had higher levels of herpes antibodies in their blood than those who were in better spirits. Since antibody levels go up during periods of reactivation, higher levels are thought to reflect a depressed immune system that is unable to keep the virus under control.[3] Meditation and positive thinking can help keep stress-induced outbreaks under control.

HIATAL HERNIA

See DIGESTIVE PROBLEMS.

HIGH BLOOD PRESSURE (HYPERTENSION)

Hypertension, or high blood pressure, is defined as systolic blood pressure above 140 mm/Hg or diastolic blood pressure above 90 mm/Hg. Between 40 and 50 million Americans, including almost 65 percent of the population over age 60, have high blood pressure. Hypertensive men outnumber hypertensive women until the age of menopause, after which women outnumber men. High blood pressure is a risk factor for coronary artery disease, stroke, renal disease, and death from all causes.[1]

Causes of high blood pressure can include constricted arteries, a heart that's pumping too hard, or tired kidneys that are retaining fluid. Hypertension can also be induced by pregnancy, most commonly in the third trimester. It may also occur in association with oral contraceptive use. Older formulations of contraceptives containing high doses of estrogen induced hypertension in 5 percent of users, but newer, lower-dose formulations cause minimal elevation in blood pressure. Hormone replacement therapy, which uses a much lower dose of estrogen than any of the oral contraceptives, does not raise blood pressure. Other drugs that can raise blood pressure include diet pills and many cold remedies.[2]

CONVENTIONAL TREATMENT

About half of all people with hypertension take medication to lower their blood pressures; once hypertension is diagnosed, the drugs usually have to be taken two or three times a day for life. Since the average age at diagnosis is 50, that means the drugs are typically taken for twenty years or more. They have such serious side effects that nearly four out of ten patients may stop taking their medications due to tolerability problems.[3] But doctors continue to recommend the drugs, even if they mean a loss of energy and sex drive, on the ground that studies have found high blood pressure to be a major risk factor for heart disease and stroke. An often-overlooked flaw in the data is that distinction has not been made between healthy subjects with low blood pressure who were that way naturally because of genes or lifestyle and those who got that way by using drugs. (See "Heart Disease" on page 133.)

A comprehensive study reported in the *British Medical Journal* in 1998 involving 30,000 Swedish men, who were followed for twenty years, found that those whose blood pressures were lowered to an average of 145/89 with drugs were 60 percent more likely to have died by the end of the study than men whose blood pressures were in that range naturally.[4] A careful review of studies in which hypertension has been lowered with drugs indicates that no overall increase in survival has resulted, except in that limited group of high-risk patients who have already suffered a heart attack or stroke, or who have unusually high blood pressure levels.[5]

For women, the outlook could be even worse. There is data indicating that *for white women with mild hypertension, treatment may actually be detrimental, causing mortality rates to increase rather than to decrease.*[6] Since women have a lower incidence of cardiovascular disease than men until later in life, they have been excluded from most of the largest studies of mild to moderate hypertension. Reanalysis of the data has raised questions about whether drug treatment confers significant benefits for women, particularly in younger age groups.

The Hypertension Detection and Follow-Up Program (HDFP) was a community-based, multicenter, randomized trial of almost 11,000 subjects. Forty-six percent were women and 44 percent were black. The HDFP resulted in the most comprehensive data collection to date on the effects of sex and race on hypertension. Overall, people receiving drug intervention had a statistically significant 17 percent reduction in all-cause mortality. Black women also had a significant decrease in all-cause mortality. But white women did not. In fact, there was a trend toward harm in treated white women with moderate to severe hypertension. The trend was considered particularly disturbing in that white women achieved the highest rate of blood pressure control of any subgroup.[7]

In several other large treatment trials enrolling women, subgroup analysis again showed that women fared significantly worse than men. The Australian Therapeutic Trial in Mild Hypertension involved 3,427 subjects (37 percent women). At four-year follow-up, men had a statistically significant 26 percent reduction in all end points; however, after control for other cardiac risk factors, women had no treatment benefit.[8] Worse, in the Medical Research Council trial, which compared three drug therapies with placebo in more than 17,000 British clinic patients (almost all white, 48 percent women), all-cause mortality rates were 15 percent lower in men receiving therapy, but 26 percent *higher* in women.[9] The study was further evidence that drug treatment of mild to moderate hypertension in white women may be dangerous, leading some experts to recommend against treatment of mild hypertension in white women.[10]

You might risk the drugs "just in case" if they made you feel better in the short term; but drugs whose side effects make you feel worse in the short term need to have some compelling and incontrovertible evidence behind them before reasonable people will take them. And all blood pressure–lowering drugs have substantial short-term side effects, which result directly from the mechanisms by which they work.

Beta-blockers are considered first-line drugs for hypertension. They cause the heart to beat more slowly by blocking nerve receptor sites called "beta receptors" that are stimulated by adrenaline and adrenaline-like chemicals to work the heart. When these receptors are blocked, the brain can't signal the heart to beat faster or the arteries to constrict. Heart function is diminished, less blood is forced through the arteries, and blood pressure is reduced. As a result, beta-blockers can cause drowsiness, dizziness, low blood pressure, nausea, weakness, diarrhea, numbness and coldness in fingers and toes, dry mouth and skin, impotence, insomnia, hallucinations, nightmares, headaches, bronchial asthma or difficult breathing, joint pains, confusion, depression, reduced alertness, and constipation.

These side effects are a direct effect of the drugs' mode of action: beta-blockers slow the heart's pump. The brain tells the heart to beat faster and pump harder for a reason. In older people, it's usually because the arteries have become corroded with deposits of calcium and fat. These narrow the arterial openings, requiring a greater pressure to push enough blood through to keep the body running at normal levels. Any artificial reduction in this pressure will at least make you feel tired. At worst, it can weaken your heartbeat enough to cause heart failure. (See "Heart Disease" section.) The depression that beta-blockers can cause is also predictable: they kill the "adrenaline rush" that makes life exciting. They can trigger bronchial asthma by suppressing epinephrine, the natural chemical that opens up the bronchi or breathing tubes. Serious problems can also result if beta-blockers are withdrawn suddenly; so once you're on them, it's hard getting off.[11]

Diuretics, another category of first-line antihypertensives, have traditionally been considered the safest and most conservative first-choice treatment. Yet in one major study, one out of three patients had to discontinue drug treatment because of intolerable side effects.[12] Diuretics can cause weakness, dizziness, sexual dysfunction, impotence, gastrointestinal distress, rash, muscle cramps, and hearing impairment. The drugs work by causing the kidneys to increase the amount of water excreted, decreasing blood volume and thus blood pressure. Diuretics can also increase blood sugar, uric acid, and serum cholesterol levels, increasing the risk of diabetes, gout, and heart disease. Diabetes frequently develops during treatment with diuretics.[13]

Lowering blood pressure by increasing fluid excretion can cause valuable minerals to be lost at the same time. Potassium is the most critical, since its loss can seriously affect the heart's electrical activity. Potassium is known to help prevent strokes, the dreaded scourge antihypertensive drugs are supposed to prevent. Drugs that deplete this mineral are therefore counterproductive, even if they do lower blood pressure. Diuretics also deplete magnesium, which is necessary to retain potassium in cells. If blood magnesium is low, cells become more permeable. Potassium leaks out, and sodium and calcium leak in. The cells become electrically unstable, producing irregular rhythms. In the worst case, this can mean sudden death.[14]

In an Australian study, mortality among hypertensives treated with thiazide diuretics was found to be twice as high as in the other treatment groups, which included the beta-blocker propanolol, simple salt restriction, or a placebo. In other words, *twice as many deaths occurred among hypertensives taking diuretics as among those receiving no treatment at all.*[15]

Problems with the old "first-line" drugs prompted the development of new types of antihypertensives. Alpha-blockers block nerve receptors in the autonomic nervous system and can cause a drop in blood pressure if you suddenly stand up. Angiotensin-converting enzyme inhibitors (ACE inhibitors) cause blood vessels to dilate by blocking the formation of a natural chemical called angiotensin II. Their most common side effect is a dry cough. Calcium channel blockers or calcium antagonists work by interfering with the normal flow of calcium to the muscles and nerves, relaxing the arteries and reducing their resistance to blood flow. Although they are generally well tolerated, they can cause dizziness or lightheadedness.

By 1995, more prescriptions were written for calcium channel blockers, the current favorites, than for any other type of drug, including antibiotics. But recent studies involving calcium channel blockers (including Procardia and Adalat) have found that the drugs *increase* the risk of heart attack and sudden death by a factor of four and the risk of death from any cause by 35 percent. This risk was found to be particularly serious for African-Americans.[16] Studies of this sort prompted the National Heart, Lung, and Blood Institute to issue a statement saying that beta-blockers and diuretics (the problematic drugs prompting the search for alternatives) should continue to be the first line of treatment. Calcium channel blockers should not be used unless the other two types proved ineffective.[17]

Studies have established benefit from treatment of hypertension in elderly patients of both sexes, but nondrug therapy is still recommended first.[18]

Side effects and risks aside, lowering blood pressure with drugs simply does not work very well. In one report, as few as 21 percent of treated hypertensives actually achieved blood pressures of 140/90 or lower by this means.[19] Natural remedies are not patentable and, therefore, cannot generate the type of profits necessary to fund FDA studies. But anecdotal evidence indicates that a range of natural remedies can lower blood pressure without side effects and at substantially reduced cost—in many cases, more effectively than drugs.[20]

Natural Remedies

Herbal Therapy

Hawthorn berry complex is a blood pressure–lowering herb that has the advantage over drugs that it will lower blood pressure to normal but not below normal. Jarrow makes a good hawthorn berry product. Take one capsule three times daily or as directed by a practitioner.

Dandelion leaf, another blood pressure–lowering herb, has been shown to have diuretic properties equivalent to those of Lasix (furosemide), a popular diuretic drug. A downside of pharmaceutical diuretics is that potassium is lost along with water through the kidneys. Dandelion is an excellent natural source of potassium, making it a safe, balanced natural alternative.[21] Dandelion comes in standardized capsule form. Take one 400-mg capsule three times daily with food or as professionally prescribed. Pregnant women should not use this herb without the supervision of a qualified practitioner.

Caution: Certain herbs including goldenseal, ginseng, and licorice raise blood pressure and should, therefore, not be taken by people with high blood pressure.

BLOOD PRESSURE LOWERED WITH HERBS

A woman whose blood pressure hovered around 190/95 reported that after she started taking Jarrow's hawthorn berry extract (one capsule three times daily), her blood pressure dropped to a healthy 122/82 without drugs. It was checked weekly and remained consistently in that range, except once when it shot back up. Questioned about what she had been doing, she said she was taking goldenseal root for a cold. She was switched to another anti-cold herb (elderberry). Her blood pressure has remained normal ever since.

Homeopathic Remedies

Homeopathic remedies can also effectively lower blood pressure. Finding the right constitutional remedy will balance out the body's energy patterns and keep the blood pressure normal. Consult a homeopath for a suitable remedy for your individual needs.

Nutritional Supplements

Nutritional supplements can also help lower blood pressure. One option is coenzyme Q_{10}. Take 1 mg per pound of body weight. Other natural blood pressure regulators available in health food stores include garlic (Super Garlic 3X by Metagenics is good) and cayenne. Use according to label directions. A form of cayenne that is gentler on the stomach than other brands is Capsi-Cool by Nature's Way.

Another important supplement is magnesium, called "Nature's calcium channel blocker." Hypertension is accompanied by low levels of this mineral, which have actually been found to be a better predictor of hypertensive disease than either sodium or calcium levels.[22] Magnesium is best taken in equal proportions with calcium (for example, 400 mg of each). A good way to determine appropriate amounts for your body is by taking note of your bowel movements. Calcium makes stools firmer; magnesium makes them loose. Increase or decrease your intake of each to suit your body's needs.

Relaxation Techniques

If your hypertension is the kind linked to tension, relaxation techniques may be your answer to beta-blockers. The sympathetic nervous system increases blood pressure as part of the fight-or-flight response to stress. Beta-blockers reduce blood pressure by blocking the activities of this regulatory system; however, the same effect can be achieved without drugs,

---

BLOOD PRESSURE LOWERED WITH HOMEOPATHIC REMEDY

Maggie, age 68, had had very high blood pressure, averaging about 180/100 or 180/110. No prescription medicine had helped. Two doses of homeopathic *Sulphur* at a strength of 200 stabilized her blood pressure for three months. When it crept back up, Maggie took a single dose at a strength of 1M. When it went back up a month later, she took another single 1M dose. In the three years since that time, her blood pressure has remained normal without medication or remedies of any sort. *Note: While that protocol worked for Maggie, treatment is very individual. You should see a licensed homeopath for guidance in your own case.*

TRACKING THE CAUSE OF HIGH BLOOD PRESSURE

Improper diet is a recognized factor in hypertension. Foods like fried fats, refined sugar, and processed salt heated to high temperatures can contribute to clogging of the arteries. Clogged arteries have narrower openings, requiring greater pressure to move blood through them. Deficiencies of calcium, magnesium, and potassium—nutrients found in fresh whole foods—have also been linked to high blood pressure.

In April of 1997, *The New England Journal of Medicine* reported the results of a landmark multicenter study sponsored by the National Institutes of Health, finding that blood pressure can be lowered as much by diet as by drugs without side effects or risks. The antihypertensive diet used was rich in fruits, vegetables, and low-fat dairy products. The study was hailed as demonstrating the most significant improvement in life expectancy of any dietary intervention to date.[23]

For eleven weeks, the volunteers, who weren't on blood pressure medication, ate standardized meals designed to stabilize their weight and salt intake. Daily servings were individualized but were along these lines: seven or eight servings of grain products; four or five of vegetables; four or five of fruits; two or three of low-fat or nonfat dairy foods; and one or two of meat, poultry, and fish. The diet also included four or five weekly servings of nuts, seeds, and legumes, and limited amounts of fat and sweets.

The effects of the diet were apparent within one week and peaked within two weeks. For people with moderate hypertension, the average reduction in blood pressure was 11.4/5.5. More moderate reductions resulted when milk products were eliminated from the diet, suggesting an important role for calcium. Researchers suggested that their simple diet, if widely followed, could reduce the risk of heart disease by 15 percent and the likelihood of stroke by 27 percent.

This American study followed a more stringent Swedish study, in which hypertensive patients who were unhappy with the side effects of their drugs switched to a salt-free vegan diet (no animal products). After one year, most of them had succeeded in abandoning their blood pressure medications entirely, while maintaining blood pressure levels that were lower than with drugs.[24]

As for the role of salt, which has long been considered a culprit in hypertension, a massive study called INTERSALT led researchers to conclude that it actually has only minor importance in the disease. In *Your Body's Many Cries for Water*, Dr. F. Batmanghelidj, M.D., maintains that the body's tendency to retain salt is an effect rather than a cause of hypertension. The underlying problem, he says, is a lack of water. When the body lacks sufficient water, it compensates by reducing the openings of its main blood vessels and closing down its peripheral blood vessels, so the scant water left can service the whole system. The body retains salt in order to reduce water losses in urine and sweat. The result is an increase in blood pressure. Treating this condition with diuretics and a no-salt diet, says Dr. Batmanghelidj, is counterproductive. The correct therapy is to drink more water—enough to equal half your body weight in ounces per day. He says you should actually *increase* your salt intake and get more exercise.[25] Unheated sea salt is preferred. Table salt, which has been heated to very high temperatures in processing, can be treated by the body as a foreign toxin. Better yet is Bio-Salt by Gilbert's Health Food Labs in England, a biochemically balanced mineral salt compound containing sodium chloride plus all the cell salts.

Other factors linked to high blood pressure include obesity; stress; lack of exercise; smoking; and alcohol, coffee, and tea intake.[26] Poisoning from heavy metals, including lead, cadmium, and mercury, is another suspect. The major source of mercury in our bodies is silver/mercury amalgam dental fillings. A study comparing fifty 22-year-olds who had mercury amalgams to fifty-one 22-year-olds who did not found that blood pressures in the former group averaged six systolic points higher than in the latter. The subjects with amalgam fillings also had a greater incidence of chest pains, tachycardia (racing heartbeat), anemia, fatigue, and loss of memory; remember, these were young adults. The difference undoubtedly gets greater over the fifty years or so that it takes to develop "essential hypertension."[27] For detoxification alternatives, see Chapter 5 and "Multiple Chemical Sensitivity" on page 185.

by simple techniques for letting go of tension.[28] Yoga, meditation, and biofeedback have all been shown to effectively lower blood pressure.[29]

What about using drugs to induce relaxation? They don't seem to be effective. The artificial relaxation resulting from sedatives and tranquilizers has not been shown to lower blood pressure, and these kinds of drugs have many side effects.[30]

The psychological factor in high blood pressure is reflected in the observation that for some people, blood pressure becomes high only while they're in the doctor's office.[31] *You should always get several readings, preferably in the security of your own home, before starting any antihypertensive drug regimen.*

HIP FRACTURES

See OSTEOPOROSIS.

HIVES

See SKIN PROBLEMS.

HOT FLASHES

See MENOPAUSE AND PERIMENOPAUSE.

HYPERTENSION

See HIGH BLOOD PRESSURE (HYPERTENSION).

HYPERTHYROIDISM

Hyperthyroidism is a condition in which the thyroid produces an excess of thyroid hormone. It is most commonly seen in those with Graves' disease, an immune system malfunction of unknown cause that is thought to have a hereditary component. Symptoms of hyperthyroidism include nervousness, irritability, sweating, and muscle weakness. Postpartum thyroiditis is an overactivity of the thyroid gland that occurs a few months after childbirth. The condition may be followed by underactivity of the thyroid (hypothyroidism) a few weeks later. Hyperthyroidism can also result from too much iodine in the diet.

CONVENTIONAL TREATMENT

Conventional treatment for Graves' disease consists of antithyroid drugs that cause hormone production to drop—methimazole (Tapazole) or propylthiouracil (PTU). The side effects of these drugs may include drowsiness and, in rare cases, a blood disease called agranulocytosis. If the drugs fail, a high-dose radioactive iodine capsule or beverage may be given that slows the thyroid by permanently damaging overactive cells. However, if too many cells are destroyed (as is often the case), the patient winds up on hormone supplements for life.[1]

For postpartum thyroiditis, some doctors prescribe drugs to relieve anxiety and nervousness. However, the condition generally goes away by itself.

HYPERTHYROIDISM CORRECTED NATURALLY

Carey, age 28, had a two-year history of thyroid problems. When her condition was first diagnosed, she was told she had *hypothyroidism* and was put on Synthroid (pharmaceutical thyroid hormone). At a later visit, however, her doctor found that she had hyperthyroidism. She vacillated from one extreme to the other for two years. Her frustrated doctor finally proposed surgically removing her thyroid and keeping her on medication permanently. Carey avoided surgery by using a homeopathic product called Thyroplus by Deseret. She took it for one month (ten drops three times daily) to balance her thyroid function. Then she took CompliMed's homeopathic Thyroid for a further two months. When her thyroid function was subsequently checked by a thyroid endocrinology specialist, he said he couldn't understand it. All Carey's lab tests were perfectly normal. The tests were still normal a month later, although the homeopathic remedies were by then no longer needed and had been discontinued.

NATURAL REMEDIES

Hyperthyroidism can be a function of the same hormonal imbalance that produces an underactive thyroid. The same homeopathic remedies effective for that condition can rebalance a hyperthyroid condition, eliminating the need for drugs. Lycopus by Marco Pharma International is particularly effective at balancing thyroid levels. Take according to label directions for two or three months to stabilize the thyroid. For other remedies, see "Hypothyroidism" on page 150.

HYPOGLYCEMIA

Hypoglycemia (low blood sugar) is the flipside of diabetes (high blood sugar). Both conditions are seen in women more often than in men. Hypoglycemia can be precipitated by a diet high in sugary foods, which cause the body to secrete large amounts of the hormone insulin. In the hypoglycemic person, the sugar is used up before the insulin is, causing the concentration of sugar in the blood to drop too low. Symptoms include fatigue, mood swings, and depression.

CONVENTIONAL TREATMENT

Conventional treatment, like alternative treatment, focuses on regulating the content and timing of the diet to make sure blood glucose and insulin levels remain constant.

NATURAL REMEDIES

Hypoglycemia is corrected by the same natural blood sugar balancers as is diabetes. Chromium picolinate (200 mcg taken with each meal) can help regulate the blood sugar level. Protein should also be eaten with every meal. Almonds are particularly good. Sugar should be avoided. Apricots have a low sugar index and can be chewed like chewing gum to bring low blood sugar up. Small, frequent meals of whole foods and the avoidance of alcohol, caffeine, and cigarettes are advised.

HYPOGLYCEMIA CORRECTED WITH NATURAL REMEDIES

Karen, a 38-year-old artist, was experiencing severe blood sugar swings. When her blood sugar was abnormally low, she would get very tired, shaky, and irritable, rendering her nearly paralyzed. Her blood sugar dropped frequently and at the most inconvenient times. Testing indicated that her pancreas was extremely toxic, due apparently to the chemicals she was exposed to as an artist. She was put on Exchem, a homeopathic detoxifier, along with Pancreas-Total Endotox M17 to regenerate her pancreas (both by Apex). To temper the healing crises from detoxing, which can temporarily increase the severity of attacks of low blood sugar, she was advised to carry dried apricots with her for snacking. The apricots helped Karen get through the detoxification, after which her blood sugar was normal.

◆ HYPOTHYROIDISM

Thyroid imbalance is thought to be fifteen to twenty times more prevalent in women than in men, and 90 percent of women with thyroid problems have hypothyroidism (an underactive thyroid). Only 10 percent have hyperthyroidism (an overactive thyroid). Researchers studying 25,862 participants at a Colorado statewide health fair in 1995 found clinical hypothyroidism in 8.9 percent of women who were not already taking drugs for the condition and, for the most part, didn't suspect the problem.[1]

Symptoms of hypothyroidism include unexplained weight gain, habitually cold hands and feet, hair loss, fatigue and weakness, anemia, headaches, menstrual problems, and an increased susceptibility to infection, heart disease, cancer, premature aging, heart palpitations, and cardiac arrhythmias. Women in menopause or perimenopause who have heart palpitations should have their thyroid levels checked before considering drugs.

Other symptoms of an underactive thyroid may include flaky and itchy skin, brittle nails that continually split and layer, hair loss, slower than normal pulse, and a "foggy" mind. Hypothyroidism causes stomach acid and other digestive juices to be in short supply and intestinal movements to become weak, producing gas and constipation. A woman with hypothyroidism can be malnourished even on a good diet, because she isn't properly

THYROID PROBLEMS CORRECTED NATURALLY

Darcy had a sluggish thyroid. She was gaining weight, sleeping poorly, and losing her hair. Lycopus by Marco Pharma International, taken as directed for three months, rapidly reversed her condition. Normal thyroid levels were then maintained on homeopathic Thyroid by CompliMed (ten drops three times weekly).

Kara had been on Synthroid ever since she was diagnosed with hypothyroidism at the age of 16. Her doctor had said she would have to take the drug for life. But after nine years of this course of treatment, she asked to be switched to Armour Thyroid, and he reluctantly agreed. She took Armour Thyroid (one grain daily) for about three months, then began taking homeopathic Thyroid by CompliMed (ten drops three times daily). Over the next three months, she slowly weaned off Armour Thyroid and onto a thyroid product called Raw Thyroid, which she took only as needed. After that, she took only the CompliMed homeopathic Thyroid. Throughout this treatment, repeated lab tests showed normal thyroid levels. Remarkably, they stabilized and have remained normal without remedies of any sort.

assimilating her food. She can also gain substantial weight even when she is honestly (as she tells her friends) eating almost nothing, because she isn't burning her calories efficiently.

Hypothyroidism directly affects hormonal balance. Hormone imbalance is a leading reason that women of childbearing age have difficulty getting pregnant or carrying a fetus to term. Seventy percent of women with infertility and miscarriages have been found to have thyroid problems. For this reason, thyroid levels are routinely tested by fertility doctors. Fibrocystic breast disease, fibroids, ovarian cysts, endometriosis, PMS, menopausal symptoms, and multiple sclerosis can also be worsened by thyroid imbalance. The condition can also lead to elevated cholesterol and triglyceride levels, increasing the risk of heart disease, and can weaken the immune system, increasing the risk of infections.

One cause of hypothyroidism is estrogen dominance (an excess of estrogen in relation to progesterone), which interferes with the uptake of thyroid hormones. Estrogen dominance can result from taking birth control pills, estrogen replacement therapy, or exposure to pesticides and other environmental toxins that are powerful estrogen mimics. An imbalance of microbes in the gut can also interfere with thyroid hormone uptake, as can stress and deficiencies of nutrients such as selenium, glutathione, iodine, and zinc.

Other thyroid inhibitors include excess intake of unsaturated fats, fluoride, heavy metal poisoning, mercury amalgam fillings, low-protein diets, soy products, raw cruciferous vegetables (such as cabbage, cauliflower, and broccoli), and endurance exercise.[2] Another suspected cause of hypothyroidism is radiation, both the ionizing radiation emitted by nuclear reactors and non-ionizing radiation from the electromagnetic fields of common electrical appliances.

CONVENTIONAL TREATMENT

The usual medication for an underactive thyroid is synthetic thyroxine (levothyroxine or Synthroid). Ranked among the top ten prescription drugs in America, this drug is taken by millions of women every day; however, it never received formal FDA approval. On June 1, 2001, *The Wall Street Journal* reported that the FDA may remove Synthroid from the market, after finding that patients taking it experienced unintended variations in their

SIMPLE AT-HOME THYROID TEST

Thyroid tests in the doctor's office aren't always accurate. A simple home test is to check the body temperature on awakening. Broda O. Barnes, M.D., recommends the following procedure. Menstruating women should do this test only on the second and third days of their menstrual flow.

1. Shake down a glass oral thermometer and leave it on your night table before going to bed.

2. Upon awakening, with as little movement as possible, place the thermometer firmly in your armpit or under your tongue.

3. Keep the thermometer there for ten minutes.

4. Record the readings on three consecutive days.

A thyroid that is functioning normally should have a reading of 97.8 or higher. A reading below 97.8 may indicate low thyroid function. If low readings are found, homeopathic thyroid remedies may be tried whether or not thyroid imbalance is the problem, since they are harmless, inexpensive, and serve to correct imbalances of any sort.

doses that were "not conducive to proper control of hypothyroidism." Synthroid has other downsides as well. It is a synthetic thyroid replacement to which the body becomes accustomed, causing the thyroid gland to atrophy so you can't go without it. There is evidence that it not only shrinks the thyroid gland but also suppresses the pituitary, suppresses cellular respiration, and can cause osteoporosis. Other side effects can include heart palpitations, insomnia, nervousness, and diarrhea.[3]

For people who want to break the Synthroid habit, a more natural and less habit-forming option called Armour Thyroid, taken along with homeopathic remedies, can help wean the body from reliance on the drug. Synthroid contains only the thyroid hormone T3. Armour Thyroid also contains T4, which stimulates the thyroid to produce its own hormone. Armour Thyroid is a desiccated thyroid preparation extracted from pigs that is standardized to government specifications to allow proper monitoring. *Note: If thyroid supplementation is necessary, it should be prescribed by a competent professional. Excess thyroid hormone can be harmful. It stimulates the osteoclasts, the cells that tear down or resorb bone. An excess of bone resorption over formation results in bone loss.*[4]

NATURAL REMEDIES

Even more supportive of the body's own mechanisms than Armour Thyroid are homeopathic remedies, which work to correct the problem at its source. Hormone levels go out of balance for a reason: stress, pregnancy, menopause, radiation exposure, and so on. Homeopathy works to regulate the thyroid gland so the body can function normally without drugs. Lycopus by Marco Pharma International, taken according to label directions for two or three months, is particularly effective at balancing thyroid levels. Thyroid by CompliMed is another effective option. Take ten drops three times daily.

Other alternatives include acupuncture, which can help stimulate thyroid function; natural progesterone, which balances the thyroid-inhibiting effect of estrogen dominance; and supplementation with thyroid glandular extracts, enzyme therapy, and herbal remedies such as the Ayurvedic herb guggulipid.[5] Good guggulipid products are Jarrow's Opti-Gugul and Doctor's Best Brand Guggul. Follow directions on the label.

Supplementing with trace minerals may also help. Thyroid function is dependent on a balance of two trace minerals, manganese and iodine. Hypothyroidism could be due to a shortage of either. Manganese by Nestmann can help increase manganese levels. Take fifteen drops three times daily. Dulse and kelp are good food sources of iodine that can help stimulate the thyroid. People who ingest large quantities of soy products particularly need extra iodine, since soy taken daily in quantity can suppress the thyroid. The Asian diet, which is high in soy, is also high in kelp and seaweed. A good liquid kelp product is Kelp by World Organics. Take four drops daily in half a glass of water.

Other recommendations to support thyroid function include getting adequate protein (organic beef, poultry, eggs, fish, and cultured milk products such as kefir and yogurt) and eating foods high in B vitamins (wheat germ, whole grains, nuts, seeds, dark greens, legumes, and Brewer's yeast). Also good are wheat germ oil or natural vitamin E, and organic nonhydrogenated coconut oil.

HYSTERECTOMY

Hysterectomy, or surgical removal of the uterus, has seen a dramatic increase in the United States, where the hysterectomy rate is six times that in Europe. Twenty-five percent of American women now reach menopause prematurely and abruptly by way of hysterectomy.[1] Not only the uterus but also the ovaries are often removed, since the ovaries produce estrogen, which stimulates uterine cancers to grow.

A statistical survey of American hysterectomies performed between 1965 and 1984 published by the U.S. Department of Health and Human Services found that only 10.5 percent of these operations were medically indicated and necessary due to cancer. The others were elective surgeries performed for a variety of reasons, including sterilization and uterine prolapse. The reason for the surge in hysterectomies is a matter of speculation, but Vicki Hufnagel, M.D., who helped conduct the survey, suggests it's economic. The operation is the bread and butter surgery of OB-GYNs, who are backing away from obstetrics because of increasing medical malpractice liability. They're leaning toward the safer, easier hysterectomy.[2]

Fibroid tumors are the most frequent reason given for hysterectomy. More than 40 percent of women over age 50 have these normally benign growths, and one survey found that more than a quarter of a million uteri were removed annually to excise them. Although fibroid tumors are rarely malignant, they can cause excessive menstrual bleeding and pelvic pain that precipitates surgical removal. Endometriosis and uterine prolapse are other leading reasons for hysterectomies, which aren't reserved for older women but are often carried out on women in their twenties and thirties who have no children.[3]

DOWNSIDES OF HYSTERECTOMY

For the nearly three quarters of a million American women who now reach menopause prematurely because of surgery, the abruptness of the change wreaks havoc on hormone balance. It can bring on severe hot flashes within twenty-four hours of the operation. To counter them, most women resort to lifelong estrogen replacement. For downsides of estrogen replacement, see Chapter 2. Hysterectomy can also result in the prolapse of other organs, including the intestines, bowels, bladder, and vagina, causing pelvic pain, sexual problems, or pressure on the bowels and bladder. Other long-term complications can develop as well, including osteoporosis, bone and joint pain and immobility, chronic fatigue, urinary problems, emotional problems, depression, and increased risk of heart disease.

The Nurses' Health Study found that women who have both ovaries removed and are not on hormone replacement therapy have twice the risk of a nonfatal heart attack as other women.[4] A quarter of all women undergoing hysterectomies before age 40 have both ovaries removed. And even when they aren't removed, in more than a third of cases, the ovaries simply die following hysterectomy, and menopause follows.[5]

A less obvious problem involves sexual response. In normal women, the ovaries continue to secrete some hormones for many years after menopause.[6] One is testosterone, which encourages libido. In recent studies in the United Kingdom, 33 to 46 percent of women reported decreased sexual response after hysterectomy or oophorectomy (removal of the uterus and ovaries).[7] For some women, the cervix and uterus, which are eliminated with hysterectomy, are also major triggers for orgasm.[8]

SURGICAL ALTERNATIVES TO HYSTERECTOMY

Medical wisdom says that fibroids cannot be dissolved. Small ones may disappear by themselves after menopause, but the conventional treatment for eliminating large or painful fibroids remains surgical removal. Dr. Hufnagel maintains, however, that up to 90 percent of all hysterectomies currently performed might be avoided if other options were explored. Even fibroid tumors that are growing rapidly do not, in her view, necessarily create a need to remove the uterus. Nonmalignant fibroids can be surgically removed without removing the organ.

Dr. Hufnagel favors a modified surgery that can eliminate fibroids and correct uterine prolapse while preserving the uterus and ovaries. Called "female reconstructive surgery," the procedure involves a surgical resectioning of the organ. The abdomen is opened with a bikini-type incision and the uterus is lifted out for complete inspection. The tissue connected to the uterus is clamped off with a special clamp and a drug is injected to stop the flow of blood, which allows maximum surgical time. Fibroid tumors are then removed, or, in the case of prolapse, the ligaments and organs are restructured and resuspended.[9]

SHRINKING TUMORS BY BALANCING HORMONE LEVELS

Hormone researcher John Lee, M.D., maintains that surgery usually isn't needed at all. Uterine fibroids, along with breast fibrocysts and painful breast swelling, can be prevented as well as treated by correcting hormone imbalances. These conditions are common in the estrogen-dominant phase of perimenopause. Supplementing with natural progesterone before menopause can prevent them from developing, and supplementing with it after menopause is an effective way to protect against bone loss while avoiding the risk of fibroid development.[10] Estrogen supplementation, on the other hand, can actually lead to hysterectomies, since estrogen stimulates fibroid tumor growth. If estrogen levels are allowed to drop off naturally after menopause, existing uterine tumors will typically atrophy away by themselves; however, when the hormone is artificially supplied, uterine tumors are stimulated to grow.[11]

The heavy and irregular menstrual bleeding that can signal a uterine tumor can also be a symptom of hormone imbalance from an underactive thyroid gland. Before you resort either to hysterectomy or to hormone replacement therapy, it's a good idea to have your thyroid function tested.[12] (See "Hypothyroidism" on page 150.)

NATURAL REMEDIES

Herbal products are also available that can help shrink fibroid tumors and cysts. Chinese herbal formulas include *Laminaria 4* (for fatty type swellings), *Zedoaria Tablets* (for hard masses), and *Chih-ko* and *Curcuma* (for phlegm or blood stagnation, considered in Chinese medicine to be the cause of many fibroids). All are made by Seven Forests. Consult a licensed acupuncturist or herbalist for recommendations and dosages.

FIBROIDS AND CYSTS SHRINK WITH NATURAL PROGESTERONE

Among cases cited by Dr. John Lee was one of a woman troubled with ovarian cysts and a fibroid tumor. After three months of treatment with natural progesterone, the cysts disappeared, and the fibroid was substantially smaller. Despite these dramatic effects, the patient's gynecologist refused to believe that natural progesterone had done it, since he was not convinced that progesterone could be absorbed effectively from a cream through the skin. Dr. Lee therefore recommended a test to determine the patient's blood progesterone levels. Normal levels for a menstruating woman are in the ten to twenty range. This woman was well past menopause and her ovaries had stopped producing hormones, so her progesterone level should have been near zero. In fact, it was forty—twice that of a healthy young woman.[13]

A European herbal formula that was particularly promising before it was pulled off the market by the FDA was the over-the-counter product Petasan, made by Dr. A. Vogel's Swiss herbal company Bioforce. Petasan is composed of a combination of the herbs mistletoe and butter bur. In 1991, at the recommendation of European homeopath Jan de Vries, author Dr. Walker gave it to six women with fibroid tumors. Within a week, all six reported that bleeding and other painful symptoms had subsided. Two of the women's fibroids had shrunk from the size of a grapefruit to that of a walnut and all of the women were doing well. Then, the FDA banned the product's further sale on the ground that Petasan was not one of its accepted herbal remedies. Although the formula is no longer available in the United States or Canada, its individual ingredients (mistletoe and butter bur) can be purchased in Canada and other countries. If you're interested in trying this approach, consult an experienced practitioner for recommendations.

Homeopathic remedies can also help shrink tumors. One possibility is *Calc carb 200*. A homeopath can determine the appropriate constitutional treatment for your body and personality type.

Caution: Although the natural remedies discussed here are safe, you should not attempt self-treatment. Fewer than two in every thousand fibroid tumors are found to be malignant, but cancer still remains a possibility.[14] If you have symptoms suggesting fibroids—including abdominal swelling, pelvic or back pain, heavy or irregular bleeding, painful periods, constipation, pressure on the bladder, or frequent urination—see a gynecologist. If you are interested in exploring natural remedies, see an Eastern medical, homeopathic, or naturopathic physician.

NATURAL REMEDIES FOR POST-HYSTERECTOMY HOT FLASHES

Hot flashes and heavy sweating are more severe and more sudden in onset when hormone output has been reduced abruptly and prematurely by hysterectomy/oophorectomy than when menopause occurs naturally. For some women, hot flashes and night sweats increase significantly after hysterectomy even when the ovaries are preserved.[15] These hot flashes need immediate treatment, but prescription estrogen isn't the only choice. Natural estrogen creams made from plants are also available. One effective product is OstaDerm by Bezwecken. Use ½ teaspoon daily.

Even if you are already taking estrogen after a hysterectomy, you don't need to stay on it forever. Health writer John McDougall, M.D., states that after about age 45, when estrogen production would have fallen off anyway, you can gradually wean yourself from it.[16] The problem is that it's hard to get off estrogen once you start. Supplementing with es-

THE AUTHORS' OWN EXPERIENCES

Both authors of this book have avoided hysterectomies by using natural therapies.

Dr. Walker was only 33 years old when she was told that a large fibroid tumor was growing in her uterus and that she needed a hysterectomy. Determined to explore the alternatives before agreeing to this surgery, she went to an acupuncturist who gave her a selection of Chinese herbs and homeopathic remedies appropriate to her own case, along with regular acupuncture treatments. When these resolved Dr. Walker's problem without surgery, she was so impressed that she broadened her field of expertise from pharmacy to Chinese medicine and homeopathy. Since then, she has frequently seen Eastern and Western herbal remedies help shrink the tumors of her patients.

Ellen Brown was told she needed a hysterectomy by seven different gynecologists, first for a prolapsed uterus, then for a large fibroid tumor, and then for cysts on the ovaries. She avoided the surgery by using natural progesterone cream (ProGest) and receiving several courses of live cell therapy, a treatment that is not currently available in the United States but is available in Mexico and in Germany, where it has been researched for nearly a century.[17] See "Uterine Prolapse" on page 236.

trogen raises the set point below which you will experience hot flashes. When you are withdrawing from estrogen, hot flashes can be worse than before you started taking it. It's important to wean yourself from it gradually. Taking natural progesterone along with it can help you decrease the dose without uncomfortable symptoms.

Women who have had a hysterectomy typically aren't given progestins along with estrogen because they don't have to worry about uterine cancer. However, *natural* progesterone can still be useful to these women, not only to help them decrease the need for estrogen but also to preserve their bones. Estrogen can slow bone loss, but natural progesterone actually increases bone density. Unlike synthetic progestins, it may also reduce breast cancer risk. Progesterone combined with estrogen blocks estrogen receptors in the breasts and ovaries and seems to prevent the development of cancer at sites outside of the uterus.[18]

Eastern herbs and other plant-based natural products are other effective alternatives for quelling post-hysterectomy hot flashes. Traditional Chinese herbal formulas come in balanced combinations that avoid the side effects and risks of HRT. For recommendations, see a practitioner trained in the use of these herbs.

POST-HYSTERECTOMY HOT FLASHES RELIEVED WITH HERBAL REMEDY

Sarah came to Dr. Walker five months after she had had a hysterectomy/oophorectomy at the age of 36. Because a Pap smear had indicated cervical cancer, her doctor refused to give her estrogen. He said she would just have to suffer with her hot flashes, and this she was indeed doing. She was nervous, anxious, tired, unable to sleep, and had gained substantial weight, largely from water retention. Dr. Walker gave her the Chinese herbal formula Quiet Contemplative. Sarah was amazed by the results. Not only did her hot flashes vanish but many of her other bothersome symptoms also disappeared.

INCONTINENCE

Urinary incontinence is an inability to hold the urine. More than 13 million people in the United States experience it, and 85 percent are women. Most are also elderly. Pregnancy and childbirth, menopause, and the structure of the female urinary tract account for the gender difference. Both sexes may also become incontinent from strokes, multiple sclerosis, and physical problems associated with old age.

If coughing, laughing, sneezing, or other movements that put pressure on the bladder cause you to leak urine, you may have stress incontinence. Physical changes resulting from pregnancy, childbirth, and menopause are common causes. Stress incontinence can worsen during the week before the menstrual period or at menopause because lowered estrogen levels can lead to lower muscular pressure around the urethra, increasing chances of leakage. Incontinence can also result from overactive nerves controlling the bladder, nerve damage from diabetes and other diseases, medications, urinary tract infections, mental impairment, restricted mobility, and stool impaction (severe constipation).[1]

CONVENTIONAL TREATMENT

Conventional treatment of urinary incontinence includes Kegel exercises (contracting and releasing the pelvic floor muscles to strengthen them), electrical stimulation, biofeedback, and medications that contain hormones. Some of these medications, however, can produce harmful side effects if used for long periods. Other options are the use of a pessary (a stiff ring inserted into the vagina by a doctor or nurse), implants injected into the tissues around the urethra to add bulk and help close the urethra, catheterization (the insertion of a tubular device into the urethra), and surgery.[2]

NATURAL REMEDIES

Women who lose urine when they sneeze, cough, or blow their noses can be helped with natural estrogen products including Phyto-B, Osta-B3, Gin-yam, and OstaDerm V. All are made by Bezwecken. The difference is in the proportions of estrogen and progesterone they contain. An experienced practitioner can help you determine the correct product and dosage for you. Another product that can help is Uri-Control, a homeopathic remedy by BHI. Take one tablet two to four times daily.

INDIGESTION

See DIGESTIVE PROBLEMS.

INFECTIONS, BACTERIAL AND VIRAL

Infections are not unique to women, but high levels of environmental stress added to our fluctuating internal hormonal states can make us particularly prone to colds, influenza, and other infections. Sexually transmitted infections are another source of concern for women. Today, we have an even more alarming concern: the threat of serious disease spread intentionally through bioterrorism.

CONVENTIONAL TREATMENT

Antibiotics are the conventional answer to bacterial infection, but after more than half a century, bacteria are becoming resistant to them. Moreover, antibiotics come with unwanted side effects and are effective only against bacterial infection. Vaccines are the pharmaceutical response to viral infection, but they too come with hazards. These hazards are particularly serious for vaccines against a bioterrorist attack with anthrax or smallpox (discussed separately below).

Antibiotics were considered wonder drugs when they first came on the market. These days, however, diseases that were once responsive to them either require stronger forms of the drug or no longer respond at all.[1] Antibiotic resistance is attributed to overuse of the drugs not only in humans but also in animals. The livestock industry purchases an astounding one-half of all antibiotics sold. The drugs are incorporated into feed to kill bacteria that stunt the growth of the animals. Resistant bacteria then develop and multiply; when you eat these animals, you can become infected with the resistant strains. Cooking the meat will kill the bacteria, but the antibiotic remains in the flesh and is absorbed into your bloodstream when the meat is eaten. The doses absorbed are low but are sufficient to allow the bacteria to develop a resistance to the drug. Your risk is increased if you've taken antibiotics recently yourself, since the normal bacterial population in your intestines will have been wiped out, allowing the invading strains to take over. Another suspected source of antibiotic resistance is the use of antibacterial soaps in the kitchen, giving the organisms an opportunity to adapt to the antibacterial agents in the soap.

Even when they work, antibiotics are not the ideal response to infection. They depress the body's own immunological response, preventing the development of natural antibodies. They also permit overgrowths of resistant strains of *Candida albicans*, which then produce toxins that can weaken the immune system and further reduce resistance.[2] (See "Fungal Infections" on page 116.) Worse, homeopaths maintain that antibiotics merely suppress bacteria without actually eliminating them. The disease is therefore liable to recur.

Steroids like cortisone, contained in popular drugs for asthma, arthritis, skin conditions, and other ailments, give infections even greater opportunity to spread. Steroids suppress inflammation by suppressing the immune system. For a fuller discussion, see "Asthma" on page 57.

For preventing flu, a viral infection, flu shots are heavily promoted. However, the flu shot is specific for certain strains and won't work on "surprise" epidemics of unanticipated strains. Julian Whitaker, M.D., warns strongly against this prophylactic measure in any case. Unlike for childhood diseases, in which a single course of vaccination is considered good for a lifetime, flu shots must be repeated every year; tampering with the immune system is risky business. Fifty percent of people who get the shots, according to some studies, have complications; and for a small percentage, they can be life-threatening. In anticipation of a swine flu epidemic in 1976, a vaccine aimed at that scourge caused thousands of cases of Guillain-Barre syndrome, a very serious neurological disease that can be fatal, but the swine flu epidemic never hit.[3] Fortunately, there are safer and more effective alternatives to antibiotics and vaccines.

NATURAL REMEDIES

Nutritional Immune-System Boosters

Vitamin and mineral supplements can help boost the immune system. Dr. Whitaker observes that in a Canadian study, taking vitamins and minerals cut the incidence of sick days from flu by nearly 50 percent—more than with the flu shot, without side effects or risks.

Jarrow Pak Plus, a high-dose vitamin, mineral, and herbal supplement, is a particularly effective combination. Many people prone to colds and flus throughout the winter report that taking one packet daily has kept them healthy through those precarious months. This supplement was originally developed to bolster the immune systems of AIDS patients but is now available in health food stores.

Vitamin C is well known for its ability to reduce the duration and severity of colds. Numerous studies have found that vitamin C supplements taken at a dose of 1,000 mg daily can significantly reduce symptoms and help speed recovery, although benefits appear to be greater for children than for adults. The evidence suggests that taking vitamin C only at the onset of cold symptoms is just as effective as taking it daily for speeding recovery.

As for *preventing* colds, there is no real evidence that high-dose vitamin C is effective unless the immune system has been weakened for some reason or a deficiency of the vitamin exists. The exact dose to use for colds is debated, but a typical recommendation is 500–1,000 mg three to six times daily while cold symptoms last.[4] Too much vitamin C can cause diarrhea. There is also some evidence that high doses cause free-radical damage.[5] It is best to take moderate doses of vitamin C daily (200–500 mg) and high doses only when a cold seems to be developing.

Zinc has also been shown in clinical studies to help at the first stage of a cold. Recent studies at Dartmouth College and the Cleveland Clinic Foundation indicate that sucking on zinc lozenges can reduce the duration of colds and flu by half. The dose that helped cold and flu sufferers in the Cleveland study was 13.3 mg of zinc every two hours. Avoid products with fillers and sweeteners included to enhance palatability. Zinc gluconate or acetate is best, not zinc picolinate or citrate.[6] Because zinc is a heavy metal, this therapy should be limited to colds in their early stages.

Another nutrient shown to cut flu incidence nearly in half in elderly and chronically ill people is N-acetylcysteine (NAC). In a study reported in 1997 involving more than 200 people, the percentage getting flu symptoms dropped from 51 percent to 29 percent in those taking NAC. In people who did get symptoms, severity and duration were significantly reduced.[7] Again, Jarrow makes good product. Use as directed on the label.

Another effective immune-system booster available in health food stores is colostrum. Derived from the first milk of cows, it is now available in pill form. In many reported cases, taking colostrum capsules has kept colds from developing. Take 500 mg one to four times daily, or every hour or two at the first sign of a cold.

Herbal Immune-System Boosters

Elderberry (*Sambucus nigra*) extract is a popular herbal remedy for colds and flu that, rather than merely suppressing the body's eliminatory mechanisms, has been shown to actually halt the spread of infection. An extract of the herb was shown in an Israeli study to cut flu recovery times in half.[8] Elderberry C 1000 by Zand may be taken all winter long to boost the immune system.

Olive leaf extract is another herbal antibiotic and antiviral, widely available in health food stores, that has been shown valuable in treating not only infection but also degenerative disease.[9]

Immunity-building herbs recommended by Chinese doctors include reishi and maitake mushrooms and astragalus. These products are available at supermarkets and health food stores either as pills or food.

Echinacea can also help strengthen the immune system's ability to ward off pathogens. But while it is quite effective if used at the right stage of a cold—on the first day of symptoms—if used at the wrong stage, clinical practice suggests it may actually make symptoms worse. The Chinese explanation is that it strengthens the *wei chi*, the protective energy layer on the outside of the body that stops things from going in or out. At the first stage of a cold, echinacea stops pathogens from getting in; however, once they are in, it can trap them inside. People who complain that they've been sick with a cold for several weeks ("It just won't seem to go away") frequently turn out to be taking echinacea. The herb is good to take when you feel like you "might be coming down with something," or when others around you are sick but you're still well. At that stage, it strengthens the body's internal energy and protects it from invasion. Zand and Bioforce are good sources of echinacea.

With all of these products, use as directed on the label.

Homeopathic Remedies

Homeopathic *Oscillococcinum*, the largest-selling flu remedy in France, was shown in a clinical study to be significantly better than placebo in treating the flu.[10] The remedy comes in a package containing six small tubes of tiny granules. The best way to use it is to take one tube at the onset of symptoms, then put another tube in half a glass of water and sip it slowly over the next six hours. Boiron, the manufacturer, also recommends taking one tube every week during flu season as a preventative. A cheaper alternative that is good to take when you first feel you are getting sick is Dolisos Cold and Flu Solution Plus. Take one tablet every fifteen minutes for the first hour, then one tablet every hour for four hours, then one tablet four times a day.

The German homeopathic company Staufen also makes a number of effective influenza remedies specific for each year. Dolisos also makes a line of specific flu remedies. Other options are Influenza CM by CompliMed and Virus by Deseret. Thymactive by NF Formulas is another homeopathic product that is good for strengthening the immune system. Take five drops once or twice daily or as directed on the label.

A cell salt that is an effective immune-system booster is Bioplasma. The recommended dose is four pills three times a day. A cell salt that is good for building the blood to strengthen the immune systems of people with chronic colds is *Ferrum phos* in a 6X potency. Take three to four times daily.

HOMEOPATHIC ALTERNATIVES TO VACCINES:
FROM FLU TO BIOTERRORISM

Immunizations are controversial, can produce side effects, and have been linked to certain autoimmune diseases, including hypothyroidism, allergies, diabetes, multiple sclerosis, and, in children, autism and encephalitis.[11] Vaccines for anthrax and smallpox, the current bioterrorist threats, can have side effects that are much worse.

No vaccine is currently available for a widespread anthrax attack. The vaccine used by the military is not accessible to the public, is highly toxic, and takes eighteen months to work if it works at all. According to an Army study, adverse reactions range from 40 percent in men to 70 percent in women. They can include severe bone and joint pain, loss of vision, severe skin problems, blackouts and loss of consciousness, grand mal seizures, internal organ problems, amyotrophic lateral sclerosis, multiple sclerosis, and death. No human trials have been done using the vaccine against inhaled anthrax, and animal studies have shown only partial effectiveness.[12]

Homeopathic nosodes offer a viable alternative. Nosodes are available or can be readily developed for any pathogen, including anthrax, smallpox, and any genetically engineered new strains. Nosodes can be produced in sufficient quantities for the entire population in two days, are entirely nontoxic, and can be administered at home.

A nosode is a homeopathic remedy in which the "active" ingredient is a disease-causing entity (a pathogen rather than an inert substance). It works like vaccination to stimulate immunity. The difference is that vaccination involves viral or bacterial macromolecules that can induce unwanted side effects. Homeopathic remedies are without side effects because they are extremely dilute—at some strengths so dilute that no molecule of the original substance is likely to be left in solution. Only its vibration remains. Chemically, the remedy consists of nothing but water.

The effectiveness of homeopathic nosodes against potentially fatal pathogens has recently been verified in the laboratory. A landmark study reported in 1999 by Wayne Jonas, M.D., of the Department of Family Medicine, Uniformed Services University of the Health Sciences, Bethesda, Maryland, tested whether a homeopathic nosode could protect mice from a deadly pathogen. In fifteen trials, the nosode consistently produced decreased mortality compared to controls. Dr. Jonas concluded that homeopathic nosodes may provide an interim method of reducing disease or death from infectious agents for which vaccination is currently unavailable.[13]

INFERTILITY

See SEXUAL DYSFUNCTION.

INFLAMMATION

See PAIN AND INFLAMMATION.

INFLAMMATORY BOWEL DISEASE

See BOWEL DISORDERS.

INSOMNIA

According to a 1998 poll, insomnia afflicts more than 50 percent of women. Those in menopause or under stress are particularly affected.[1] The number of hours you sleep doesn't matter as long as you feel well rested; however, if you habitually can't sleep and don't feel well rested, you might want to see a doctor to rule out underlying factors. Besides menopause and stress, causes may include anemia, infection, and sleep apnea (a disorder in which sleep is disturbed by improper breathing).

Insomnia can also be caused by drugs. Stimulant drugs include analgesics like Anacin and Excedrin, which contain caffeine; over-the-counter diet aids; nasal decongestants; and many prescription drugs, including those for asthma; many cough and cold remedies; amphetamines; and thyroid preparations. Centrally acting adrenergic blockers, hypnotics, and diuretics taken late in the day can also worsen sleep.[2] Sleeplessness may also result when you try to discontinue the drugs intended to counteract it. For that reason, it's best not to start on them if you can help it.

If no physical problem explains your insomnia, you may simply need to retrain your body and your mind in the ways of sleep. Sleeping well is a habit. Four out of ten people with insomnia get a good night's sleep on placebos (sugar pills that they think are sleeping pills).

CONVENTIONAL TREATMENT

Prescription sleeping pills—barbiturates and benzodiazepines—are effective, but they can depress brain function, have unwanted side effects, be addicting, and cause crises during withdrawal. They also tend to lose their effectiveness after about two weeks of continuous use, so users must keep increasing the dose. Increasing the dose means increasing the buildup of metabolites (byproducts of the drug's active ingredients), along with their hangover-like side effects. Elderly people branded as senile may actually be suffering from these side effects. The sleep these medications induce is stuporlike, with insufficient time spent dreaming. Withdrawal from them can lead to insomnia, anxiety, restlessness, headache, shaking, and visual disturbances. Prescription sleeping pills can be fatal in people with certain health problems, and you can't necessarily tell ahead of time if you're one of them. The drugs suppress breathing, so can be hazardous to women with breathing problems; and they cause grogginess and dizziness, precipitating falls in the elderly. The drugs can also be fatal if mixed with other drugs, or with narcotics or alcohol.

These concerns have made doctors leery of prescribing sleeping pills. In 1979, the FDA found that no over-the-counter sleeping pills on the market were safe or effective for treating insomnia and, therefore, banned the sale of all of them. Resourceful drug manufacturers then turned to antihistamines, which have the *negative side effect,* officially recognized by the FDA, of inducing drowsiness in some people. Originally marketed for the relief of allergies, antihistamines thus became the main ingredient in over-the-counter insomnia remedies like Nytol and Sominex. But antihistamines can have other side effects besides insomnia, including nausea and vomiting; dizziness; dryness in the mouth, throat, and nose; ringing in the ears; frequent urination; fatigue; and double vision. Dizziness and confusion are particularly likely in elderly people who take these drugs. In children, these drugs can produce restlessness and insomnia, the very problems they're supposed to prevent. In pregnant women, certain antihistamines can produce birth defects. Moreover, breast-fed infants can experience adverse effects from the antihistamines taken by their mothers.[3]

Natural Remedies

Resetting Your Biological Clock: Herbal and Homeopathic Alternatives

A safer, more natural alternative to sleeping pills is melatonin, a hormone secreted by the pineal gland when darkness falls. In pill form, melatonin has been touted as a wonder remedy that will soon make sleeping pills obsolete. While melatonin is definitely an advance over the barbiturates, it does have limitations. Ten percent of people with insomnia report no effects at all from its use, and another 10 percent complain of side effects, including nightmares, headaches, morning grogginess, mild depression, and low sex drive. Anecdotal evidence suggests that melatonin works better for men than for women, and it isn't recommended for habitual use for people under age 40.[4] Supplementing too often with melatonin can cut off the body's natural supply and make you dependent on it.

An alternative without side effects is homeopathic Melatonin 12X by Dolisos. Unlike the drugstore variety, it works by stimulating the body to produce its own melatonin, the hormone that puts you to sleep and resets your body clock so you continue to sleep. Take two pellets in the evening and again at bedtime.

Another effective homeopathic remedy for insomnia is *Passiflora* 3X or 6X. It eliminates the anxieties and worries of the day, allowing you to get a good night's sleep, and also helps to reset your sleep patterns. Take two pills in the evening (around 8 or 9 P.M.), then two before going to bed. Leave two on your nightstand and take them if you awaken before morning. Users report that in a few days, they are sleeping through the night and waking refreshed, not drowsy.

There are also many effective combination homeopathic remedies for insomnia, including Pineal Essence by PCH, and Quietiva and Insomnia Plus by CompliMed. Take ten drops or one tablet in the early evening and again right before bed. An effective protocol is to take Quietiva or another of these combination remedies in the evening to relax, then a second dose at bedtime along with homeopathic *Melatonin*.

The Eastern Approach

Chinese doctors recognize different forms of insomnia. The type of sleep and the time you awaken in the night are considered important diagnostic indicators. Some people have restless sleep; some can't fall asleep; some fall asleep, then wake up and can't go back to sleep; and some say they haven't slept through the night in years. In Chinese medicine, these are different ailments that require different remedies. For people who can't fall asleep in the first place, a Chinese patent formula called *Anmien Pien* can help by calming the mind. For other types of insomnia, other herbal remedies are indicated. For the correct remedy in your case, see a practitioner of Chinese medicine.

SLEEPING PILLS TRADED FOR NATURAL REMEDIES

Wendy, age 49, said she had been taking Restoril prescription sleeping pills for more than three years and could not sleep through the night without them. She was advised to discontinue the pills and start taking three homeopathic *Passiflora* pellets at 8 P.M. and three Melatonin 6X pellets at bedtime. If she woke in the night, she could take three more *Melatonin* 6X pellets. The first few nights she needed the extra dose, but in a week, she was sleeping through the entire night. The next week she dropped the *Passiflora* and just took two pellets of the *Melatonin*. Within a month, she was sleeping well without supplements of any sort.

Western Herbs and Nutrients

Western herbs are also available that can help induce sound sleep, including valerian, passion flower, and skullcap. Skullcap Oats by Eclectic Institute is a particularly good product. Follow label directions.

Evening primrose oil helps promote production of the body's own hormones. Two capsules totaling 2,600 mg taken before bed (not earlier) can help promote deep sleep. An added benefit is that evening primrose oil softens the skin and improves hair and nails. *Note: Women should not take evening primrose oil during their menses, as it promotes bleeding. For the same reason, it should not be taken by people on Coumadin or other anticoagulant therapy.*

Other Sleep Aids

Rescue Remedy is a Bach flower combination that can bring on the relaxation required to fall asleep. Five Flower Essence by FES is also good. Most health food stores carry these products, along with printed information on how to use them.

If you are prone to leg cramps that keep you awake at night, try Hyland's homeopathic Leg Cramps. Follow label directions. Potassium or calcium can also help. Emer'gen-C is a good source of potassium. Take one packet before bed. For calcium, Jarrow's Bone-Up is good. Take 1,000 mg before bed.

Another simple home remedy is to walk barefoot in the grass before bed. Dr. John R. Christopher, a renowned herbalist, maintained that static electricity that has built up in the body prevents people from getting a good night's sleep. This is a problem particularly for people who wear rubber-soled shoes.

The traditional hot bath, good book, and hot drink remain viable aids. A good meditative habit once in bed is to stop thinking and simply be present. Follow the breath or "watch" the thoughts. As they come in, slow them down by categorizing and putting labels on them ("memory," "plan," and so on). The act of analyzing the thought stops it from flowing.

INTESTINAL WORMS

See PARASITIC INFECTION.

IRREGULAR HEARTBEAT

Arrhythmias, dysrhythmias, fibrillations, and palpitations are all forms of irregular heart-beats. They are of concern to doctors mainly because they can warn of an impending heart attack. But irregular heartbeats aren't necessarily cause for alarm. They are also common side effects of thyroid imbalance, a problem from which many women suffer, particularly at menopause. Other possible causes of irregular heartbeats include emotional stress, in-fections, hypertension, and drugs, including nicotine, caffeine, diet pills, and other stimulants.

CONVENTIONAL TREATMENT

Cardiac arrhythmia is a known risk factor for subsequent sudden death in people who have already had a heart attack. Conventional practice was, therefore, to treat this symptom routinely with antiarrhythmic drugs, until an upsetting major study raised questions about the practice. The study found that the popular antiarrhythmics flecainide (Tambocor) and encainide (Enkaid) not only did not forestall a second attack in arrhythmia patients but also actually doubled the chances of bringing one on.[1] Correcting the symptom, it seems, aggravated the underlying disease. Tambocor is no longer on the market, but it has been replaced with other drugs that are also suspect.

Paralleling the use of antiarrhythmic drugs to prevent heart attacks, anticoagulant drugs used to prevent strokes have routinely been prescribed for atrial fibrillation (rapid randomized contractions of the heart, causing a totally irregular rate). However, a 1987 study, published in *The New England Journal of Medicine*, found that atrial fibrillation unaccom-panied by other symptoms is associated with a very low risk of stroke, at least in patients under age 60. Again, the researchers concluded that routine medication is probably unwarranted.[2]

If irregular heartbeats are due to some cause other than heart disease, as is often the case in women, the drugs are clearly unwarranted and can only make matters worse.

NATURAL REMEDIES

Women with heart palpitations who are in menopause or approaching it should have their thyroid levels checked before considering antiarrhythmic drugs. For a simple home test and natural remedies for thyroid imbalance, see "Hypothyroidism" on page 150.

Herbs, nutrients, and homeopathic remedies can help regulate cardiac arrhythmias. A homeopathic remedy called *Cactus*, used in conjunction with the herb hawthorn berry and the nutrient coenzyme Q_{10}, has been found to effectively normalize non-life-threatening cardiac arrhythmias. Hawthorn berry is an herb that supports the heart. Coenzyme Q_{10} is a nutrient that strengthens the heart. Homeopathic *Cactus* is now available only by pre-scription, but combination homeopathic formulas containing it are available over the counter, including Irregular Pulse and Heart Drops by Professional Complementary Health. See a homeopathic practitioner for recommendations and dosages.

Magnesium is another nutrient that helps. Magnesium depletion is known to cause rapid or irregular heartbeats. Take 400 mg two to three times daily.

ARRHYTHMIAS CURED WITH NATURAL REMEDIES

Terry, age 35, was concerned about repeated bouts of heart palpitations. She would wake up short of breath, her heart beating too fast. Her doctor had put her on drugs, but the drugs had only made her tired without eliminating the frightening palpitations. She sought help from Dr. Walker and went home with homeopathic *Cactus.* She didn't come back for a year and a half. When she did, she said that she had taken the remedy only one day. She hadn't had a single episode of palpitations since and hadn't felt so well in years.

Beverly, age 44, had heart palpitations associated with low thyroid levels, along with weakness and a lack of energy. She began taking homeopathic Cactus Comp along with homeopathic Thyroid, and from the first dose she too never had another palpitation. As her thyroid got back in balance, her energy level also rose.

For other natural alternatives for strengthening heart function, see "Heart Disease" on page 133.

IRRITABLE BOWEL SYNDROME

See BOWEL DISORDERS.

ITCHING

See SKIN PROBLEMS.

JET LAG AND JET TRAVEL

Women have joined the business frequent fliers, adding stress to their bodies and their immune systems. Frequent air travel ages the body and increases the risk of illness from exposure to an onslaught of germs as a result of poor air circulation, jet stress, the low oxygen content of recycled air, and exposure to free radicals. While airplanes once used 100 percent fresh air that was circulated every three minutes, newer model airplanes save fuel by using half recirculated air that is freshened every six or seven minutes or longer.[1]

Jet lag is a syndrome of fatigue, weakness, sleepiness, and irritability caused by a disruption in the normal cycle of sleeping and waking, as when traveling across several time zones in a short time. Adapting to a time zone can take five to fifteen days. Frequent air travel can throw off not only your sleep patterns but also your immune system.

CONVENTIONAL TREATMENT

You can coerce your body into sleeping on cue by taking a sleeping pill, but the drug may leave you drowsy during the day. Halcion is a popular sedative. Taking it before a flight, however, can be dangerous, resulting in some cases in an incapacitating condition called "traveling amnesia."[2]

NATURAL REMEDIES

A natural alternative for correcting a disturbed sleep pattern is melatonin, a hormone secreted by the pineal gland in response to light hitting the eyes. Melatonin determines when we sleep and wake up. Five milligrams of supplemental melatonin taken nightly has been shown to help airline employees adjust to new time zones. Better yet is to take homeopathic Melatonin 12X. For this and other natural sleep inducers, see "Insomnia" on page 162.

For countering the onslaughts to the immune system wrought by air travel, herbal and homeopathic remedies are available. The following recipe for immunity is particularly effective: put one dropperful of the homeopathic formula Geopathic Stress by Deseret in an 8-ounce bottle of water, and add one tablet of Cold and Flu Solution PLUS by Dolisos. Sip this mixture the entire time you are aloft. It is also a good idea to add a few drops of the homeopathic remedy Radiation to an 8-ounce bottle of water and sip it on the plane.

To counter the free radicals to which fliers are exposed, heavy doses of antioxidants are recommended. Good options are OPC grapeseed extract (100–200 mg daily), alpha lipoic acid (100–200 mg daily), and Jarrow's Antioxidant Optimizer (one tablet up to three times daily).

It is also effective to wear a device called a Diode that counteracts harmful radiation emanating from low-frequency electromagnetic fields. New research shows that the body has an electrical field of its own, which protects the body's rhythms and keeps it functional.[3] When harmful electromagnetic radiation is passing through the body, the body's own electrical system is disturbed. The Diode is said to work by giving the body's electrical system the extra boost it needs to stay in balance. The device is a small, square piece of lightweight, nontoxic material projecting forty-seven different frequencies. When worn on the left side of the body, it balances the body's own electrical energies and counteracts conflicting energies (for example, microwaves) within the airplane. The Dio-Pad, a large pad on which you sit during flight, works on the same principle. The Diode can also be used to counteract harmful radiation emanating from computers, televisions, fluorescent lights, and X-ray machines. It may either be attached to the radiation-producing machine or worn directly on the body. It is nonmetallic and should pass security checkpoints at airports.

OTHER HELPFUL TIPS

1. Drink plenty of water to avoid dehydration. It's best to avoid alcohol and coffee; however, if you don't wish to avoid these beverages, drink even more water to replenish the water losses they induce. Carry your own bottled water; airplane water isn't fresh.

2. Reduce food intake.

3. Wear comfortable clothing.

JET LAG CONQUERED

Polo traveled frequently for the movie industry, but she complained that she had trouble sleeping and typically lost nearly a day of work getting readjusted after a long plane trip. She was delighted to discover homeopathic Melatonin 12X and Deseret's Geopathic Stress. She put a dropperful of the Deseret remedy in a bottle of water and sipped it throughout the flight. These two remedies got her back on track immediately after a flight. She felt fine as soon as she arrived and was more efficient at her work.

4. For sleeping on the plane, bring eyeshades, earplugs, and an inflatable neck pillow.

5. Resist the urge to go to sleep immediately upon arrival in a country where it's still daylight, even if your own body clock says it's the middle of the night. Try to hold out until the locals are going to sleep. Go for a walk in the sun to stimulate your pineal gland and reset your internal clock.

LIVER DISEASE, HEPATITIS, AND JAUNDICE

Many women's diseases can be traced to an overburdened liver, which has to deal with the breakdown products of female hormones and stress hormones along with other toxins. The liver's chief function is to detoxify the body. Besides the harmful byproducts of metabolism, it has to detox pesticides, pollutants, drugs, and toxic chemicals. Alcohol contributes to the liver's load, precipitating cirrhosis (chronic inflammation and degeneration) of the liver in the chronic alcoholic. Constipation and the habitual use of pharmaceutical drugs can also overburden the liver, leading to its degeneration over time.

Jaundice is a yellowish discoloration of the skin and eyeballs resulting when toxins accumulate in the blood. Jaundice may indicate hepatitis, inflammation of the liver caused by a viral infection.

Hepatitis A, the least dangerous form of hepatitis, does not cause long-term liver damage. It is usually transmitted through fecal matter from food or water (for example, from restaurant workers who don't wash their hands). Besides jaundice, symptoms include loss of appetite, fatigue, mild fever, muscle or joint aches, nausea, vomiting, abdominal pain, and dark urine.

Hepatitis B is the most widespread of the hepatitis viruses, affecting 300,000 Americans annually. It can be passed from mother to child or through sexual contact, blood

HEPATITIS C VICTIM STABILIZED WITH SIMPLE REMEDY

Diane, in her early forties, came in to Dr. Walker's office quite distraught after she had been told by her medical doctor that she had tested positive for hepatitis C. She was given homeopathic Hepatitis C series therapy by the German company Staufen and Mixed Hepatitis by Deseret. She called back six months later, quite excited to report that she had tested negative for hepatitis C.

BACK TO WORK IN A WEEK ON GREENS

A 35-year-old nurse diagnosed with hepatitis A was concerned about the two to six months of lost work the disease would entail. To the nurse's delight, three days after starting on the Liver Cleanse Diet, consuming generous doses of green leafy vegetables and green drinks, and taking the German homeopathic remedy Hepatitis A, all hepatitis symptoms were gone.

transfusions, or the shared needles of IV drug users. Most victims recover completely, but some develop chronic hepatitis and possibly cirrhosis of the liver.

Hepatitis C is the most frightening hepatitis virus. Usually spread through blood transfusions or contaminated needles, it can have no or only mild symptoms for ten or twenty years, while the liver is insidiously being destroyed. The victim may feel exhausted, but the disease is detected only by a blood test showing that liver enzymes are abnormally high. A definitive diagnosis requires a biopsy (a test in which a piece of the liver is cut out and analyzed).

CONVENTIONAL TREATMENT

Conventional medicine has little to offer for hepatitis. Certain drugs like interferon have been tried experimentally, but none are clearly effective. Hepatitis B vaccines are available but are so controversial that doctors themselves often refuse to take them. As for diet, most doctors say it has nothing to do with recovery. The patient can eat whatever she wants.

NATURAL REMEDIES

Alternative practitioners, on the other hand, maintain that diet is key to clearing liver disease. A diet heavy in greens can clean the liver and reduce recovery times dramatically. The liver also needs to be given a rest from proteins, which are hard for it to handle and should be eaten only in very small amounts if at all. The Liver Cleanse Diet is described in detail in Chapter 4.

Herbal supplements useful for cleaning the liver include milk thistle and yellow dock. Homeopathic remedies can also be remarkably effective. Dr. Walker has seen Hepatitis series therapy (by Deseret or Staufen) clear cases not only of hepatitis A but of hepatitis B and hepatitis C. See a practitioner for products and use.

LIVER STAGNATION

See MULTIPLE CHEMICAL SENSITIVITY.

LUPUS

Lupus is a chronic autoimmune disease in which the immune system attacks the body's own connective tissue. One type, discoid lupus erythematosus affects only skin exposed to sunlight. Systemic lupus erythematosus (SLE), the most serious form of lupus, is a chronic multisystem autoimmune disease affecting not only the skin but other vital organs. Although it was once uncommon, SLE has increased in incidence over the last fifteen years by a factor of somewhere between 4 and 15. (The figure is uncertain because the condition is frequently misdiagnosed.) In the United States, between 500,000 and 1.5 million people are thought to have SLE, and it strikes women ten times as frequently as men. Common symptoms include a butterfly-shaped skin rash across the cheeks and nose, anemia, joint inflammation, kidney inflammation, abnormal antibodies in the blood, and chronic fatigue. The condition can produce quite serious complications that often lead to death.[1]

It is not clear why SLE favors women so much more than men, but hormones undoubtedly play a role. In one study, the ratio of females to males with the disease increased dramatically after puberty, from 3:1 in adolescence to 10:1 in adulthood. In another study, women with SLE were interviewed to determine menstrual, sexual, and reproductive history prior to SLE diagnosis. Eighty-seven percent of those with SLE who had been pregnant had a history of miscarriage.[2]

Although the specific cause of lupus is unknown, an estimated 10 percent of American cases are drug-related. Known offenders include the drug procainamide, an antiarrythmic drug used to regulate erratic heartbeats; the antiarrhythmic quinidine; the blood pressure–lowering drugs hydralazine and methyldopa; the tuberculosis drug isoniazid; and the tranquilizer chlorpromazine. A probable association has also been shown with the antipsychotic lithium, many anticonvulsant agents, antithyroid drugs, penicillamine (used to treat rheumatoid arthritis), sulfasalazine (used to treat ulcerative colitis), and the beta-blockers (used to lower blood pressure). A possible association has been shown with estrogens, the antibiotics penicillin and tetracycline, para-aminosalicylic acid (used to treat tuberculosis), gold salts (used for arthritis), griseofulvin (used for fungal infections), and reserpine (used to lower blood pressure).[3] Intentional poisoning has also produced elusive symptoms diagnosed as lupus, fibromyalgia, depression, and chronic fatigue syndrome.

CONVENTIONAL TREATMENT

The usual treatment for lupus is corticosteroids, especially prednisone. The drugs suppress symptoms by suppressing the immune system, but they can have quite serious side effects. Long-term steroid use can cause weight gain and facial fullness, hypertension, diabetes, osteoporosis, cataracts, intestinal bleeding, and increased susceptibility to infections. Side effects on the central nervous system can include sleeplessness, memory loss, anxiety, and depression. After taking steroids for prolonged periods, a serious condition known as adrenal insufficiency can develop if withdrawal isn't tapered very carefully to give the body a chance to recover its own ability to produce natural steroids.

NATURAL REMEDIES

On the face of it, the immune systems of patients with lupus and other autoimmune diseases appear to have gone awry and to be attacking themselves. But the fact that drugs and poisons induce lupuslike symptoms suggests that the problem is not in the mechanisms of the body (a brilliantly efficient machine) but in what it has been forced to deal with. The body is reacting to toxins that have been incorporated into the structure of its cells along with fats. The body knows the toxins are foreign chemicals but can fight them only by fighting itself.

Whether drug and chemical toxicity actually causes lupus or merely mimicks its symptoms, a better approach than suppressing the immune system is a detox program to elim-

LUPUS TRACED TO DRUG AND CHEMICAL TOXICITY

In *Cured to Death,* British authors Arabella Melville and Colin Johnson report the case of Mary, a healthy woman in her late twenties who had been under a lot of stress. She started suffering heart palpitations, for which her doctor prescribed a beta-blocking drug called practolol. The heart palpitations stopped, but Mary's periods became very heavy and she was often dizzy. When she went completely blind for several hours, her doctor prescribed tinted glasses. When it got to the point that Mary ached all over and was in constant pain, her doctor prescribed painkillers. When she got a severe pain in her neck that kept her in bed for three days, he prescribed a surgical collar and more painkillers. Yet Mary's eyes continued to hurt, her ears ached and rang, her skin itched, she cried frequently, and she couldn't sleep. Her doctor prescribed a battery of sleeping pills. Her stomach became upset and her nose and throat were sore and dry. When her stomach pains became severe, her doctor finally took her off practolol. The rash cleared up, but her other troubles persisted. Her stomach grew huge. She had a hysterectomy, and a grapefruit-sized mass of fibrous tissue was removed. She tried to hold down a job but couldn't, because she kept falling. She was given medicines for vertigo, along with sleeping pills, painkillers, and tranquilizers. She had to undergo another operation, after which she was kept in the hospital for six weeks for extensive testing. Her doctors diagnosed multiple sclerosis. Mary was convinced she did not have this disease, and her suspicion was subsequently confirmed. Her condition was finally diagnosed as lupus resulting from her treatment with the drug practolol, which caused her body to reject its own tissues as foreign.[4]

Shirley's lupus was also drug-related. When she came for help with a complex of symptoms that had been diagnosed as lupus, Dr. Walker took her history. It revealed that she had developed the symptoms after being put on a prescription drug for trigeminal neuralgia (severe pain in a facial nerve). Dr. Walker, who is also a pharmacist, observed that that particular drug had been linked to lupus. Shirley was surprised, saying her doctor hadn't mentioned it. She stopped taking the drug and started taking homeopathic *Arsenicum alba* and a constitutional remedy specific to her. Her facial pain is now much relieved, and her lupus is no longer progressing.

A more dramatic case involved the 38-year-old wife of a prominent medical doctor, who called Dr. Walker in a hysterical condition after seeing a score of doctors including some of the top medical doctors in New York City. She said she had been diagnosed with a severe kind of lupus that affects the heart and was told that if she did not immediately take a number of powerful drugs, her heart would be destroyed. Before that, she had been declared psychotic and was put on antidepressants. Laboratory testing indicated that she had unusually high levels of toxic chemicals in her urine. Dr. Walker therefore started her on a very strong detox program. (See Chapter 5.) When she went back to her New York City doctor only a month later, he was amazed to find that all her lab values were normal and her "lupus" was completely gone. No residual toxins were found in her heart, which was fine. She was still far from healthy, however. She was abnormally tired, and her face was pallid. After two more months on a strict detox program including intravenous chelation with EDTA, she became completely well. The case eventually wound up in court, where poisoning by her doctor/husband was proven. The evidence included arsenic in the victim's urine, very high levels of organophosphates in her blood, poison found on her clothes, and proof that carbon monoxide was leaking into her car from a deliberate cut that allowed it to flow from the engine. A police commissioner involved in the case said the poisoning of wives by their husbands is a quite common crime.

inate the cause. The true case histories in the inset below illustrate the link with drugs and poisonous chemicals. For a range of effective detox alternatives, see Chapter 5 and "Multiple Chemical Sensitivity" on page 185.

LYME DISEASE

Lyme disease (*Lyme borreliosis*) is a flulike bacterial infection, once thought to be carried only by a few species of black-legged ticks, but now known to be carried by fleas and gnats as well. Lyme disease has been called a "hidden epidemic" and possibly "the most insidious—and least understood—infectious disease of our day." While the official count of cases is relatively low, some doctors who work with the disease feel it may affect as much as 25 percent of the population.[1] Animal studies have shown that the Lyme spirochete (*Borrelia burgdorferi*) can be deeply embedded in muscles, tendons, tissue, and the heart and brain in less than a week after infection occurs. It is also transmissible across the placenta at birth.[2]

JoAnne Whitaker, M.D., Research Director of the Bowen Research & Training Institute in Palm Harbor, Florida, specializes in advanced testing methods for Lyme disease. She suspects an enormous number of people in the United States are infected with the disease because the hundreds of tests she performs every year now come out positive. She believes that Lyme disease is at the base of both chronic fatigue syndrome and fibromyalgia (all three illnesses were "discovered" around the same time in the 1980s), and that in more than half of chronically ill people, Lyme disease may be a factor in their conditions. Besides fibromyalgia and chronic fatigue, Lyme disease has been suspected as contributing to the symptom complexes of multiple sclerosis, Alzheimer's disease, and other degenerative diseases to which women are particularly prone.[3]

DIAGNOSIS

In cases that come to the practitioner without a diagnosis, the first problem is determining what the disease is. Although Lyme disease can be detected with a blood test, the usual lab test is very unreliable, and practitioners often don't think to test for it. Lyme disease symptoms are elusive and imitate other diseases. The complaints of victims tend to change from day to day. They can feel great one day and wretched the next. The illness is liable to be misdiagnosed or to be branded as "psychological." The clearest early sign is usually a bull's eye–shaped rash appearing within weeks of the tick bite; this sign is often missed, however. Other early symptoms of Lyme disease include muscle and joint aches and swelling, headache, stiff neck, overwhelming fatigue, fever, facial paralysis (Bell's palsy), meningitis, and (less commonly) eye problems and heart abnormalities. Late-stage symptoms include intermittent or chronic arthritis and neurological conditions such as confusion and memory loss.[4] For women, testing around the time of the menses has been found to increase the probability of discovering the presence of Lyme bacteria. The decline of estrogen and progesterone at the end of the menstrual cycle is associated with a worsening of the symptoms of women with the disease.[5]

CONVENTIONAL TREATMENT

Standard drug treatment consists of a month-long course of intravenous antibiotics, which must sometimes be repeated. Intravenous antibiotic treatment can be quite disruptive and toxic to the body. Doctors caution that it should be used only when the case is advanced and the diagnosis is definitive. The problem, again, is that diagnosis is difficult. Misdiagnosis can subject the patient to quite toxic drugs for the wrong underlying condition.

NATURAL REMEDIES

One solution for dealing with Lyme disease is homeopathic treatment, which can be used without a definitive diagnosis because the remedies have no dangerous side effects. If the remedy is not the correct one for the patient's condition, it will simply have no effect. Experimentation with these remedies can be used, in fact, to establish an otherwise tentative diagnosis. Homeopathic remedies are not only nontoxic but also have proven effective in cases where antibiotics failed.

Hundreds of cases of Lyme disease have been referred by a medical office to Dr. Walker after the patients' symptoms returned following treatment with antibiotics. The drugs simply had not worked. They had suppressed rather than cured the disease, and had thrown off the natural balance of the body. The remedy that resolved these patients' symptoms was a formulation of homeopathic *Borrelia* by the German company Staufen (now available in the United States as series therapy from Deseret). The recommended protocol was a single dose in potencies varying from 200X to 5X taken every three days for a month. As is typical of homeopathic treatment, the symptoms tended to get worse before they got better (the "healing crisis"). Then, they generally disappeared permanently.

If you've been bitten by a tick and catch the problem in the first few days, taking ten drops three times daily of a homeopathic remedy by Deseret called LYM can help ward off the disease. If more time has elapsed, however, the full series therapy is required.

MASTITIS

See BREAST PAIN AND TENDERNESS, BREAST LUMPS, AND FIBROCYSTIC BREASTS.

MELANOMA

See SKIN CANCER AND SUNBURN.

MEMORY LOSS

Although gradual memory loss comes to everyone with age, the fact that memory can be enhanced with detox therapies suggests that this symptom is related to an accumulation of toxins in the brain over time. A different sort of memory loss that women can find quite

---

MEMORY RETURNS WITH NATURAL HORMONE REPLACEMENT

Lynne had such a good memory that she didn't need an appointment book. She remembered it all. Then at age 47, her estrogen level fell off; suddenly, her memory was virtually gone. She tried gingko biloba, but it didn't help. She added soy products to her diet and began using Osta-derm natural estrogen cream. On the days that she used the cream, her memory was back. Too much of the cream gave her a bloated feeling, but when she properly adjusted the dose to meet her body's demands, she experienced definite improvement in both her memory and her sense of well-being. For her, ¼ teaspoon daily proved to be about right. DMAE capsules helped her as well.

---

alarming is the sudden lack of recall of ordinary facts well known to them, a symptom that is liable to hit at menopause. Fortunately, this symptom is hormone-related and goes away when fluctuating hormones reach equilibrium again.

CONVENTIONAL TREATMENT

No drug is of proven effectiveness in reversing memory loss. For detailed discussion of drugs used to slow the degenerative process, see "Alzheimer's Disease" on page 40.

NATURAL REMEDIES

A number of herbs and supplements are specifically recommended to slow memory loss, including ginkgo biloba, gotu kola, phosphatidylserine (PS), omega-3 fatty acids (Efalex is a good product), choline and other B vitamins, amino acids (especially L-glutamine and L-phenylalanine), acetyl-L-carnitine (ALC), antioxidants (especially coenzyme Q_{10}), di-methylaminoethanol (DMAE), pregnenolone, *Bacopa monniera* (an Ayurvedic herb), and nicotinamide adenine dinucleotide (NADH).[1] All are available at health food stores. Combination products for the brain containing a selection of these nutrients and herbs are also available. Use as directed on the labels. For other remedies, see "Alzheimer's Disease" on page 40.

The memory loss associated with hormone fluctations at menopause can be relieved with natural hormone creams. For their advantages over the pharmaceutical varieties and for recommended brands, see "Menopause and Perimenopause" on page 174. Adding soy products to the diet can also help, although soy can be overconsumed, since too much soy can suppress thyroid and iron levels. See "Hypothyroidism" on page 150 "Anemia" on page 44.

MENOPAUSE AND PERIMENOPAUSE

Menopause, or the cessation of monthly menstrual periods, occurs in Western women at around age 50. Perimenopause is a transitional period when menopausal symptoms may be experienced although menses have not yet ceased. Hot flashes are suffered by more than two-thirds of menopausal women and are the most common reason they seek medical attention for menopausal complaints. Hot flashes may or may not be accompanied by profuse sweating, which is likely to occur most heavily at night. Clothing and bedding can become so wet that they must be changed several times. Other disturbing symptoms of menopause can include loss of interest in sex, depression, moodiness, crying, anger, irritability, shortness of breath or difficult breathing, dizziness, fatigue, indigestion, constipation, diarrhea, gas, headaches, heart palpitations, insomnia, muscle and bone aches and tingling, shoulder and hip pain, cramps in the legs and feet, numbness in the arms, painfully sensitive skin, urinary problems, memory loss and mental sluggishness, dryness of the skin and vaginal tissues, breast tenderness, and weight gain. The risks of osteoporosis (bone loss) and heart disease go up significantly after menopause.

All of these problems have been blamed on diminishing levels of female hormones. However, women in other cultures who eat natural diets and follow holistic lifestyles often manage to escape menopausal symptoms.[1] Nature seems to have intended this passage to be a gradual process of reduced hormone output by the ovaries, which belong to a complex of glands under the control of the pituitary. As ovarian function falls off and hormone levels drop, the pituitary sends signals to the adrenals to increase their hormone output. When this backup hormone system is working properly, menopause should come with few or no side effects. The reason it fails for Western women has been blamed on adrenal exhaustion, caused by stress, low blood sugar, and poor diet. Many women report breezing through menopause until some crisis hits at work or at home, after which they suddenly get crippling hot flashes and night sweats.

CONVENTIONAL TREATMENT

The conventional solution for diminishing hormone levels is to supplement with pharmaceutical hormones. Hormone replacement therapy (HRT) consists of pharmaceutical estrogen and synthetic progesterone, most popularly Premarin (derived from mare's urine) and Provera. Premarin is one of the most widely prescribed drugs in the country, but accompanying its rising popularity has been a precipitous rise in breast cancer, to which it has been linked. For a fuller discussion on hormone replacement therapy, see Chapter 2.

Pharmaceutical hormones also come with a long list of disturbing side effects. Adverse reactions to Premarin listed in the *Physician's Desk Reference* or *PDR* (the standard medical reference on drugs) include PMS-like symptoms; breast tenderness, enlargement, and secretion; nausea, vomiting, abdominal cramps, and bloating; skin and eye sensitivities; headaches, dizziness, and depression; weight gain and water retention; bleeding between periods or missed periods; changes in libido (sex drive); and enlargement of uterine fibroid tumors. Provera's listed side effects include bloating, water retention, nausea, insomnia, jaundice, mental depression, fever, masculinization, weight changes, breast tenderness, abdominal cramping, anxiety, irritability, and allergic reactions. Fluid retention can exacerbate asthma, migraines, epilepsy, and heart and kidney problems.[2]

NATURAL REMEDIES

For women who feel they need hormones but want to avoid the side effects and risks of the prescription versions, estrogen and progesterone are available in natural plant form.

Herbal and homeopathic remedies can also help balance hormone levels and relieve menopausal symptoms. Hot flashes, night sweats, and heart palpitations can be the result not only of adrenal imbalance but also of thyroid imbalance. Women in menopause or perimenopause who have heart palpitations should have their thyroid levels checked before considering drugs. (See Chapter I and "Hypothyroidism" on page 150.)

Natural Hormone Creams

Both plants and animals produce hormones that regulate cell metabolism and growth. In fact, the sterols of plants such as soybeans and yams are the basis from which many inexpensive, commercially available hormones are made. They are also the basis of natural estrogen and progesterone creams available at health food stores.

For many women, natural progesterone cream alone can control hot flashes, without the use of estrogen. Their bodies apparently synthesize estrogen from it as needed. Progesterone is a hormone precursor, from which other hormones are made in the body. Studies show natural progesterone to be as effective as synthetic progestins in protecting against uterine cancer, without the drugs' side effects. Studies of oral natural progesterone have found that it not only eliminated the side effects of synthetics but also lowered blood pressure and significantly reduced the rate of bleeding as compared to women on synthetic progestins.[3] Many women on HRT have found that substituting natural for synthetic progesterone allowed them to reduce their estrogen dose by at least half. After six months, women taking natural progesterone who are well past menopause can often give up estrogen altogether.[4]

A particularly effective over-the-counter natural progesterone cream, containing 3 percent natural progesterone, is ProGest by Transitions for Health. The recommended protocol varies depending on hormonal status. For premenopausal women, rub ⅛ to ¼ teaspoon of the cream on the abdominal area each night for the fourteen days before your period, stopping a day or so before the period starts. For postmenopausal women without menses, use the cream for twenty-five days out of the month. Relief from hot flashes can take up to several months, since the hormone gets to the blood by way of the fatty layer under the skin and builds up only gradually. Herbal and homeopathic remedies can be used to reduce hot flashes while the progesterone is kicking in.

Natural estrogen creams derived from plants are also available. Although these creams have not been studied directly, plant estrogens have been studied. Preliminary research suggests that unlike animal and synthetic estrogens, plant estrogens are not associated with increased rates of cancer of the breast and uterus and may even afford protection against those diseases. Research also indicates that plant estrogens are as effective as pharmaceutical estrogen in increasing HDL ("good" cholesterol), lowering LDL ("bad" cholesterol), and causing arteries to constrict and dilate when they should.[5] Particularly effective products are made by Bezwecken (OstaDerm and Osta-B3). Use ⅛ to ½ teaspoon as needed, once or twice daily. Bezwecken's OstaDerm V is applied vaginally and is particularly good for vaginal dryness. The dosage is ⅛ to ½ teaspoon as needed three times weekly.

Hormone levels can also be boosted with the precursor hormones DHEA and pregnenolone. Natural forms are better than synthetics. Human growth hormone (hGH) is another currently popular option, but the product is quite expensive and may not live up to its claims. A cheaper and more natural alternative is to take homeopathic remedies that stimulate the body's own production of hormones.

Homeopathic Remedies

Growth Hormone Plus by Deseret Biologicals is an effective hormone stimulant. Hormone Combination, also by Deseret Biologicals, is another excellent homeopathic product, which helps to balance the hormones in the brain and stimulates the body to increase hormone production. It works not only for perimenopausal, menopausal, and postmenopausal women but for men. Both men and women with low sex drive often report increased interest in sex and increased sexual function after using this remedy for just a few weeks. Follow label directions.

The effectiveness of homeopathic remedies in alleviating hot flashes was shown in a study reported in 1992 involving a German homeopathic remedy called *Mulimen*, including homeopathic doses of *Vitex angus castus* (chasteberry), *Cimicifuga racemosa* (black cohosh or black snake root), *Hypericum perforatum* (St. John's wort), and *Sepia* (cuttlefish ink). Half the women who took the remedy were relieved of their hot flashes, an objective result unlikely to be the product of suggestion.[6]

Individual constitutional remedies specific to the personality and body type can also effectively quell hot flashes. *Lachesis*, the most popular choice, is an excellent hot flash remedy for many women. *Sepia*, another common choice, works for a woman with hot flashes who is completely exhausted. The table on page 179 details other constitutional remedies for menopausal complaints and their constitutional types. For all of these remedies, you can start with a potency of 30C, increasing as needed. Take three to five pellets one to three times daily.

A gemmotherapy effective for relieving hot flashes and night sweats is a homeopathic version of the herb red raspberry leaf called *Rubus idaeus* (the Latin name for the plant), manufactured by Dolisos. Gemmotherapies are a special form of homeopathic made from the plant's immature roots, which are believed to have more life force than other plant parts. Take fifty drops in half a glass of water every morning.

Women who can't or don't want to take conventional doses of estrogen can also take it in homeopathic doses. Little information is available on homeopathic estrogen because it's too inexpensive to be worth promoting, but practitioners who use it report that it's generally effective for women who need it.[7]

Other homeopathic remedies address the adrenal stress underlying hot flashes and other menopausal symptoms. The effects of unusual stresses can be relieved by taking homeopathic remedies to support the adrenals. Good options include Adrenal/Spleen by CompliMed, and Norepinephrine, Neuro I, and Neuro II by Deseret. Isocort by Bezwecken can provide herbal support for exhausted adrenals, although homeopathic solutions are safer. If used, see a practitioner for dosages. Adrenal stress can also be relieved by curtailing coffee and sugar intake, and ensuring that sleep is adequate.

For the bone loss accompanying the menopausal decline in hormones, a calcium and silica homeopathic product called Calcium Absorption is good. It helps stabilize the bones and prevent calcium loss by signaling the body to stop pulling calcium off the bones. In combination with evening primrose oil (up to 2,600 mg at bedtime), this product also helps provide the substrate necessary to manufacture better quality hormones. Take two pills three times daily.

HOT FLASHES AND NIGHT SWEATS MINIMIZED WITH HOMEOPATHIC REMEDIES

Valerie, age 51, complained of such severe hot flashes that they struck 200 times a day. She had tried everything, including the estrogen patch and pharmaceutical progesterone, without success. Questioning suggested that her major problem was mental and emotional stress. She had not had hot flashes until she pushed herself too hard at work getting ready to go on vacation, but this was just the last straw collapsing a burden of stresses. She was very unhappy with her job, her marriage, and her life in general. Her husband had had an affair two or three years earlier. She said she had forgiven him, but in her heart she still carried resentment. She was continually suspicious and worried that her marriage would break up. Because her problems were on many levels, her treatment was too. She was given natural progesterone (ProGest cream, ½ teaspoon daily), Osta-B3 natural estrogen replacement (two to four tablets three times daily), and homeopathic *Lachesis* (three pellets twice daily). Within a month, the frequency of her hot flashes had dropped substantially; in eight months, there was real progress in her life. She acquired the drive and strength of will to quit her job and risk becoming a writer. She is now crazy about her husband and is happier than ever in her life. *Lachesis* was the key; it opened her to express and eliminate her feelings of jealousy and worry, allowing her to change her focus to what she really wanted to do.

Barbara, age 38, complained of night sweats so severe that she had to change her nightgown four or five times every night. Barbara's doctor diagnosed her condition as early menopause and wanted to put her on hormones, but she was very young. Dr. Walker tested her and found that her thyroid levels were off, throwing all her hormones out of balance. Homeopathic Thyroid by CompliMed (ten drops three times daily) rebalanced her thyroid. The remedy worked so well that Barbara got pregnant, an unexpected but happy result that clearly indicated she was not in menopause. Thyroid imbalance is a leading reason women of childbearing age are unable to conceive.

Chinese Herbs

Herbal remedies can also effectively relieve menopausal complaints. The components of the traditional Chinese formulas for menopause include hormones derived from plants. Plant estrogens are effective but do not have the strong side effects of prescription estrogen because they are weaker and are more easily absorbed and used by the body. Chinese doctors, who consider menopause to be a deficiency of blood and yin (the fluids of the body), also treat symptoms with natural remedies that strengthen and build the blood. The advantage of this approach over drugs is that you don't have to take the remedies forever. You need them only until your yin is built back up and your body is back in balance. However, you may want to continue to take different Chinese herbs as your body's needs change.

Dong quai or tang kwei (*Angelica sinensis* root) is a highly effective remedy for hot flashes, although its estrogen content is only 1/400th that of drugstore estrogen. Clinical and laboratory studies have shown dong quai to be effective in stimulating uterine contractions, resolving blood clots, increasing the metabolism of the body and the oxygen consumption of the liver, lowering blood pressure, protecting the cardiovascular system, fighting bacteria and viruses, and reducing water retention.[8] When used in combination with other herbs, dong quai is an effective antidote for menopausal anxiety, depression, nervousness, and insomnia. Results may take a week or two, but homeopathic remedies can be used in the meantime for relief of symptoms. Ginseng, another common Chinese herbal component, naturally stimulates estrogen production in menopausal women without risk.

Paeony (*Radix paeoniae lactiflorae*), a Chinese herb that nourishes the blood, is used for deficient blood patterns including menstrual dysfunction, leukorrhea (vaginal discharge),

POPULAR HOMEOPATHIC REMEDIES FOR HORMONAL COMPLAINTS

Homeopathic Remedy	Selected Symptoms and Indications
Aconite	Complaints begin after a fright or sudden shock; great thirst for cold drinks; anxiety states; panic attacks.
Apis	Marked aggravation from heat; flushes of heat; made better by cold applications; severe menstrual cramps.
Belladonna	Affected by change of temperature; all symptoms worse around menstrual period; intense heat in affected parts.
Calcarea carbonica	Heavy bleeding; uterine fibroids; sensation of inner trembling; perspiration on head or back of neck; craves sweets (pastries and ice cream).
Caulophyllum	Arthritis of fingers or toes, worse before menses; vaginitis; infertility; vaginal discharge; painful menstruation.
Chamomilla	Feet feel hot and must be put outside covers; oversensitive to pain; complaints of anger, great irritability, aversion to being touched.
Cimicifuga racemosa	Hot flashes worse at the onset of menstrual flow; severe headaches; changeable mood; talkative; jumps from one subject to the next.
Ignatia	Perspiration only on face; lump in throat; sighing; easily offended, defensive.
Kali carbonicum	Wakes at night, especially 2 to 4 A.M.; wakes four hours after falling asleep.
Lachesis	Hot flashes better at onset of menstrual flow; suspicion, even paranoia; flushes of heat; aggravated by heat; irritable; jealous; depressed.
Phosphorus	Tremendous thirst for cold drinks; bleeding bright red blood; ovarian cysts; uterine prolapse.
Pulsatilla	Weeps easily; headaches; worse with heat, exertion, or after emotional stress; better in open air.
Sabina	Gushing flow of bright red blood, worse with motion; back pain with bleeding; thigh pain.
Sanguinara	Migraine headache on the right side; hot flashes; hay fever; heartburn.
Sepia	Involuntary weeping; symptoms worse from 2 to 4 P.M. or from 3 to 5 P.M.; flushes of heat with perspiration; worse at night.
Sulfur	Worse with heat; worse after bathing; craves sweets, chocolate, fats; insomnia.

and uterine bleeding. It is also used for spontaneous sweating and night sweats, caused in Chinese medical terminology by deficient yin that allows the fiery yang to surface.[9]

Bupleurum is used in Chinese herbal formulas to reduce liver inflammation and congestion. The liver is where female hormones are converted into usable compounds.

Classical Chinese formulas contain these and other herbs in traditional combinations that have been proven safe and effective over centuries. A patent formula that is particularly good for menopausal complaints is Relaxed Wanderer (*Hsiao Yao Wan* or *Xiao Yao Wan* in Chinese). It works particularly well for women with a tendency to be cold (for example, to have cold hands and feet). For restlessness and hot flashes, a formula called *Zhi Bai Di Huang Tang* is effective. The Zand version of this formula is called Anem-Phello and Rehmannia Formula. The K'an Herb version is called Temper Fire. Herbal formulas vary among manufacturers; follow label directions.

Western Herbs

The European and Native American herbal traditions also include excellent botanicals for premenstrual and menopausal complaints.

Red raspberry leaf (*Rubus idaeus*) is one of the most popular Western herbs for correcting hormone imbalances. A member of the rose family, it is best taken in the form of a simple infusion or tea. It restores and harmonizes uterine functions and helps rebuild uterine tissue, making it one of the few herbs that can actually be recommended throughout pregnancy. It also arrests bleeding and discharge and is useful in the treatment of uterine prolapse and mild digestive complaints, including diarrhea and constipation.

Black cohosh or black snake root (*Cimicifuga racemosa*) is an estrogen stimulant traditionally used for quelling hot flashes. The mechanism for its observed benefits was confirmed in a controlled study in which the levels of luteinizing hormone (LH) of 110 menopausal women treated with extracts of the herb declined. An elevation of LH has been linked to hot flashes.[10]

Another useful Western herb is chasteberry or monk's pepper (*Vitex agnus castus* root). It works whether hormones are deficient or in excess, by stimulating the pituitary gland to harmonize hormone imbalances and make its own progesterone; the herb won't force production of more hormone than the body needs. *Warning: Chasteberry is a strong uterine stimulant and, therefore, should not be used during pregnancy.*[11]

Wild yam (*Dioscorea villosa*) contains a substance that converts to the steroid hormones progesterone and cortisone. It is used to treat inflammation, menstrual problems, and (in small amounts) morning sickness.[12] Mexican yams are the source of the progesterone in the available natural progesterone and estrogen creams.

Diet and Lifestyle Factors

Hormone precursors can also be obtained from specific foods. Plant sterols in foods are easily converted to human estrogen and progesterone in the body. The difference between getting hormones from pills or hormone-fed animals and getting them from fruits and vegetables is that in the plant form, you're getting only the precursors. Your body can take from these building blocks and make whatever it needs. You don't have to worry about pushing your estrogen levels to dangerous heights.[13]

Studies suggest that the lack of menopausal complaints in women in certain non-Western cultures may be due largely to the high amounts of plant sterols in their diets. In one study, Japanese women were found to excrete 1,000 times the amount of phytoestrogens (plant estrogens) as women in Finland.[14] Another study found that menopausal symptoms were significantly reduced in British women who ate a diet high in phytoestrogens (furnished in that study as soya flour, red clover sprouts, and linseed or flaxseed oil).[15]

So far, some 300 plants with estrogenlike activity have been identified, including carrots, corn, apples, barley, and oats. Soybean products like tofu seem to pack the strongest hormonal wallop. But not everyone likes tofu, and not all concentrated soy products contain the requisite isoflavones. If the soy protein in your soy burger, for example, has been extracted using alcohol rather than water, the isoflavones will largely have been lost. Eating large amounts of soy products isn't recommended for other reasons. They can impair iron absorption, leading to anemia and iron deficiency in women, and they can suppress thyroid function. As usual, moderation is the key. It is best to limit soy to one product daily (for example, one cup of soymilk or one tofu dish). Jarrow's Isoflavone 50 combines genistein, daidzein, and puerarin, the active components of soybeans. One or two capsules may be taken daily. Kelp or seafood can help balance thyroid levels.

Besides soy products, good food sources of estrogen-containing bioflavonoids include citrus fruits, cherries, and grapes. Bioflavonoids have been found effective in controlling hot flashes, anxiety, and irritability, even though they're only 1/50,000th as strong as drugstore estrogen. They also help in strengthening the capillaries and preventing heavy irregular menstrual bleeding. Other foods high in plant hormones include yams, papayas, peas, cucumbers, bananas, bee pollen, raw nuts, seeds, sprouts, and certain herbs (alfalfa, licorice root, red clover, sage, sarsaparilla, and sassafras).

Nutritional Supplements

Vitamin E has been shown in medical studies to be quite effective in reducing hot flashes.[16] It also helps relieve other menopausal symptoms, including breast tenderness and vaginal dryness. When buying vitamin E, look for the natural product (d-alpha tocopherol or d-alpha tocopheryl), which is absorbed better from the digestive system and retained in the body longer than synthetic vitamin E (dl-alpha tocopherol or dl-alpha tocopheryl).[17] Vitamin E is also absorbed better when taken with meals than on an empty stomach. It should not be taken with iron supplements, which destroy it. Iron-rich foods like raisins and spinach, on the other hand, can be eaten without harm to the vitamin E. Vitamin E is one of those vitamins you can get too much of, but for hot flashes, 400–600 IU daily is considered safe.[18] For quelling intractable hot flashes, some doctors prescribe up to 1,600 IU of vitamin E per day; these levels aren't recommended without first consulting a doctor.[19] *Caution: If you experience blurred vision while taking vitamin E supplements stop taking them.*

Estrogen production can also be maintained and hot flashes relieved by taking evening primrose oil (two capsules at bedtime, totaling 1,300 mg). The oils of seeds and nuts have other benefits as well, including helping to counteract the dry skin, dry hair, and dry vaginal tissues that plague menopausal women, symptoms that can indicate a lack of essential fatty acids (EFAs). To counteract dry skin, two teaspoons of linseed or flaxseed oil daily are recommended. Also good is Ultimate Oil by Nature's Secret, which contains a blend of oils. Take two capsules at bedtime or as directed on the label.

Antistress vitamins involved in progesterone production include vitamin A (10,000 IU of the water-soluble beta-carotene form is recommended daily), vitamin C (200–500 mg daily), and pantothenic acid (50–100 mg daily). Other helpful supplements are an-

HORMONE THERAPY AVOIDED WITH TOFU SHAKE

A 44-year-old woman whose hormone level was a low 28 said her doctor wanted her to start on pharmaceutical HRT, but she was reluctant to start taking hormones so early in life with no real symptoms. Instead, about four mornings each week, she drank a shake consisting of tofu, soymilk, and fruit mixed in a blender. When her hormones rose from 28 to 154 over a four-month period, even her doctor was impressed and agreed she did not need the drugs.

tioxidants, including grapeseed extract and Coenzyme Q_{10}. Take one milligram per pound of body weight of each.

Good combination supplements are also available for menopause. One is Dr. Christopher's Change-O-Life by Nature's Way. Take one or two capsules up to three times daily.

MENSTRUAL PROBLEMS

For younger women, the bane of their monthly periods is liable to be painful cramping. For women near menopause, a common menstrual problem is flooding or prolonged bleeding that can lead to anemia. Bleeding can be so heavy and draining as to propel women to get hysterectomies. While their doctors may have promised that their problems would then be over, many women say they wished they hadn't rushed into these surgeries. Natural remedies are available that can slow heavy bleeding without surgery.

Other premenstrual complaints are discussed under "Premenstrual Syndrome (PMS)" on page 215.

CONVENTIONAL TREATMENT

For menstrual cramps, the conventional approach is painkillers such as Midol and Advil (ibuprofen). The problem with these drugs is that they merely mask the symptom without addressing the real problem, and women often find they need more and more of the drugs to get the same results. Sarafem, heavily marketed for a rare form of premenstrual syndrome, is identical to Prozac and comes with the same side effects. See "Premenstrual Syndrome (PMS)" on page 215.

For persistent hemorrhage-like flooding in an older woman, surgical removal of the uterus may be recommended. "You don't need that organ anymore," her gynecologist may say. "Let's just solve the problem by getting rid of it." But hysterectomies can lead to a host of other, unanticipated problems, including osteoporosis, bone and joint pain and immobility, loss of libido, chronic fatigue, urinary problems, emotional problems, depression, prolapse, and increased risk of heart disease. (See "Hysterectomy" on page 153.) It is better to address the underlying hormone imbalance with natural remedies.

NATURAL REMEDIES FOR EXCESS BLEEDING OR FLOODING

Effective herbal tonics are available for correcting hormone balance. A good choice is Female Tonic by Marco Pharma. (Take ½ teaspoon twice daily or according to label directions.) Another is Female Balance by Apex. (Take ten drops three times daily.)

Women who experience flooding may have red blood cell counts in the low but normal range as shown on lab tests; however, in Chinese medical theory, what counts isn't the absolute level but the change from high to low. A woman whose red blood cell levels are normally high will feel weak and experience palpitations and nightmares if her levels suddenly drop. Chinese herbal remedies are aimed at correcting the resulting blood deficiency. A three-step approach is necessary: 1) stop the immediate bleeding, 2) build the blood back up, and 3) correct the underlying hormone imbalance. For remedies to correct iron loss and build the blood, see "Anemia" on page 44.

Natural remedies that provide quick relief from excess bleeding include Bleeding by BHI and Trillium by Marco Pharma. A good start is to take one tablet of Bleeding every fifteen minutes until bleeding has slowed. Then take one tablet four times daily until menstruation ends. For more severe bleeding, try mixing twenty drops of Trillium in half a glass of water with I tablespoon of luvos earth (a form of clay). Drink this mix three times daily.

For bleeding from fibroids, an effective herbal tincture is *Thlaspi bursa*. Drink twenty drops mixed in water every fifteen minutes for the first hour, then twenty drops every hour until bleeding has stopped. This remedy may also be taken over several months to help reduce fibroids.

The herb capsicum (cayenne pepper) also stops bleeding. CapsiCool by Nature's Way is easier on the stomach than other forms and is a remedy many women swear by. Take one or two capsules every hour as needed, not to exceed eight in a twenty-four-hour period.

The Chinese have a very effective patent formula to stop bleeding called *Yunan Paiyao*, used either orally or topically. In an emergency, capsules of this formula can be taken by mouth. Products vary; follow directions on the label.

Hormone imbalance is the usual cause of excess bleeding, particularly if it involves bright red blood, when estrogen is likely to be too high in comparison to progesterone. This often occurs after a period of stress: the adrenaline released will cause a deficiency of progesterone relative to estrogen, producing very long and heavy periods. A permanent solution requires rebalancing the hormones. This can be done with natural progesterone cream (ProGest) along with remedies to support the adrenal glands. (See "Adrenal Stress" on page 36.)

NATURAL REMEDIES FOR CRAMPS

Menstrual cramps vary in degree and type. When the blood is dark with clots, Chinese doctors say that last month's blood has stayed in the tubes. The more stagnation there is in the body and the darker and more clotted the blood, the worse the cramps. Relief requires "moving the blood." The Chinese patent formula to achieve this result is *Hsiao Yao Wan*. Take eight pills three times daily from ovulation to menstruation.

SEVERE FLOODING CORRECTED NATURALLY

Becky, age 46, was desperate. She had been bleeding heavily for more than six weeks. She was weak, couldn't sleep, and was very tired. She worked at a very high-stress job and couldn't take time off. Just having to rush to the bathroom every hour was stressing her out. Bleeding by BHI slowed her bleeding, but not enough. More effective was Trillium combined with luvos, which stopped her bleeding in about four hours. But Becky still had problems. Blood loss had caused her to be severely anemic, her hair was falling out, she was having nightmares, and her hormones were still out of balance. She began a daily regimen of ProGest cream along with Female Tonic by Marco Pharma; by the time of her next period, she reported that her bleeding level was normal and she felt like her old self again.

For Debbie, also in her mid-forties, the problem was traced to overdosing on products that increased her estrogen levels. She was taking a number of hormone products, including soy, OstaB3, ProGest, and DHEA, which had worked to send her estrogen levels skyrocketing. She had been bleeding bright red blood for nearly three weeks and had become anemic and suffered from weakness, sleeplessness, and memory loss. The bleeding was slowed with Bleeding by BHI (one tablet four times daily), but not sufficiently. Trillium (used as directed on the label) stopped the bleeding after one day's use. To get her estrogen levels back in balance, she had to discontinue the soy and hormone products. She gradually added the ProGest back into her regimen (¼ teaspoon daily fourteen days out of the month). Her periods then became normal.

SEVERE CRAMPS RELIEVED

Indi had such severe cramps that she usually missed a day from work every month. Cyclease by Boiron and homeopathic *Mag phos* helped, but she was still uncomfortable. A constitutional homeopathic remedy specific for Indi's personality and constitution called *Veratrum* 30C (for cramps that radiate to the back and up the thighs) did the trick. Taking three pills four times daily during her period not only relieved her pain that month, but also made her cramps much more tolerable the following month. This is, in fact, how the right homeopathic remedy should work: not just symptomatically at the time but also over the long term.

In the homeopathic line, Cyclease by Boiron has many satisfied users. Follow label directions. *Mag-phos* 6X by Hyland's, a cell salt, is also good. Take four tablets three to four times daily from the day before until the second day of the menstrual period. If these don't work, consult a homeopath for an appropriate constitutional remedy.

MIGRAINE HEADACHES

See HEADACHES.

MONONUCLEOSIS

Infectious mononucleosis (mono) has been linked to chronic fatigue syndrome (CFS), a long-term condition with a similar disease pattern that affects women twice as often as men. The Epstein-Barr virus (EBV) has been suspected in both conditions, but it now seems clear that CFS cannot be caused exclusively by EBV or by any single recognized infectious disease agent.[1] In fact, the infectious nature of mono has also been questioned. Although it has been called "the kissing disease" and frequently occurs in adolescents and young adults living together, researchers have been unable to successfully transmit it from one volunteer to another.[2]

Symptoms of mono come on gradually. They include fever, sore throat, general discomfort, loss of appetite, and headache that can be severe. The lymph glands gradually swell, and the spleen and liver are frequently enlarged. The disease can last from one to eight weeks, after which the patient may feel abnormally weak and tired for weeks or months. Symptoms may then recur, or may develop into chronic fatigue syndrome, which can persist for years. At least 100,000 cases of mononucleosis occur in the United States each year.[3]

CONVENTIONAL TREATMENT

There is no conventional cure for mononucleosis. The usual recommendation is to wait it out, with bed rest, a soft diet, fluids, and aspirin. While antibiotics don't affect the course of the disease, they often get prescribed before the diagnosis has been clearly established. The result can be repeated courses of different and stronger antibiotics, with a corresponding weakening of the body's immune defenses.

> ### LINGERING MONO KICKED IN TWO WEEKS
>
> A 14-year-old girl who had contracted mono was still tired, pale, and missing school four months later. Dr. Walker started her on the series therapy Mononucleosis. Although the full course of treatment with Mononucleosis this series therapy takes a month, after two weeks on the remedy she was back in school and quite healthy. Her mother still drops in to Dr. Walker's office to express her gratitude for her daughter's remarkable recovery.

Natural Remedies

Homeopathic series therapy called Mononucleosis, by Staufen or Deseret, has consistently knocked mono out early and permanently. Homeopathic treatment is recommended even for people who have had mono years earlier, to keep the disease from developing into chronic fatigue syndrome. People are amazed at how much better they feel after taking this series therapy, even when they thought they were well before. Directions for use are on the label, but a practitioner should be consulted for products and guidance.

MORNING SICKNESS

See NAUSEA AND VOMITING.

MOTION SICKNESS

See NAUSEA AND VOMITING.

MULTIPLE CHEMICAL SENSITIVITY

Food and chemical sensitivities can mimic so many other diseases that they are often misdiagnosed and may be labeled emotional or psychosomatic conditions. Women seem to be more troubled by them than men, perhaps because their livers have more to deal with. All of the toxins that come into the body have to be broken down by the liver before they are excreted. The liver also has the task of breaking down hormones. In women, hormone levels are highest from ovulation to the menses, so the liver is hardest worked at that time. Stress makes the situation worse, by throwing the stress hormone cortisol and its breakdown products into the mix. When extraordinary environmental toxins and drugs are added to the normal metabolic load, the liver can be overwhelmed. The woman who is "environmentally ill" typically complains of being enormously tired, run down, and barely able to function, but medical testing finds nothing. Only after careful questioning is the problem revealed: the liver has become so overburdened with accumulated toxins that it can't "keep up." The diagnosis is established when detoxification measures reverse the problem.

Toxic chemicals that women are routinely exposed to include those in cosmetics, hair products, contraceptive creams, household cleaning products, chemically treated fabrics, and drugs. Other unsuspected immune-system assailants include pesticides sprayed in the house, on the lawn, or on a nearby golf course; formaldehyde and other chemical fumes from the upholstery in a new car, new carpeting, paint, fire retardants in a new mattress, or dry-cleaning fluid; petrochemicals in perfumes, dyes, plastics, synthetic rubber; the chlorine in swimming pools; and the metals and plastics in dental materials. Sensitivity to these stressors can produce not only the commonly recognized symptoms of allergy (rash, hives, nasal congestion, and gastrointestinal problems) but also more elusive symptoms, including depression, anxiety, "brain fog," fatigue, hyperactivity, attention deficit disorder, joint pains, migraines, irritable bowel syndrome, and food cravings.[1] An accumulation of toxic chemicals and metals in the body has also been linked to more serious diseases with unknown causes. Cases of Parkinson's disease, multiple sclerosis, lupus, and Alzheimer's disease have been traced to pesticide exposure, pharmaceuticals use, and heavy metals accumulated in brain tissues.

DETOXIFYING FROM CHEMICAL TOXINS

A new line of homeopathic remedies is specifically designed for detoxifying particular chemicals in the body. CompliMed's products include Enviro-Pest for pesticides, Enviro-Chem for chemicals, and Enviro-Met for heavy metals. Apex makes Exchem for chemical sensitivity. Deseret makes Addiclenz for sensitivity to food additives, Enviro-I and Enviro-II for environmental chemicals, Chemtox for chemicals in general, and a line of remedies called phenolics for specific chemical sensitivities. For example, one called Acetaldehyde is good for formaldehyde sensitivity—women who react to new carpet or car upholstery, or to the chemicals in treated fabric.

Molecular Biologics makes a remedy called Household Chemicals for people who are allergic to household cleaners. When used together, household cleaners can release chlorine gas that actually burns the lungs. Even the chlorine acquired from swimming in a chlorinated pool can be toxic and result in symptoms. Mediral makes Chlorex for chlorine detoxification, good for use after swimming in a chlorinated swimming pool.

A remedy called Beautex by Mediral can help you detoxify from the chemicals in hair and other beauty products. It's particularly good if you dye or perm your hair.

Sulphuricum-acidum 30C is a single homeopathic remedy that is good for detoxing from perfumes and exhaust fumes.

For all homeopathic detox remedies, begin slowly with one drop daily, increasing gradually to ten drops three times daily. If you experience cleansing reactions (nausea, headaches, and so on), decrease the dose.

DETOXIFYING FROM MOLDS AND FUNGI

An increasing but unrecognized problem is sensitivity to molds and fungi, which can linger after the rainy season and blow into the house from musty basements through heating and air-conditioning systems. A cluster of infant deaths from lung disease was recently

CHEMICAL POISONING AND FUME SENSITIVITY REVERSED HOMEOPATHICALLY

A woman sought help for symptoms following a good deed done for a neighbor, which involved cleaning off the growth of black mold and fungus on a closed-in patio. She had diluted chlorine bleach with water and applied it directly to the mold. Thereafter, her lungs and skin felt as if they had been burned. She also had become dizzy, lightheaded, and nauseous. She was given Chlorinex to eliminate excess chlorine from her system (beginning with one drop in half a glass of water daily, increasing gradually to ten drops three times daily), along with *Cantharis,* the homeopathic remedy for burns (three pills as needed for pain). When she returned several days later, she happily reported that her symptoms had disappeared.

A second woman was so heavily affected with "environmental illness" that she would feel quite sick if she merely breathed in someone's perfume. At night, she would sweat the perfume onto the sheets and the sheets would make her feel sick. As a result, she was severely limited in what she could do. She was afraid to be around other women who might be wearing perfume, and she was unable to walk into stores where perfumed candles were sold. When testing indicated that she was extremely toxic, she was given homeopathic *Sulphuricum acidum* 30C. She had to be detoxed very slowly; a dose of even one drop was too much for her. She had to put the drop in an 8-ounce glass of water and take a teaspoon of this dilution, working up to a whole drop at a time. Over the space of about a year, however, she became much less sensitive to environmental insults. She still has to be careful about what she eats or drinks, but she is relieved to be able to do ordinary activities now like going shopping and associating with other women.

linked to a toxic fungus found in the home.[2] There is no known conventional treatment, but homeopathic remedies are available that are specifically designed to address the problem. Mold and Fungus by Molecular Biologics is a good product. Another is Mold/Yeast/Dust by CompliMed. For both, take ten drops three times daily.

DETOXING FROM HEAVY METALS AND TOXIC DENTAL WORK

Another new line of combination homeopathic products is designed specifically for neutralizing heavy metal poisoning from dental work and other environmental exposures. Oratox by Deseret is recommended for two or three weeks after dental work. Other Deseret combination homeopathics include Enviroclenz and Metox. A remedy by Apex called Mercury Antitox helps clear mercury from body tissues after its removal from the teeth.

BAFFLING FAMILY AILMENT REVERSED

A mother complained that her whole family was continually sick. Despite the usual preventive measures, Sam, her 9-month-old baby, got repeated colds. On questioning, the mother said they were living in a condominium converted from an old hotel in Sun Valley. In its dilapidated former state, the roof had leaked water into the walls. The walls had been painted, but black mold was still evident. Worse, the family was using a humidifier every day. The windows would get wet with water from it, making the baby's room a breeding ground for toxic molds and fungi. Mold and Fungus by Molecular Biologics was recommended for the family, and all felt better after taking it. They felt better yet after they finally broke their lease and moved.

Other combination products are Dental Detox and Amalgam by PHP. Begin with a single drop in half a glass of water daily and work up to ten drops three times daily.

Homeopathic *Alumina* is also good for metal detoxification and is particularly indicated in cases of senile dementia. Take three pills three times daily.

For chemical and nutritional chelation techniques, see Chapter 5.

DETOXIFYING THE LIVER

Chinese doctors say that when the liver gets so overloaded that it can't do its job, the internal movements of the body stagnate. The Chinese patent remedy for moving liver stagnation is *Hsiao Yao Wan* (or *Xiao Yao Wan*). For use, consult a practitioner.

Particular foods can also stimulate drainage of the liver and help detoxify the system. Foods high in sulfur and selenium act as antioxidants, while foods high in inositol and choline help the liver eliminate excess fat. Good choices include watercress, mustard greens, red and black radishes, wheat grass juice, dandelions, parsley, apples, artichokes, beet and beet greens, carrots, Brussels sprouts, horseradish, garlic, cabbage, cranberries, Swiss chard, kale, and celery.

The Liver Cleanse Diet is a detox program specifically designed for cleaning the liver. For protocol, see Chapter 4.

Skin brushing, described in Chapter 5, is a detox technique recommended by naturopathic pioneer Dr. Bernard Jensen. It involves brushing your skin before bathing with a dry brush to remove dead skin, stimulate circulation, and help the body release toxins.

REVERSING AUTOIMMUNE DISEASE

Multiple sclerosis, fibromyalgia, lupus, rheumatoid arthritis, and other autoimmune diseases involve what *appears* to be an immune system gone awry and reacting to the body itself. The fact that drugs and poisons can induce the symptoms of these diseases, however, suggests that the body is actually reacting to toxins embedded in the system. There is evidence that petroleum and other toxic chemicals in makeup, skin-care products, and hair dyes are incorporated into the structure of cells along with fats. The body knows they are foreign invaders but can fight them only by fighting itself. The problem is not in the mechanisms of the body but in what it has been forced to deal with. Author Dr. Walker has reversed a number of cases of autoimmune disease using homeopathic detox remedies. See "Lupus" on page 170, "Fibromyalgia" on page 113, and "Multiple Sclerosis" on page 189.

ACETALDEHYDE SENSITIVITY REVERSED BY DETOXIFYING THE LIVER

Virginia, in her late twenties, was under tremendous stress. She'd recently started two new businesses and was doing well financially. She used some of her earnings to buy a new car, paint her bedroom, and buy a new bed. Suddenly, she got quite ill and couldn't sleep. No medical cause could be found. After questioning, her problems were determined to be stress and sensitivity to the chemicals in the new car upholstery, paints, and new mattress. The recommended treatment was the Chinese herbal formula *Hsiao Yao Wan* (or *Xiao Yao Wan*), the Liver Cleanse Diet, and a homeopathic remedy called Acetaldehyde by Deseret (beginning with one drop in half a glass of water, increasing slowly to ten drops three times daily). After two weeks on this program, Virginia reported that her energy level and sleep habits had returned to normal.

MULTIPLE SCLEROSIS

Multiple sclerosis (MS), a disease of the nerves of the brain and spinal cord, affects women twice as often as men. "Sclerosis" comes from the Greek word *skleros,* meaning hard. Multiple sclerosis refers to multiple areas of patchy scarring, or plaques, that result from destruction of myelin, a fatty insulation covering the nerve fibers. As the myelin sheath is destroyed, signals transmitted through the central nervous system are disrupted. MS is considered an autoimmune disease, in which the immune system appears to be attacking the body's own tissues—in this case the myelin sheath in the brain. The immune system is evidently unable to distinguish between pathogens and the body's own myelin and produces antibodies that attack the myelin. In effect, the body becomes allergic to itself.

The symptoms, severity, and course of MS vary widely. Inflammation of the nerves in the eye (optic neuritis) is often the first symptom. Vision becomes unclear or doubled, and there may be shimmering, pain, or nystagmus (involuntary jerking). Other early symptoms include fatigue, heaviness or clumsiness in the arms and legs, tingling sensations, poor coordination, and Lhermitte's sign (an episode in which bending the neck causes an electrical sensation down the back and legs). Late symptoms can include spasticity, imbalance, tremors, incontinence, constipation, sexual dysfunction, hearing loss, vertigo, facial pain, memory loss, and difficulty concentrating and problem solving. Very severe cases may result in paralysis. Depression is common, along with memory loss and other changes in mental function. Up to a third of patients have a very mild form of the disease, with little disability, no need for drugs, and a normal life expectancy.

Conventional medicine has no cure for MS and does not know its cause. It can only treat symptoms. The most likely antigens triggering the autoimmune response are thought to be viruses, but no one virus has emerged as a proven trigger. Genetic factors are known to play a role, since children of MS patients are thirty to fifty times as likely as other people to develop the disease.

CONVENTIONAL TREATMENT

No known medications can repair the nerve defects or change the course of the disease. Treatment for MS is limited to addressing symptoms, including fatigue, spasticity, bladder and bowel dysfunction, tremors, facial and other pain, sexual dysfunction, and emotional disorders. Corticosteroids including methylprednisolone, prednisone, and ACTH (which stimulates production of natural steroids) can reduce the underlying inflammation and the immune system's attack on its own nervous system. But steroids have substantial side effects and are usually restricted to severe attacks. Their long-term use can cause weight gain and facial fullness, hypertension, diabetes, osteoporosis, cataracts, intestinal bleeding, and increased susceptibility to infections. Side effects of steroids on the central nervous system, including sleeplessness, memory loss, anxiety, and depression, can be particularly problematic for MS patients. Oral prednisone can actually exacerbate the optic neuritis that is often an early symptom of multiple sclerosis. Steroids and ACTH do not improve the long-term course of the disease and can lose their effectiveness if overused. After taking steroids for a prolonged period of time, a serious condition known as adrenal insufficiency can develop if withdrawal isn't tapered very carefully to give the body a chance to recover its own ability to produce natural steroids.

MS RELIEVED WITH HOMEOPATHY

Lenora had been diagnosed with MS four years earlier. She had many health problems, all aggravated by the MS, and her condition was deteriorating rapidly. The numbness and tingling in her legs were getting worse and she had periods of complete paralysis in her left leg. Dr. Walker began her treatment by suggesting she switch to a gluten-free diet and the addition of supplements to build up her strength, including CoQ$_{10}$ (200 mg daily), spirulina (five tablets three times daily), evening primrose oil (2,600 mg at bedtime), and a good all-natural multivitamin. Lenora began the gluten-free diet and supplements with reluctance, but within three weeks, she was completely sold on the program. She said she was feeling better than she had for years. She was ready to proceed to phase two, which involved remedies to limit the damage caused to her nerves and reverse the numbness and tingling. The remedies included a constitutional remedy specific for her body and personality type, along with Myelin Basic Protein Drops by Molecular Biologics and MS Myelin by Jarrow, all taken according to label directions. In just a few weeks, Lenora called back to say how much better she was feeling. She had twice as much energy as previously and felt much stronger.

Betsy came for treatment for asthma, not knowing there was anything that could be done for her MS of almost eight years. Her case history revealed years of grief and heartbreak; she always wore a smile, however, not showing the world the deep sadness within. Betsy seemed to be subconsciously "holding her breath," creating her own asthma. She was given homeopathic remedies for her MS, but the steroids she was taking for her asthma prevented them from working as effectively as they might have. She was still very tired and had to take long naps daily. After a few months on the constitutional homeopathic remedies and a low-fat diet without wheat or dairy, however, her asthma was so much better that she was able to stop taking the steroids. The MS treatment then began working much better. It included Adrenal/Spleen by CompliMed, Deseret Serotonin drops, *Natrum muriaticum* (*Nat mur*), Myelin Basic Protein Drops, Myelin-MS, green tea extract, shark liver oil, lymphomysot, CoQ$_{10}$ (1 mg per pound of body weight), and homeopathic *Phosphorus* (a constitutional remedy specific for her body and personality type). Her MS symptoms are now greatly relieved. She has much less tingling and numbness, is stronger and more stable, and has more energy, often skipping her naps.

Jamie was newly diagnosed with MS, but she had been having problems for years. An examination traced the cause to her teeth, which had cracked so that mercury from her fillings was sitting directly on her gums. An experienced dentist removed her mercury fillings and repaired the poor-quality dental work. For several weeks prior to and after that dental revision, Jamie took homeopathic Amalgam by PCH and Protomer by Apex to help eliminate mercury residues from her body (beginning with a single drop in half a glass of water and increasing to ten drops three times daily for both). She watched her diet carefully and ate a lot of greens. She also increased her intake of nutritional supplements, including CoQ$_{10}$ and antioxidants. This regimen was followed by treatment with the Hyland's cell salt *Nat mur* 6X (four pills two to three times daily) and a constitutional homeopathic remedy specific for her. Jamie says she is now feeling better than she has for years.

ALTERNATIVE THEORIES

The conventional theory attributes autoimmunity to an error in the immune system itself. An alternative theory, however, points to drugs, chemicals, and heavy metals as likely culprits. When these toxins become incorporated into body cells, the immune system winds up attacking those cells along with the invaders. On that theory, the immune system is functioning as it was designed; the toxins are at fault. Environmental toxins linked to MS include mercury amalgam dental fillings (see below), vaccines, and the artificial sweetener aspartame. (See "Aspartame, Adverse Reactions To" on page 56.)

MS and Toxic Dental Work

A number of studies have linked MS to mercury amalgam dental fillings.[1] In a study reported by Colorado State University researcher Robert Siblerud in 1992, MS patients with amalgam fillings were compared to MS patients whose amalgams had been removed. The

MS RELIEVED BY DENTAL OVERHAUL

In December of 1990, *60 Minutes* featured the amalgam issue. Among other testimonials, a woman on the segment asserted that she had had multiple sclerosis so severe that she was unable to walk unassisted, could not hold a pencil, and could not speak properly. The day after she had five mercury amalgam dental fillings removed, her voice returned and she went out dancing. "It was that quick," she said.

former group was found to have had 33 percent more flare-ups of their symptoms during the previous year. They also significantly lower levels of red blood cells, hemoglobin, hematocrit, T+ lymphocytes, and T-8 suppressor cells (indicating lowered immunity).[2]

Siblerud points out that MS was first described by a French doctor in the mid-1830s, less than a decade after silver/mercury fillings were first promoted in Paris. In the late 1940s, acrodynia, a childhood version of multiple sclerosis, was traced to poisoning from the mercury in teething powder and laxatives; however, no one seems to have linked the adult form of the disease to the amalgam fillings that were the most widespread source of mercury in adults. It wasn't until 1966 that a Swiss neurologist recognized the possibility that amalgam fillings could be such a source. Mercury poisoning, like MS, is associated with depression and a general deterioration in mental health. Other mental symptoms attributed to mercury poisoning include lack of interest, poor concentration, forgetfulness, headaches, fear, excitability, indecisiveness, hopelessness, insomnia, delusions, and mania.[3]

The relationship between mercury amalgam and autoimmune disorders like MS has been explained by mercury's high affinity for the sulfhydryl groups in the molecules composing collagen and other tissues. When mercury alters these groups, "self" molecules appear as "non-self" and become targets for autoimmune recognition.[4]

Another theory for the link involves distortions in the brain's electromagnetic field caused by the "battery effect" arising between dissimilar metals in the teeth. The standard "silver" amalgam that composes 75 percent of all dental fillings is actually a collection of metals—silver, copper, tin, and zinc dissolved in a solution of mercury. An electrical current results when electrons move from one metal with a high electrical potential to another metal with a low electrical potential. When two or more dissimilar metals are placed together in the mouth, the metals interact with the liquid medium of the saliva—an alkaline fluid—to form an alkaline battery that produces a small electrical current. This current competes with the electromagnetic field generated by the brain.

Heavy Metal Detox

MS symptoms have been relieved by following careful protocols to replace mercury amalgam fillings in the teeth and by using detox therapies to remove heavy metals from the tissues. One effective detox technique is chelation.[5] For a discussion of chelation and protocols, see Chapter 5. Another option is sweat therapy to eliminate heavy metals through the skin. Interestingly, the original description of multiple sclerosis was that it was caused by the suppression of sweat.[6] One of the primary modes for excreting mercury is through the skin by sweating. Options include hot baths, saunas, steam baths, and perspiration through exercise.[7] Another detox treatment involving elimination through the skin is the "niacin flush," also discussed in Chapter 5. *Note: Detox therapies should be undertaken by people with MS and other serious conditions only under professional supervision.*

NATURAL REMEDIES

Homeopathic remedies have also shown dramatic effectiveness in relieving MS symptoms. A remedy specific for MS is *Natrum muriaticum* (*Nat mur*) 6X taken as a cell salt, four pills two to three times daily. Homeopathic remedies that help eliminate heavy metals from the tissues include Enviro-Met by CompliMed and Heavy Antitox by Apex. For others, see "Multiple Chemical Sensitivity" on page 185. For all homeopathic detox remedies, begin slowly with one drop in water daily, working up gradually to ten drops three times daily. Homeopathic remedies that help rebuild nerve tissue include Myelin Basic Protein Drops by Molecular Biologics, MS Myelin by Jarrow, and *Hypericum* 6X or 30X. *Note: MS is a long-term systemic disease that needs to be treated by an experienced homeopath.*

Nutritional support is also important for rebuilding nerve tissue. Antioxidants are highly recommended. Options include CoQ_{10} and oligomeric proanthocyanins or OPCs (1 mg per pound of body weight for each), green tea extract (fluoride- and caffeine-free), and greens and green supplements, including spirulina (take according to label directions). Sunlight and vitamin D have also been shown to help.

MUSCLE CRAMPS AND SPASMS

In young people, muscle pains and cramps tend to follow a day of physical exercise and are caused by an accumulation of lactic acid (a breakdown product of muscular activity), reducing oxygen in cells, or by microscopic tears in the muscles. In older women, however, muscle cramps are liable to be a symptom of menopause and of low serum calcium or potassium levels.

A charley horse is a cramp in the leg muscles (usually the calf), which typically occurs at night. In young people, it is usually caused by the sudden tearing of muscle fibers after excessive athletic activity, causing fluid retention in the leg. In older people, mineral deficiency hormone imbalance, calcium deposits in the muscles, or dehydration are more likely causes.

CONVENTIONAL TREATMENT

Drug treatment of common muscle cramps is not required. For frequent, severe muscle cramps, however, you should see a doctor because they may indicate a more serious illness.

NATURAL REMEDY ELIMINATES MUSCLE CRAMPS

Mandy, age 45, got excruciatingly painful muscle cramps each night before bed. Homeopathic *Cuprum metallicum* 6X was recommended for relief. She took three pills at 7 P.M. and again right before bed. If she felt muscle twinges, she took another dose. She had only slight muscle cramps for a short time after beginning the remedy, and then they eventually disappeared.

NATURAL REMEDIES

The homeopathic remedy for relieving leg spasms is *Cuprum metallicum* 6 or 30 (two pills three times daily). Effective combination homeopathics are also available. Dolisos makes one called Leg Cramps. Hyland's also makes one by that name. Follow label directions.

To relieve muscle cramps from low potassium levels, the solution is more potassium; to relieve muscle cramps due to insufficient calcium, the solution is to increase calcium intake, either in foods or from supplements. *Calc carb* 30X, the homeopathic alternative, has the advantage that it will not cause constipation like many calcium supplements will. Take three pills three times daily. To help relieve muscle spasms occurring at night, take your usual calcium supplements right before bed, or take potassium before bed. Emer'gen-C is a good source of potassium; take one or two packets nightly. A remedy that works over the space of about a half hour to relieve charley horses in the calves is to take 500 mg of magnesium at the onset of the cramp. Liquid magnesium supplements work faster than tablets.

NAIL HEALTH

Fingernails that are brittle and weak may be an inherited trait or may be due to misuse or to exposure to harsh chemicals (including too much nail polish remover). They may also be due to underlying biochemical imbalances. According to Chinese medical theory, the condition of your nails reflects the condition of your body. Their strength indicates the strength of your bones. Their shape may indicate the condition of your heart.

CONVENTIONAL TREATMENT

The nails can be painted cosmetically with nail hardener. This superficial solution, however, fails to address the underlying problem.

HOW TO STRENGTHEN NAILS FROM THE INSIDE OUT

Naturopathic and homeopathic doctors view fingernails that split, break, or are concave instead of convex as symptomatic of underlying nutritional deficiencies. Nutrients particularly important to nail health include calcium, silica, zinc, and protein.

A homeopathic combination formula called Calcium Absorption by Bioforce helps increase the amount of calcium absorbed from food and alters how the body uses the calcium it has. Take two pills three times daily or according to label directions.

A mineral product that increases nail calcium is BioSil by Jarrow. Six drops are taken daily in juice. Since one bottle contains 600 drops, it lasts for more than three months. By the time the bottle is gone, users report that their nails are longer and stronger than they have been in years.

With-in by Trace Minerals is a complete daily mineral supplement that emphasizes the growth of strong, healthy hair and nails. Follow label directions.

Another natural recipe for strengthening nails comes from the Golden Door Spa in Southern California. A whole egg (shell and all) is allowed to sit for twenty-five minutes in the juice of one lemon, which dissolves the eggshell. The eggshell residue is then removed and the juice is drunk. Taken three times a week, this remedy can make nails remarkably hard.

A secret of Flamenco guitar players who use their nails as guitar picks is to dissolve a packet of unflavored gelatin in juice and drink it. The gelatin is taken twice daily. Capsules called Beef Gelatin are also available from NOW Foods.

The herb horsetail, which contains silica, is another natural nail strengthener.

White spots on the nails can indicate a deficiency of zinc. Zinc levels can be checked with Metagenics' Zinc Tally. The homeopathic remedy is *Silicea* 12X or 30C (three pills three times daily).

For nail fungus, see "Fungal Infections" on page 116.

NAUSEA AND VOMITING

Nausea and vomiting usually represent the body's attempt to get rid of harmful bacteria or other toxins, but in women, these symptoms can also be linked to hormone changes. They can be symptoms of pregnancy or menopause, or side effects of birth control pills or hormone replacement therapy. Other common causes include motion sickness, stress, migraine headache, and allergies. Drugs can also cause nausea and vomiting, including cancer chemotherapy, antibiotics, certain heart medications, narcotic painkillers like codeine, and prescription asthma medications. Iron supplements and salt substitutes are other culprits.

Note: Nausea can indicate something more serious, including ulcers, colorectal cancer, diabetes, an impending heart attack, Crohn's disease, meningitis, mononucleosis, or gallstones. If you are vomiting up blood or have abdominal pain, headache, dizziness, fever, or a racing heartbeat, or if the vomiting lasts more than four hours, or if you are aged or debilitated, consult a doctor.

CONVENTIONAL TREATMENT

Nausea and vomiting that represent the body's attempt to get rid of harmful bacteria and other toxins should not be suppressed with drugs, since the result will be to retain harmful poisons in the system. There are drugs that will suppress vomiting, but they either require a prescription or the FDA permits their over-the-counter sale only to treat motion sickness. Motion sickness isn't caused by something your body is trying to get rid of, so suppressing it with drugs doesn't involve retaining potential poisons. The downside of over-the-counter motion sickness drugs is that they make you tired and drowsy.

NATURAL REMEDIES

For nausea and vomiting caused by indigestion, effective homeopathic remedies are available. One is *Carbo veg* 6C. Take three tablets every fifteen minutes. For severe upset, up to six doses may be taken.

For cramps, nausea, vomiting, and pain caused by food poisoning, try *Arsenicum album* 6X. Take two pills every fifteen minutes, up to six doses. Another option is *Salmonella* 200X. Often a single dose will relieve severe cramping and nausea.

In the herbal line, ginger may be taken for nausea, either as capsules or drunk as a tea.

Pill Curing is an excellent Chinese herbal remedy for settling the stomach after a large meal or when the food feels stuck in your midsection. Take one or two vials after eating or as needed. This remedy can also effectively quell motion sickness without making you drowsy.

Other effective motion sickness remedies are ginger and a Chinese formula called *Bao Ji Wan*. Chinese patent remedies are made by different companies and are available at Chinese pharmacies or from Eastern medical practitioners. Follow directions on the box.

A particularly good homeopathic remedy for motion sickness is Travel Sickness by Dolisos. Take two pills three to four times daily.

The Sea Band is an elastic band that is placed on the wrist. It effectively relieves motion sickness by putting pressure on one of the major acupuncture points of the body.

Safe, Effective Remedies for Morning Sickness

Homeopathic remedies are the only remedies that can be recommended during pregnancy with absolute confidence in their safety. Homeopathic remedies are safe because they work on a vibrational rather than on a chemical level. They are so dilute that at higher strengths, they consist of nothing but energized water. (See Chapter 3.) The one homeopathic remedy for which caution is advised is *Pulsatilla*. In theory, it could precipitate a miscarriage if something were wrong with the fetus, although this hasn't been proven.

A great homeopathic remedy for morning sickness is *Symphoricarpus racemosa* 12X or 30C. Take ten drops before bed as needed, to relieve symptoms in the morning. Another effective remedy that is quite safe during pregnancy is a homeopathic combination by Molecular Biologics called Nausea. Follow label directions. Like with all homeopathic remedies, when the discomfort is gone, the drops should be discontinued.

No herbs should be used during pregnancy with the possible exception of red raspberry leaf, which can be sipped as a tea during morning sickness and is good for use during the last six weeks of pregnancy to strengthen and tone the uterus and prepare it for giving birth.

Other Helpful Tips

Contrary to popular belief, liquids—especially carbonated drinks—are hard to keep down on an upset stomach. A cracker or other dry food is better. You can drink colas or ginger ales, but they should be flat, at room temperature, and taken in small sips. Other good fluids are apple and grape juices drunk at room temperature. Citrus juices are not as good, since their acidity can irritate the stomach and they often contain solid pulp that is hard to digest.[1]

MORNING SICKNESS RELIEVED NATURALLY

Terri had a severe case of morning sickness. She was sick all day and losing time from work. *Symphoricarpus* followed by Nausea drops completely took her nausea away in only two days. She remained on the *Symphoricarpus* for a week or so, then discontinued all remedies and was no longer troubled with nausea.

NERVOUSNESS, STAGE FRIGHT, AND LACK
OF SELF-CONFIDENCE

More than ever, women are coming to center stage and voicing their opinions in public. But nervousness can ruin a speech, an artistic performance, or a business presentation. Women conditioned from birth to be dependent and insecure may have trouble feeling their own self-worth and demonstrating their competence in other situations as well. Women are naturally more shy, sensitive, and emotional than men.

CONVENTIONAL TREATMENT

Valium calms the nerves but can inhibit performance and has other side effects, including drowsiness, dizziness, and incoherence. Some performers take the blood pressure–lowering drug propanalol before going on stage and report that it works, but it too is a prescription drug with side effects, slowing the heartbeat, decreasing breathing, and aggravating asthma. Prozac and other SSRIs will calm the nerves but must be taken for weeks before having an effect and have other downsides (detailed under "Depression" on page 95).

NATURAL REMEDIES

Homeopathic remedies can help you overcome stage fright without side effects. *Gelsemium* retunes the emotions on a vibrational level. Another effective product is the combination homeopathic remedy Nervousness by Natra-Bio. For people who blush or embarrass easily, homeopathic *Ambra grisea* 30C can be a face saver. Take three pellets three times daily.

Rescue Remedy, a Bach flower remedy, is also excellent for calming the nerves. Put four drops in half a glass of water and sip throughout the day.

Homeopathic and Bach flower remedies are also available that can help boost self-esteem and self-confidence. The Bach flower remedy for self-confidence is Larch. Add four drops to a 16-ounce bottle of water and sip throughout the day. A good homeopathic

---

CONFIDENCE REGAINED WITH HOMEOPATHICS

Alice, a 38-year-old massage therapist, wanted to give classes using her new herbal and massage expertise, but she was afraid to get up in front of a group. With the help of *Gelsemium* she got the confidence she needed to begin lecturing and become a success with the people in her local area.

Sixteen-year-old Jamie was so terrified about her impending piano recital rehearsal that she couldn't hold her hands steady on the keys. She took Nervousness, fifteen drops hourly for several hours before the performance, and played her complicated piece flawlessly at the recital.

Pam was quite unhappy with her job and her marriage, but she lacked the confidence to speak up or stand up for herself. She was easily confused and controlled, and her memory was poor. She asked the same questions over and over. Homeopathic *Brita carb* 1M, a constitutional remedy specific for her personality and body type, made Pam more decisive and less confused. She took charge of her life and began making changes in it.

and essential flower combination is Self-Esteem by Apex. Constitutional remedies specific to the patient can also help.

NIGHT SWEATS

See MENOPAUSE AND PERIMENOPAUSE.

OBESITY

See OVERWEIGHT.

OSTEOARTHRITIS

See ARTHRITIS.

OSTEOPOROSIS

Osteoporosis, or age-related bone loss, is a condition in which calcium is lost faster than the body can replace it, leading to weak, porous bones that are subject to fracture. Bone loss speeds up during the first three to seven years after menopause, then slows down again. The increased loss at menopause is attributed to the loss of hormones necessary to retain calcium. Osteoporosis causes an estimated 1.3 million fractures annually in the United States, at a national cost approaching $10 billion. The most damaging consequence is hip fractures, particularly in elderly women, who are seven times as likely to suffer from them as elderly men. Each year, 60,000 women die within six months of their fractures, and the numbers are going up. For the survivors, coping with hip fractures may require care in a nursing home.[1] Among other risk factors for osteoporosis are a low vitamin D and calcium intake, a family history of osteoporosis (fractures or rounding of the upper back), early menopause or hysterectomy/ovariectomy, and low hormone levels.

CONVENTIONAL TREATMENT

Until recently, the only FDA-approved drug treatment for osteoporosis was estrogen therapy. But estrogen is not a cure. The package insert for Premarin (the most popular prescription estrogen) concedes that "[t]here is no evidence that estrogen replacement therapy restores bone mass to premenopausal levels." At best, it just slows down bone loss; and new research questions that benefit for older women. (See fuller discussion in Chapter 2.) The dose considered necessary to slow bone loss is higher than the dose needed to control other postmenopausal symptoms, increasing the breast cancer risk that comes with synthetic hormone replacement. Moreover, to keep receiving any benefits estrogen may provide, it has to be taken for life.[2] Researchers have found that within four years of discontinuing estrogen replacement therapy (ERT), there is no detectable difference in bone mineral content between women who have never taken the drug and those who began treatment but gave it up.[3] Even if you keep taking estrogen, it's not clear that it will keep reducing bone loss. A review in *The American Journal of Medicine* concluded that "administration of this hormone six years or more after menopause may no longer be effective."[4]

A new line of designer estrogens called selective estrogen receptor modulators (SERMs), including raloxifene (Evista) and tamoxifen (Nolvadex), has been promoted as reducing the risk of osteoporosis without some of the downsides of conventional estrogen replacement therapy, including irregular uterine bleeding. But the drugs do come with side effects. Tamoxifen increases the rate of endometrial cancer in postmenopausal women by 300 to 400 percent. It can also result in troublesome hot flashes and serious "thromboembolic" events in which blood clots break free inside blood vessels and cause emergency circulation problems that can be life threatening. For that reason, current research is directed at raloxifene. Although raloxifene also increases hot flashes and thromboembolic events, researchers hope that it does not increase the risk of endometrial cancer.[5] That too is questionable, however, since Evista caused ovarian cancer in laboratory mice in studies by its own manufacturer, Eli Lilly and Co. Based on that data, Dr. Samuel S. Epstein, Professor of Environmental Medicine, University of Illinois School of Public Health and author of several books on cancer, has called for its worldwide withdrawal from the market.[6]

As for the effects of SERMs on the bones, in a large trial involving women with osteoporosis, raloxifene significantly decreased the incidence of spinal fractures but did not have a significant effect on other fractures. That means it wasn't much help in preventing the hip fractures that are most likely to incapacitate older women.[7]

Two other drugs currently approved by the FDA for treating osteoporosis are alendronate (Fosamax), a nonhormonal product, and a salmon calcitonin nasal spray (Miacalcin). Again, however, these pharmaceutical options are not very effective and are quite expensive. In one review of osteoporosis treatment trials, bone density in the lumbar spine *decreased* by 0.2 percent in patients using nasal spray calcitonin. Adding calcium supplements improved these results, but only moderately: bone density increased by 1.15 percent.[8] Alendronate has been found to increase bone mineral density by 7 to 8 percent over a three-year period, but it does this by killing the osteoclasts, the cells that tear down old bone. The old bone is left, but no new bone is built. Four years later, the bone is actually weaker, even though it is more dense. The drug is also expensive and comes with side effects. Alendronate and calcitonin are more than five times as expensive as Premarin, which already costs up to $30 per month.[9] Provera (synthetic progesterone) has also been shown to modestly increase bone mass, but it too comes with a long list of side effects, as discussed in Chapter 2.

NATURAL REMEDIES

Natural Hormone Therapy

While the increased bone loss of elderly women is generally attributed to loss of estrogen after menopause, new research suggests that progesterone is actually the missing catalyst. Progesterone, like estrogen, is produced by the ovaries and falls off at menopause. An eight-year study conducted by John R. Lee, M.D., reported in the *International Clinical Nutri-*

tion Review in 1990 and in *Medical Hypotheses* in 1991, showed that *natural* progesterone not only retards age-related bone loss but actually reverses it. Within a three-year period, bone density was brought back to safe levels in 100 percent of the patients treated, something not even estrogen therapy can do.[10] The product used in this study, however, was not the synthetic progesterone found in pharmaceutical hormone replacement therapy. It was a natural progesterone cream (ProGest) derived from Mexican yams. The women rubbed the cream on their skin at bedtime for twelve days out of the month (or the last two weeks of estrogen use, if estrogen was being used). One-third to one-half of a one-ounce jar of progesterone cream was used per month, applied to the softer skin under the arms or on the neck and face, alternating sites each night.

The women were also instructed to take the following measures known to counteract bone loss: they were to get sufficient exercise, vitamins, and minerals, including calcium; eat a low-protein diet high in calcium-rich leafy green vegetables and low-fat cheeses; avoid cigarettes, excess phosphates (especially in soft drinks), excess protein, and certain drugs (excess thyroid hormone and corticosteroids); and limit alcohol intake. The following nutritional supplements were taken: vitamin D (350–400 IU), vitamin C (2,000 mg in divided doses), beta-carotene (15 mg or 25,000 IU), and calcium (800–1000 mg through diet and/or supplements). In addition, a modest exercise routine was prescribed (twenty minutes per day, or thirty minutes three times a week). While these other factors were necessary, said Dr. Lee, they were not sufficient to explain the impressive results, which were unequaled in studies not using natural progesterone.[11]

Expected bone loss in the women over a three-year period was 4.5 percent. At best, estrogen would have slowed this loss down, but the natural progesterone regimen actually put bone back on. In the sixty-three tested patients, bone density over three years increased by an average of 15.4 percent—double the results of the best of the prescription osteoporosis drugs. The women's bones typically got 10 percent thicker in the first six to twelve months and increased 3 to 5 percent every year thereafter. Several patients' bone densities jumped 20 to 25 percent during the first year. This increase occurred regardless of age. In fact, the patients who started out the worst improved the most. Bone density also increased regardless of whether estrogen supplements accompanied the progesterone.

In many of the women, bone density eventually stabilized at the levels of healthy 35-year-olds; in all of them, it stabilized at safe levels. Osteoporotic bone pains were relieved, muscle and bone strength and mobility increased, osteoporotic fractures dropped to zero, and regular fractures healed unusually well. The women also lost weight and had more energy, and many volunteered the observation that their lost libido (sex drive) had returned. Blood pressures dropped, and there were anticancer effects. Unlike in studies with synthetic progesterone, cholesterol levels did not rise. In fact, no unwanted side effects were reported.[12]

Besides estrogen and progesterone, other hormones decline with age, including DHEA and growth hormone. Research in this area is new, so there are no long-term studies establishing the effects of supplementation on bone density. Studies do show, however, that blood levels of DHEA are significantly correlated with bone density. Very low blood levels are seen in patients with osteoporosis.[13] For women, the hormone precursor pregnenolone is recommended along with DHEA to help keep hormone levels in balance. See a qualified practitioner for dosages.

Human growth hormone (hGH) and testosterone are also important in bone remodeling. Growth hormone is a popular nutritional supplement now being touted for everything from keeping you young to helping your skin and nails to improving your sex drive. The product is quite expensive, however, and the results may not live up to the claims. A cheaper and more natural option is to take homeopathic remedies that stimulate the body's own production of these hormones. Two excellent products are homeopathic Growth Hormone Plus and Hormone Combination. Both are made by Deseret Biologicals and are available at homeopathic pharmacies or from practitioners.

Estrogen is also available in natural form, as a cream derived from plants. Bezwecken makes OstaDerm and other plant estrogen products that are safe and effective. The recommended OstaDerm dosage is ¼ to ½ teaspoon once or twice daily. The products are available at health food stores and pharmacies or from practitioners.

Calcium Supplementation

Supplementing with calcium alone is not sufficient to prevent bone loss.[14] But getting sufficient calcium is important, and the type of calcium used is important. Only a few studies have shown any effect of calcium supplementation on bone density; in those few studies, the calcium sources were particularly bioavailable (available for use by the body).[15]

Calcium carbonate is a cheap form of calcium contained in certain antacids, including Tums and Maalox, which are advertised as filling women's calcium requirements. The problem is that calcium carbonate is an inorganic form of the mineral that is only about 5 percent absorbed, and stomach acid is needed to metabolize calcium, so taking it with something that neutralizes stomach acid further impairs its absorption. Inorganic calcium that is not absorbed may simply settle out in the joints, contributing to arthritis. Other forms of calcium that are inorganic and poorly absorbed include calcium from oyster shells and dolomite (a rock).[16]

A more bioavailable source of calcium is animal bone. The ideal bone meal is a cold-processed product that has not been heated above 125°F. A downside of bone meal is that it may be contaminated with lead. This problem is avoided, however, in a highly bioavailable bone calcium called microcrystalline hydroxyapatite compound (MCHC), the organic protein calcium matrix found in the raw young bones of cattle and sheep raised on insecticide- and pesticide-free pastures. It differs from bone meal in that it is not heated in the reduction process or washed with chemical solvents. In studies comparing MCHC with calcium gluconate and a placebo in the treatment of osteoporosis (age-related bone loss), only the MCHC groups experienced a significant increase in cortical bone.[17] Bone-Up by Jarrow Formulas is a particularly good product. Cal Apatite by Metagenics is also good.

Even these products, however, may not be absorbed well in huge quantities. It is best to take 500–1,000 mg of bioavailable calcium along with a calcium-rich diet and a product that aids the body in assimilating the calcium it takes in. Calcium Absorption by Bioforce is a homeopathic remedy effective for this purpose (take two or three pellets three times daily). Red Spruce by Dolisos is a gemmotherapy that helps increase calcium absorption (take fifty drops in half a glass of water each morning). Both are available at health food stores.

BONES STRENGTHENED WITH NATURAL REMEDIES

Gaye, in her early fifties, was quite concerned because her mother had had osteoporosis, and a bone density test done by her doctor had found Gaye's bone density to be very low. Dr. Walker recommended Bone-Up and ProGest cream. Eight months later, Gaye went for another bone density test and was pleased to report that her calcium was now in the normal range for her age. The doctor was duly impressed and told her to continue whatever she was doing.

Marsha, age 45, had been diagnosed with osteopeny, a rare form of osteoporosis in which bone density is lost in the hips, causing the bones to break very easily. She began using ProGest cream, Bone-Up, and Calcium Absorption. A year later, to her delight and the surprise of her doctor, a bone scan showed that not only had her bone loss ceased but also that her bone density had increased a significant 3 percent.

Other Nutrients Important for Bone Health

Besides calcium, vitamin D is necessary to aid calcium absorption, and magnesium is necessary to help move calcium out of the bloodstream and into the skeleton.

The typical recommendation for vitamin D is 400 IU per day, but neither foods nor vitamin supplements are ideal sources. Vitamin D is produced in the body only after exposing the skin to sunlight, which initiates a series of reactions.[18] The vitamin D produced commercially, called vitamin D_2 (ergocalciferol), is not the same as the vitamin D manufactured by the body (vitamin D_3). Studies show that blood levels of the vitamin are only weakly correlated with dietary intake. A much stronger correlation has been shown with exposure to sunlight.[19] Fortunately, to satisfy your vitamin D requirement, you needn't stay out in the sun long enough to risk skin cancer. Researchers at Tufts University have shown that in the summer, minimum vitamin D requirements are met by exposure of just the hands, face, and arms for ten to fifteen minutes a day, three times a week. These recommendations were made specifically for the elderly.[20]

Magnesium is also important for bone health. When magnesium is out of balance with calcium, the calcium you eat may never make it to your bones. Guy E. Abraham, M.D., a research gynecologist in Torrance, California, succeeded in increasing bone density in postmenopausal women by 11 percent in one year, by *decreasing* their calcium intakes to 500 mg per day and *increasing* their magnesium intakes to 600–1,000 mg per day. These results were significantly better than the results of studies involving calcium alone.[21] Magnesium is abundant in whole grains, beans, nuts, seeds, and vegetables, but fertilizers reduce its content in the soil, and sugar and alcohol increase its excretion through the urine. Although the RDA for magnesium is only 350 mg for women of all ages, Dr. Mildred Seelig, Executive President of the American College of Nutrition, suggests that older people who eat a good diet can benefit from magnesium supplements of 700–800 mg per day.[22]

Dietary and Lifestyle Factors

Women in some non-Western cultures manage to escape the increased rate of hip fractures experienced by Western women after menopause, although they don't take estrogen and their calcium intakes are below those of American women.[23] The solid bones of non-Western women have been attributed to regular exercise, low intakes of protein and meat, and a high intake of potassium. A too-high protein intake leaches calcium from the bones.[24] A too-low protein intake is also hazardous, however, because protein is necessary for the liver to detoxify estrogen.[25] The RDA for protein for women is 44 grams.

Excess phosphorus has also been linked to bone loss. Each phosphorus atom in the bloodstream must be accompanied by a calcium atom. The calcium pulled out of the blood to pair up with this phosphorus is replaced with calcium from the bones. Phosphorus is also antagonistic to potassium, a mineral found in the unprocessed vegetables, fruits, and whole grains that are abundant in traditional non-Western diets. Calcium- and potassium-robbing phosphorus is supplied in the Western diet by meat and by a worse offender, the carbonated soft drink. To protect your bones, avoid soft drinks and be moderate with your meat intake.

Women in underdeveloped countries also tend to get more exercise than Western women. Clinical studies show that weight-bearing exercise like brisk walking, jogging, low impact aerobics, and trampoline-jumping improves the density of the bones and prevents osteoporosis, among other benefits (including forestalling cardiovascular disease and preventing or relieving obesity, muscle weakness, and depression).[26]

THINGS TO AVOID

Besides excess protein and phosphates, bone loss has been linked to fluoridated water and to mercury amalgam dental fillings.[27] These can be avoided by drinking bottled water and seeking the help of a "biological" or holistic dentist in having fillings changed to more biocompatible materials.[28]

Drugs that cause dizziness, sedation, and fuzzy thinking can also be responsible for the falls that produce fractures. In one study, older people were found to be about twice as likely to suffer hip fractures if they were taking tranquilizers with long half-lives, such as flurazepam (Dalmane); tricyclic antidepressants, including amitriptyline (Elavil), doxepin (Sinequan), and imipramine (Tofranil); or antipsychotics, including thioridazine (Mellaril), haloperidol (Haldol), and chlorpromazine (Thorazine).[29] Diuretics can also contribute to hip fractures, by prompting elderly women to get up to the bathroom in the middle of the night. For natural alternatives, see individual disease categories, including "Insomnia" on page 162, "Depression" on page 95, "Anxiety and Panic Disorders" on page 46, and "High Blood Pressure" (Hypertension) on page 142.

Other drugs linked to bone loss are aluminum-containing antacids. Aluminum displaces calcium from the bones, causing them to be brittle and to break easily, and antacids

BONE DEMINERALIZATION LINKED TO ANTACIDS

The hazards of antacids were suggested in a study in the *Annals of Internal Medicine* involving two 42-year-old women with liver failure requiring liver transplants. Both women had serious bone demineralization, which was linked on x-ray examination to heavy deposits of aluminum in their bones. Both also had long histories of taking aluminum hydroxide-containing antacids (Amphojel and Mylanta) for the prevention of peptic ulcer. One woman died before a liver donor could be located. Bone staining at autopsy was strongly positive for aluminum. In the other woman, bone pain completely disappeared after the aluminum was removed by chelation therapy, a treatment involving the injection of a solution that chelates, or binds, heavy metals, which are then excreted in the urine. (See Chapter 5 for a detailed discussion.)[30]

inhibit calcium absorption by neutralizing stomach acid, raising the pH of the stomach. Calcium can be absorbed only in its soluble ionized form, which requires a low pH. For a detailed discussion of antacids and their natural alternatives, see "Digestive Problems" on page 104.

OVARIAN CANCER

See CANCERS, HORMONAL.

OVARIAN CYSTS

Ovarian cysts are fluid-filled sacs that develop in or on the ovaries. They result when the liver is not breaking hormones down properly or hormone levels are otherwise out of balance. They come and go and are usually cyclic, getting worse around ovulation or before the period. A cyst found by ultrasound may be gone two weeks later. The pain of an ovarian cyst is usually limited to the left or right side and is often confused with appendicitis. Ovarian cysts are common near menopause, when ovulation is erratic. The ovaries produce progesterone with ovulation; without ovulation, the hormones become unbalanced.

CONVENTIONAL TREATMENT

The conventional medical treatment of ovarian cysts is immediate abdominal surgery, on the theory that the cysts might rupture or, in the rare case, that they may be cancerous. The problem with surgery is that new cysts tend to continue to form, and the procedure leaves painful scar tissue and can result in infertility. A recent study from Italy found that more than one-third of women with ovarian cysts don't need surgery or even a biopsy. The problem spontaneously regresses without any medical intervention.[1] Those figures were for women who got no treatment at all. If they were to get alternative treatment to balance their hormone levels, many more would probably find that their cysts spontaneously regressed.

NATURAL REMEDIES

Alternative practitioners maintain that the problem to be attacked is not the cyst itself but an underlying hormone imbalance. Correcting this imbalance can make cysts go away for good.

John Lee, M.D., author of *What Your Doctor May Not Tell You About Menopause,* asserts that most ovarian cysts are due to failed ovulation and can be successfully treated with natural progesterone. Each ovary acts as if the other is supplying progesterone and takes a rest.

A product called Female Tonic by MarcoPharma is also quite effective for balancing the hormones. Follow label directions. Acupuncture and hormone-balancing herbs can help as well. (See "Menopause and Perimenopause" on page 174.)

Deseret makes a homeopathic progesterone and a homeopathic estrogen that may be used to restore hormone balance, the choice depending on which of those two counter-

THE AUTHORS' OWN EXPERIENCE

Both authors of this book were at one time advised to get hysterectomies for cysts on the ovaries and for fibroid tumors. Both pursued natural therapies instead and have had no problems since.

Dr. Walker was diagnosed by ultrasound with a large fibroid tumor and cysts on her ovaries at the tender age of 33. When her doctor recommended a hysterectomy, she went to an older, more conservative doctor for a second opinion. He frankly advised her that if she did nothing, she would probably be fine. Even if the cysts burst, which was unlikely, the fluid would merely be reabsorbed into her body. She decided to try alternative remedies before resorting to surgery. Homeopathy, acupuncture, and Chinese herbs caused both the fibroid and the cysts to be painlessly reabsorbed. The cysts went away without bursting and Dr. Walker avoided a hysterectomy. For Ellen Brown's success story, see "The Authors' Own Experiences" under "Hysterectomy" on page 153.

balancing hormones is in short supply. If you aren't sure, see a homeopath or other practitioner.

Whether your hormone levels are right for you can't always be determined from a blood test. What is "normal" varies considerably. Women with obvious symptoms of hormone imbalance often report that their doctors drew blood and said their levels were in the normal range. The balance between estrogen and progesterone levels is more important than absolute numbers. Symptoms typically result when estrogen levels are too high relative to progesterone levels. If your body usually has high hormone levels and they suddenly drop, you will not "feel like yourself." Problems can also result when either hormone is given in synthetic pill form without the other. Natural progesterone can be converted to estrogen by the body as needed, but synthetic progesterone doesn't convert well and can throw the hormones out of balance. (See Chapters 1 and 2.)

For recurring cysts, homeopathic series therapy called Ovarialcystom is available from the German company Staufen. Use as directed on the box.

For relieving the pain of ovarian cysts, homeopathic *Phosphorus* works well. Take two pills two to three times daily as needed for pain.

OVERWEIGHT

A study reported in 1997 found that 35 percent of Americans are overweight enough to be unhealthy. This figure is up from 25 percent in 1980. Besides the clinically obese (those 20 percent or more over their ideal weights), millions of people keep bingeing, dieting, and bingeing again, in a vicious cycle that has made dieting a $35 billion industry.[1] Women have a harder time losing weight than men do, for several reasons, including the following:

1. Women have slower metabolisms than men, due to a lower muscle-to-fat ratio. The less muscle tissue there is, the slower the resting metabolic rate (RMR) will be; the lower the RMR is, the fewer calories will be burned at rest.

2. Women have far higher levels of estrogen, a fat-building hormone. Excess estrogen production can cause excess weight gain.

3. Women's typical diets are more likely than men's to cause weight gain. Eating the wrong foods can cause overproduction of estrogen and insulin, both of which can cause weight gain.[2]

CONVENTIONAL TREATMENT

The medical trend is to view obesity as a disease that should be treated with drugs. One weight-loss drug after another has hit the market with much fanfare, only to be pulled off the shelves when their dangerous side effects have become known. In the 1930s, when the weight-loss craze was ushered in with the invention of the bathroom scales, the drug of the day was a derivative of the industrial poison dinitrophenol. Besides weight loss, it could cause rashes, fever, blindness, and sometimes death.[3] In the 1960s, you could readily get a prescription for amphetamines if you wanted to lose a few pounds. But the psychoticlike side effects and addiction potential of these drugs, as well as their failure to take pounds off long term, eventually made doctors very circumspect in their use.

In 1996, the FDA approved dexfenfluramine (Redux), the first prescription weight-loss drug to be approved in twenty-three years. Redux was a variation of another diet drug, fenfluramine (Pondimin), which had been on the market since the 1970s. Pondimin created a stir only in the 1990s, however, when a study showed weight-loss benefits in combination with a third drug, phentermine (Ionamin, Fastin, Adipex-P), a combination popularly called Fen-Phen. Fen-Phen is chemically similar to amphetamines, while Redux is chemically similar to the antidepressant drug Prozac. By 1997, when more than 2 million Americans had taken Redux and more than 6 million had taken Pondimin, the drugs were suddenly pulled from the shelves after the FDA analyzed heart tests on 291 dieters using them. Although most had no symptoms, almost a third of these users had damaged heart valves.[4]

Over-the-counter diet drugs are weaker than amphetamines but have ingredients with similar chemical structures and reactions in the body. They typically contain combinations of phenylpropanolamine (PPA), ephedrine derivatives, and caffeine. They stimulate the sympathethic nervous system, the "flight-or-fight" emergency system; in high doses, they can produce psychoticlike side effects and hypertensive crises, similar to the effects of amphetamines. In one reported case, a 35-year-old woman developed a brain hemorrhage after taking only one tablet of the popular over-the-counter diet aid Dexatrim, Extra Strength.[5] The ephedrine has now been taken out of Dexatrim, and phenyl-propanolamine was recently taken off the market, but the stimulants in over-the-counter options remain suspect.

NATURAL REMEDIES

Natural Uppers: Ephedra/Ma Huang

Though less hazardous than the pharmaceutical variety, some herbal diet pills also carry risks. The natural stimulant ephedrine (under the names Ma huang, ephedra, or epitonin) has replaced amphetamines not only in "natural" diet aids but also in herbal combinations that are advertised as producing a "natural high." These herbal combinations are often popular among young people. But overdosing on natural ephedra, as with synthetic ephedrine, can raise blood pressure and has been linked to heart attack, stroke, and sudden death. This has led the FDA to consider banning or limiting the use of all ephedrine products both as weight-loss and as bodybuilding aids. New York and Florida banned their sale after a 20-year-old college student died following an overdose of an ephedrine-containing herbal product called Ultimate Xphoria.[6] Opponents of the ban, however, counter that herbal ephedra is safer than the synthetic ephedrine and amphetamine products it has replaced both as diet aids and as "street drugs," and that the key is simply moderation.

For weight loss, both ephedra and caffeine are natural thermogenic agents, increasing body temperature, circulation, and the burning of fat and suppressing appetite. A Swedish study comparing obese women given caffeine and ephedrine three times daily with women given a placebo found that the caffeine/ephedrine group lost significantly more fat and maintained more lean body weight after eight weeks.[7] But taking ephedra for long periods isn't advised. Ephedra depletes certain chemicals in the brain, causing depression. Like with amphetamines, the dieter initially feels enormously energetic; however, when the brain chemicals have been depleted, she can crash overnight, becoming physically and emotionally drained.

Other Herbal Options

Safer herbal dieting products that are reported to be effective include herbal Fen-Phen, which consists of amino acids, and HCA, a plant extract (*Garcinia cambogia*), which is found in Citrimax and other products. Directions are on the labels. Citrimax works well for a woman who is normally lean but has gained a little extra weight. Results require patience. Typically not much effect is noticed for the first three to four weeks; then, you suddenly start eating less and consequently lose weight.

Homeopathic Diet Aids

Homeopathic remedies can also help with weight loss. Weight OFF by Professional Complementary Health suppresses the appetite. Metaboslim by CompliMed is said to speed up metabolism and burn calories faster. For both, take ten drops three times daily. To correct depressed thyroid function, which can be a cause of weight gain, CompliMed suggests taking homeopathic Thyroid in combination with Metaboslim. Thyroid normalizes thyroids that are either underactive or overactive. For many overweight people, the problem seems to be a very deep *Candida* infection that causes them to crave sugar and to overeat. For them, homeopathic Candida 1M by Deseret can take away the sugar cravings, changing their eating habits on a subconscious level. The dosage is two drops daily.

DIET-RELATED DEPRESSION RELIEVED

For months, Sherry had been taking E'ola, a popular multilevel marketing product containing ephedra, to keep her weight down. Her weight was under control and her life was going well, yet she was so depressed she was thinking about suicide. When it was suggested that the ephedra was her problem, she said she was afraid to stop taking it for fear she would put on weight and become even more depressed. But she was finally persuaded, and after two weeks without the drug, her depression went away as suddenly as it had appeared.

WEIGHT LOST WITH HOMEOPATHIC REMEDIES

Marta, age 32, would not have been considered overweight, but she was carrying an extra 10 pounds around her middle that made her feel uncomfortable and that she couldn't seem to lose. The homeopathic remedy Weight OFF in combination with Metaboslim helped redistribute her weight. Although the difference on the scales was a mere 10 pounds, her whole body shape was different. She looked and felt so good that she referred many other women to Dr. Walker for Metaboslim. These women also reported good results.

Alyce was quite unhappy with her weight and decided to try homeopathic remedies. She took Weight OFF drops, Metaboslim, and homeopathic Candida 1M. In the first few months, she noticed little difference but was determined to persist. By the third month, she lost 20 pounds. Thereafter, her weight loss continued fairly rapidly. Once the remedies started working, they *really* worked. Overall, she lost about one-third of her body weight, putting her at a weight she felt was good for her. This weight loss was effortless—it just seemed to fall off—and she's like a different person now. She is not stressed out. She doesn't overeat anymore and doesn't think about it. She felt that all the remedies helped but that the Candida 1M was most important.

Dietary Solutions

Weight can be lost without drugs or herbs, just by exercising your body and your willpower. Dieting is as popular as ever, but many popular diets are of dubious merit. The low-calorie, low-fat diet is the most common weight-loss plan. Ideally, it consists of cutting out junk foods and concentrating on fruits, vegetables, whole grains, and lean meats. Problems arise when dieters try to trick their taste buds with artificial sweeteners and artificial fats (such as Olestra). The Calorie Control Council reports that four out of five Americans now consume low-calorie, sugar-free, or reduced-fat food and beverages containing these altered substances; however, Americans have gotten heavier, not lighter, since artificial sweeteners became popular. Another problem with artificial sweeteners is their side effects. See "Aspartame, Adverse Reactions to" on page 56.

In 1996, Olestra was conditionally approved by the FDA for marketing as a "fat-free fat" in the United States—the only country in which it is approved; in 2000, Canada declined to approve it. Virtually identical to mineral oil, Olestra is a laxative that depletes the body of fat-soluble vitamins and other essential nutrients if used habitually. It also can cause diarrhea and cramping. Artificial fat isn't liable to work any better than artificial sugar for producing weight loss. Low-fat food products often contain more calories than high-fat foods; the fat is simply replaced by sugar.[8] In any case, you need some fat in your diet. Hormones including estrogen, progesterone, and testosterone are all made from cholesterol. (See Chapter 1.) Cholesterol is a form of fat found only in animal foods, but you don't necessarily need to ingest it in that form, because your body can make its own. You do, however, at least need some vegetable fat.

Beyond Calorie-Counting: Foods That Encourage Weight Loss
Metabolic conditions and types of food eaten may be more important than the calorie count in determining weight status. If the body contains excess estrogen and insulin, it will not burn body fat because these two hormones induce lipogenesis—the production and retention of fat. One-third of Americans suffer from insulin resistance, in which cells do not adequately accept insulin. The food sent to the muscles to be burned as fuel is turned away and sent instead to the fat cells.

Certain types of food can increase metabolism and weight loss. They include foods high in fiber, which helps lower the levels of the fat-building hormones estrogen and insulin; omega-3 fats, which can improve insulin sensitivity even in the presence of sugars; and lean complete proteins, which can increase the production of glucagon, a fat-burning hormone.[9]

Another approach to food selection is recommended by Dr. Peter D'Adamo in *Eat Right 4 Your Type*. Dr. D'Adamo maintains that the right diet for your body is determined by your blood type, which reflects hereditary factors. "A" blood types do better on vegetarian diets. "O" blood types need meat. "B" types are in between. Although the scientific basis for this diet has been challenged, Dr. Walker has concluded it has merit after hearing many enthusiastic women claim painless weight loss following the protocol.

Diet books like *The Beverly Hills Diet* and *Fit for Life* follow the food combining theory of the earlier Natural Hygienists: eat fruit only for breakfast, and don't eat protein and starch in the same meal. Again, researchers question the scientific basis for the theory, but these authors know many people who have lost weight on it. People with a tendency to have digestive problems swear by it, too. The plan at least is well balanced and includes ample portions so it can be followed indefinitely. It's a lifestyle rather than a crash diet.[10]

A diet that one of this book's coauthors (Ellen Brown) has found particularly effective and rejuvenating is described in the 2002 book *The pH Miracle* by Robert and Shelley Young. Besides food combining and an essentially vegan diet, it stresses vegetable supplements and chlorine dioxide or hydrogen peroxide drops to alkalize the body and eliminate *Candida,* viruses, and other pathogens. For details, see "Fungal Infections" on page 116.

Eliminating the Cause of Food Cravings

We can force dietary restriction with drugs or grueling willpower, but if the cause of overeating is not addressed, the weight is liable to come right back when the "heat is off." A real cure requires eliminating the underlying cause. The question is, why do we crave food? One factor is the *Candida* problem: Because *Candida* fungi crave sugar, you will too. An alkalizing diet (stressing vegetables and raw foods, minimizing sugars, animal foods, and processed foods) helps eliminate *Candida* overgrowth and associated cravings.

Another factor involves toxic buildup. When we don't eat for a few hours, our bodies switch into cleansing mode and start dumping toxins into our bloodstreams. The result is a headache and feeling of weakness. To dispel these uncomfortable feelings, we reach for more food.

We may also keep reaching for food because we are malnourished. Although we may be eating plentifully, we may not be eating the *right* nutrients. Artificial fats and sugars can fool the taste buds, but our bodies know they need real ("good") fats and carbohydrates and will continue to crave them. To be well nourished, we need essential fatty acids, complex carbohydrates, protein, fiber, and a wide range of vitamins and minerals.

A more fundamental problem may be that we are not properly absorbing the nutrients we ingest. Absorption is prevented by the buildup of a slimy sludge of toxins that coats the intestines as a result of poor elimination. For some remarkable photos of the tissuelike intestinal sludge eliminated during supervised fasting, see Dr. Bernard Jensen's classic, *Dr. Jensen's Guide to Better Bowel Care.*[11] His proposed solution is a regime of detoxification to eliminate this toxic buildup. He recommends fasting along with coffee enemas to clean the colon so that it can make better use of nutrients. Although not recommended for long-term use, coffee enemas used in moderation in conjunction with fasting can be quite beneficial.[12]

Despite fasting's long history, it remains controversial as a method of weight control. Some authorities maintain that the tendency after famine is to feast. But fasting enthusiasts point out that when the body has been scrubbed from the inside out, your ability to absorb nutrients from foods is increased and the taste buds are sharpened. Recent research indicates that people who are overweight have *less* sensitive taste buds than people who are thin. The more sensitive your taste buds, the less food you require for satiation. Simple, whole foods suddenly become sufficient and delicious. Fasting expert and Natural Hygienist Dr. Herbert M. Shelton wrote that he found nothing so satisfying after a fast as half a head of plain lettuce. For fasting protocols, see Chapter 4.

PAIN AND INFLAMMATION

A recent Gallup survey found that for 46 percent of women and 37 percent of men, pain is a daily experience. One in three women cited the stress of balancing work and family life as a significant causal factor, compared to only one in four men.[1] Women also take more painkillers than men, and the drugs seem to work differently on them. In a 1999 study of the effects of ibuprofen on men and women, only the men reported significant relief, suggesting women have different pain pathways that require different remedies for treatment.[2] Pain is closely linked to inflammation, the body's response to injury. Nutrients are carried to the site and toxins are carried out, swelling the blood vessels, which press on the nerves.

CONVENTIONAL TREATMENT

One-fourth of over-the-counter drug purchases are analgesics (painkillers), a market principally divided among aspirin, acetaminophen, and ibuprofen. Aspirin, the oldest analgesic, has been around in pill form since 1899. It has been estimated that Americans take about 80 million aspirin tablets a day, or 29 billion a year, not to mention what's contained in many combination drugs. That works out to 117 aspirin tablets per person annually—actually a misleading statistic, since 20 percent of users consume 80 percent of the drug.[3] Aspirin's ability to reduce inflammation makes it a leading drug recommended for arthritis, in which pain comes from the movement and stress of inflamed joints. Aspirin is also used to relieve simple tension headaches, reduce fever, retard blood clotting, and "thin the blood." The latter property underlies its use as a preventative for heart attacks. (See "Heart Disease" on page 133.)

Aspirin was on the market for more than seventy years before the mechanism for its effects was discovered. The mechanism involves natural substances called prostaglandins. One called PGE2 alerts the body to disturbances in normal function by increasing the awareness of pain. Other prostaglandins contribute to the heat and swelling of inflammation and promote the coagulation of blood. Released when cells are injured or stimulated, prostaglandins can cause tissue damage themselves. Aspirin interferes with the body's biosynthesis of these prostaglandins, suppressing inflammation and the awareness of pain.

Other drugs in the aspirin group work the same way. They are collectively called non-steroidal anti-inflammatory drugs (NSAIDs)—as opposed to steroid drugs, which also reduce inflammation but have more serious side effects. NSAIDs include ibuprofen (Motrin and Advil), indomethacin (Indocin), naproxen (Aleve and Naprosyn), piroxicam (Feldene), and sulindac (Clinoril), among others.

Like all drugs that work by suppressing natural processes, NSAIDs can have unwanted side effects, which can be quite serious if the drugs are used for long periods. Besides failing to address the cause of pain, the drawback of this approach is that prostaglandins have normal body functions that are suppressed along with inflammation. Some prostaglandins help to regulate the flow of blood through the kidneys and the filtration and excretion of sodium and toxins. When aspirin and other NSAIDs inhibit these functions, the result can be fluid retention and the buildup of nitrogenous wastes in the blood.[4] Other prostaglandins have a direct action on stomach cells. They inhibit acid production and prevent acid damage to the lining of the stomach. When these prostaglandins are suppressed, acid can eat holes in your stomach and intestines. Ulcers and gastrointestinal bleeding caused by NSAIDs have become the most common serious adverse drug reactions in the United States. A recent Stanford study attributed 107,000 hospitalizations and 16,500 deaths yearly to these drugs.[5] Aspirin overdose can also cause dizziness, ringing in the ears, impaired hearing, nausea, vomiting, diarrhea, and confusion. It also can increase the bleeding resulting from wounds, tooth extraction, surgery, and childbirth. *Caution: Because aspirin keeps blood platelets from sticking together normally, it should be avoided by pregnant women, newborns, and people with clotting disorders or ulcers.*

Some of aspirin's drawbacks are avoided by its competitor acetaminophen (Tylenol, Datril, Anacin-3, Panadol, and Liquiprin). Acetaminophen won't reduce the pain associated with inflamed joints, but it's easier on the stomach lining than aspirin. It is, therefore, considered safer, but it also comes with risks. Overdoses of aspirin are unlikely to be fatal to adults if treated in time, but large doses of acetaminophen can cause irreversible liver damage and death; and normal doses can cause liver damage if given daily for long periods.[6]

The side effects of ibuprofen are similar to aspirin's but their incidence may be lower. According to a Vanderbilt University study, elderly people who take ibuprofen are four times as likely to die from ulcers and gastrointestinal bleeding as those who don't take it.[7] Like all NSAIDs, ibuprofen also tends to cause sodium retention and to inhibit kidney function. *Note: Ibuprofen isn't recommended for women who are pregnant or nursing, for alcoholics, or for people who have stomach problems or are allergic to aspirin.*

For a discussion of prescription drugs for pain relief, see "Arthritis," "Headaches," and "Surgical Trauma."

NATURAL REMEDIES

While conventional medicine uses one pain reliever for all types of pain, alternative practitioners treat pain according to its cause. Headache pain, pain from a trauma or muscle injury, or chronic pain from a disease such as cancer all have different causes and different treatments.

For migraine headaches, the herb feverfew has been touted as a miracle cure that can eliminate the need for drugs and their concomitant side effects. British researchers have found that feverfew not only cuts the number and severity of headaches but also reduces the nausea that goes with them. For more about this and other natural headache relievers, see "Headaches" on page 128.

For arthritis, the nutrients glucosamine and chrondoitin sulfate have been shown to relieve pain without the side effects of aspirin. They take longer to work, but it's because they are addressing the cause. These nutrients are the building blocks of cartilage and evidently work by stimulating the production of new cartilage cells and reducing the action of enzymes that harm cartilage. For quicker pain relief, DMSO cream applied topically works well. For specifics on this and other arthritis alternatives, see "Arthritis" on page 50.

The herbal form of aspirin is willow bark. Used by Chinese physicians as long as 2,500 years ago, it contains salicin, nearly the same pain reliever as in aspirin. Another herbal aspirin is meadowsweet tea. These herbal options can be just as effective as aspirin at much lower risk.[8] Many conventional drugs are extracted from plants, but naturopathic doctors maintain that the whole herb is more therapeutic than its isolated ingredients and is less likely to result in side effects. Extraction unbalances the remedy and makes it a toxin in the body.

Antioxidants reduce pain by reducing free-radical formation. Antioxidants include vitamins E and C, beta-carotene, selenium (found in garlic and onions), Pycnogenol, bioflavonoids, coenzyme Q_{10}, and alpha lipoic acid. The herbs ginkgo biloba and bilberry also have antioxidant properties. Many products are available; follow label directions.

Other nutrients are natural anti-inflammatories, which reduce pain either by decreasing local fluid levels or because of diuretic properties that reduce inflammation. They include vitamins C and B_6, potassium, and many herbs.

Magnesium is another natural pain reliever. Too low levels of magnesium increase nerve cell excitability and pain.[9] To replenish this mineral, take 400 mg one to three times daily.

In the homeopathic line, there are also natural pain relievers. *Hypericum* 30C can work as well as aspirin for reducing inflammation, without the risk of side effects. Take three pills four times daily.

For dental pain, effective homeopathic remedies include Gunpowder 6X (three pills four times daily) and *Bacticin* (ten drops every hour). *Pyrogenium* 6X or 12X expels pus. Take two pills every couple of hours as needed. If pus or a bad taste appears in the mouth, don't worry; it means the remedy is working.

For relief from the swelling and pain of dental abscess, homeopathic series therapy called Corynebacterium Anaerobius Nosode by the German company Staufen is excellent. Comparable series therapy is available in the United States from Deseret Biologicals. Directions for use are on the label.

Herbal remedies for temporary relief from toothache include oil of clove applied directly to the painful tooth. Another herbal remedy reported to work is to apply a few drops of a liquid extract of echinacea and goldenseal directly to the tooth. Leave for a few hours or overnight, freshening periodically.

Pain can also be relieved by improving circulation with physical therapies to help eliminate pain-response chemicals and exhausted immune-system cells. Effective therapies include massage, acupressure, heat treatments, stretching, and exercise.[10]

PAIN AND THE MIND

Recent research suggests that the painkilling abilities of analgesics may be largely in the mind. Painkilling drugs are particularly subject to the "placebo effect," a trick of the mind by which an anticipated effect is produced although the drug contains no active properties known to produce it. A Mayo Clinic study found that for 21 percent of patients tested as much pain relief resulted from a placebo—a "dummy" pill without active painkilling properties—as from either aspirin or a stronger drug. The study also found that for pain relief, aspirin was as good as or better than any other drug tested, over the counter or prescription, including Darvon, the prescription drug favorite.[11]

Up to one-third of prescription drugs, and a much higher percentage of nonprescription drugs, are thought to act primarily as placebos.[12] Patients get better because they expect to. Placebos apparently work by triggering the release of endorphins, the brain's own chemical pain relievers, which function like opiates in the body. Pure placebos—pills that have no physiological effect at all—can be effective pain relievers, but drugs that have actual physiological effects work better. This is true although their physiological effects are unrelated to the patient's condition. Thus, anxious patients will feel more relaxed if given a placebo that causes them to be lightheaded or dry-mouthed than if given one that does nothing at all. Patients feel the drug is "working" and, having been told it will work to relax them, feel more relaxed.[13]

The ideal analgesic would trigger this trick of the mind without pills and their side effects. Certain biofeedback and meditation techniques are reported to work by triggering the release of natural endorphins. Acupuncture is an effective analgesic that is thought to work the same way. In China, major surgeries are done with only acupuncture for an anesthetic. Exercise (the "runner's high") and yoga-type breathing also release endorphins. Even the pain of cancer has been reduced by nondrug analgesic therapies, including biofeedback, relaxation training, hypnosis, and behavior modification. Simply laughing or staying calm and happy can produce natural painkilling endorphins.[14]

PALPITATIONS

See IRREGULAR HEARTBEAT.

PANIC ATTACKS

See ANXIETY AND PANIC DISORDERS.

PARASITIC INFECTION

Parasites are hidden assailants that can cause bloating and add to the toxic liver load underlying a wide range of women's complaints. Toxins from protozoan parasites (usually *Amoeba* or *Giardia*) can cause gastrointestinal permeability, leading to allergies and other autoimmune diseases. Parasitic infection can also lead to adrenal shock, pancreatic shock, decreased levels of serotonin and other neurohormones, stomach acid and pepsin insufficiency, microorganism overgrowths, and general energy disturbances in the body. Parasite toxins readily get into the blood and can affect any organ. The liver and pancreas may get overloaded from having to deal with them. The brain may also be affected, resulting in depression, anxiety, schizophrenia, paranoia, and autism.[1]

Amoebas and intestinal worms were once considered problems mainly in the under-developed world, but the Centers for Disease Control now documents fifteen to twenty outbreaks of waterborne parasites each year in the United States. Experts speculate that the true number of outbreaks is in the hundreds, since parasitic illnesses are often mistaken for stomach flu and other intestinal disorders. A 1994 study put the hidden parasite epidemic at 2 million U.S. cases per year.[2] Potential uninvited guests include hookworms, pinworms, roundworms, tapeworms, heartworms, various flukes, *Amoeba, Entamoeba histolytica, Endolimax, Giardia, Blastocystis, Trichomonas vaginalis, Toxoplasma gondii, Cryptosporidium muris, Pneumocystis carinii, Strongyloides, Trichinella,* Anisakine larvae, Filaria, Cestoda, and Trematoda. Symptoms of infestation include gas and bloating, irritable bowel syndrome, joint and muscle aches and pains, skin conditions, granulomas, nervousness, sleep disturbances, anemia, allergy, constipation, diarrhea, teeth grinding, chronic fatigue, and immune dysfunction.[3]

Giardia is a protozoan resident of the intestinal tract that infects more people than is realized. The common assumption is that to have *Giardia,* one must be violently ill and vomiting; however, *Giardia* can be living in the systems of apparently healthy people. Their immune systems are strong enough to keep the parasite at bay so they don't get seriously ill from it, but they may have vague abdominal complaints. The main symptoms are gas, bloating, abdominal discomfort, and alternating diarrhea and constipation. The symptom complex is compounded when the parasites and their host stress each other. When the host is stressed, the pH of the intestines drops, causing parasites to become more active and the person to feel more bloated and miserable. When the parasites living in the body get more active, the person gets more irritable, edgy, and emotional.

Food poisoning is often confused with parasites or worms, while conditions diagnosed as more serious intestinal diseases like Crohn's disease or colitis sometimes turn out to be simply parasitic infections.

CONVENTIONAL TREATMENT

The standard treatment in the United States for intestinal parasites is metronidazole (Flagyl), an expensive drug required by law to bear the warning, "carcinogenic in rodents. Avoid unnecessary use." The drug is of limited effectiveness and can have troubling side effects. Those listed in the *Physician's Desk Reference* include convulsive seizures, numbness in the extremities, nausea and vomiting, headache, and intestinal distress. *Warning: Metronidazole should not be combined with alcohol, even the alcohol in cough syrup or in herbal or homeopathic remedies.*

To avoid giving this toxic drug unnecessarily, testing for parasites is always prescribed in the United States before the treatment is. But stool tests are notoriously unreliable, so parasites often go undetected and untreated. In Central America, this problem is avoided because the available remedies are much less toxic and less expensive. People therefore don't worry about stool tests. Parasite-eliminating herbs are incorporated into the local diet, and mothers routinely give their children over-the-counter deworming drugs preventatively, the way veterinarians regularly deworm dogs and horses. These remedies aren't available in the United States, evidently because demand for them is not great enough to prompt their European manufacturers to leap the $100 million hurdle to FDA approval. Levamisole (Ketrax), which can be purchased in Central America for about $2.50 for a full course of treatment, is available in the United States as a treatment for colon cancer, but the prescribed regimen costs $1,200 a year. The drug is classified as a "biologic response modifier" that, like interferons and interleukins, potentiates the immune response.[4]

Although over-the-counter antiparasite drugs aren't available in the United States, a number of effective herbal and homeopathic remedies are.

NATURAL REMEDIES

Homeopaths maintain that the antiparasite drug Flagyl doesn't actually kill parasites but merely pushes them deeper into the system. The patient keeps coming back with parasites, which are even harder to get rid of after the drugs have driven them deeper into the body. Homeopathic and herbal remedies can bring the infestation to the surface for elimination. How well they work and how long they take, however, depends on how deeply the parasites have gotten embedded into the system. A year's treatment may be required to eliminate a deeply embedded infestation.

Amoebas and *Giardia* are relatively easily treated with homeopathic remedies, but roundworms usually require herbal remedies. To rout out parasites that have been in residence for some time, a four- to six-week course of herbal treatment is generally necessary. The best protocol seems to be an herbal parasite combination developed by Marco Pharma that includes an antiparasitic called Para A, an antimicrobial remedy, luvos to heal lesions, and other remedial agents. Marco Pharma products are available only from practitioners.

Also good is Parastroy by Nature's Secret, a combination herbal product for killing parasites and balancing the intestines that comes as a complete kit with instructions. Another herbal solution for a variety of parasites is Clarkia 100 by Bio-Nutritional Formulas.

Antiparasitic herbs, including wormwood, black walnut, cloves, and valerian, may also be purchased individually. They can be mixed in half of a glass of water with a teaspoonful of luvos mineral earth (available from health food stores) and taken at a dosage of two droppersful three times daily.

Homeopathic remedies are good for prevention when traveling abroad or eating out frequently, or when you come home from a trip abroad or a meal at an exotic restaurant with an upset stomach, diarrhea, or other symptoms of parasitic infections. For parasites that have been in the body awhile, the remedies will give only symptomatic relief; however, they can be used to relieve occasional stomach upset while other remedies have time to work. Good homeopathic options include Worms and Amoeba by CompliMed, and Parasite Complex, Ver, and Dia-Verm by Deseret Biologicals. Dosages for all of them are ten

HYSTERECTOMY AVOIDED WITH SIMPLE WORM REMEDY

In Guatemala (where one of the authors previously lived), the wife of an American foreign service officer was emotional, agitated, depressed, and suffered from severe abdominal pains. Her gynecologist, suspecting uterine problems, had scheduled a hysterectomy. The woman called off the surgery after she took the local worm remedy mebendazol and eliminated a bowl full of tiny worms. Her symptoms disappeared with the parasites.

PARASITES ELIMINATED WITH NATURAL REMEDIES

A woman complained that she was unable to eat fats, mayonnaise, or dairy products without getting quite ill. Tests revealed that she had *Giardia,* and she was given Giardia/Lamblia homeopathic series therapy by Deseret. She had an upset stomach for a few days while taking the remedy, but afterward, to her delight, she could once again eat the offending foods without a problem.

A second woman had deeply embedded parasites from multiple trips to India and Puerto Rico. She knew she had them but didn't know how to get rid of them. She had tried conventional drug treatment without success. Dr. Walker recommended the Marco Pharma Para A and luvos earth, which worked to clear them up when nothing else had.

drops three times daily. When traveling, take ten drops daily throughout the trip for prevention.

For *Giardia,* homeopathic series therapy is particularly effective. The Deseret Biologicals product is called Giardia. The Staufen product is called Lamblia. The prescribed regimen is one ampule every three days for one month. A vibrational remedy called Giardia by Kroeger Herbs is also good, but it works on newly acquired *Giardia* only. The recommended dose is ten drops three times a day until the bottle is empty.

For pinworms, the homeopathic remedy is *Cina* 30C, three pills twice daily for a month, then for four or five days around the full moon for a year.

For toxoplasmosis—an infestation of a parasite carried by cats—Staufen has an effective homeopathic series therapy called Toxoplasmosis, including ampules in varying doses from 200X to 5X. Directions are on the label. Professional Complementary Medicine also makes homeopathic drops for toxoplasmosis.

Caution: To avoid acquiring toxoplasmosis and transmitting it to the fetus, pregnant women should not change cat litter boxes.

PERIMENOPAUSE

See MENOPAUSE AND PERIMENOPAUSE.

PREMENSTRUAL SYNDROME (PMS)

Premenstrual syndrome (PMS) is a cluster of uncomfortable symptoms that sets in seven to ten days before a woman starts her period. They can include headaches, abdominal bloating, breast swelling, fluid retention, increased thirst, increased appetite, cravings for sweet or salty foods, and emotional symptoms including anxiety, irritability, mood swings, depression, hostility, crying, and loss of self-confidence. The condition normally begins sometime in a woman's thirties, when hormone production is slowing down. Once thought to be merely psychological, PMS gained recognition as a true physical syndrome when British gynecologist Katharina Dalton found that nearly half the women admitted to a hospital for accidents or psychological illnesses were in their premenstrual week. Other studies showed that about half the crimes for which women were responsible were committed during this period. PMS is now thought to plague from 25 to 90 percent of all women, depending on who defines it.

Dr. Dalton was personally interested because she was a chronic sufferer of premenstrual migraine headaches herself. She noticed that her symptoms went away, however, during the last six months of her pregnancy. Knowing that progesterone levels are twenty to thirty times higher during that time than at other times, she proceeded to treat herself with daily injections of progesterone after her baby was born. Her migraines did not come back. Since then, the link with progesterone levels has been verified in thousands of other women.

PMS symptoms are now thought to be due to a hormone imbalance before menstruation. During the normal menstrual cycle, immediately after ovulation, levels of both estrogen and progesterone rise, and they continue to rise until menstruation. The progesterone acts as an estrogen antagonist, keeping estrogen levels from going too high. But progesterone stores can be depleted by stress (emotional, dietary, or environmental), causing progesterone to be converted to the stress hormone cortisol. Without enough progesterone, estrogen levels get too high. Excess estrogen can then produce salt and fluid retention, low blood sugar, blood clotting, breast tenderness, thyroid problems, and weight gain. These physical imbalances produce the mood swings and other psychological effects associated with PMS.[1]

CONVENTIONAL TREATMENT

In theory, progesterone supplementation should correct estrogen imbalances by normalizing estrogen levels. But doctors have been slow to credit progesterone therapy with helping PMS, because controlled trials of several different synthetic progestins have failed to show a significant benefit on PMS symptoms.[2] Critics point out that these studies were flawed, since they used synthetic copies of the hormone. Provera (medroxyprogesterone acetate) and other chemically altered forms of progesterone not only don't work on PMS but can make it worse, by inhibiting natural progesterone production and lowering its concentration in the blood. Synthetic progesterone performs some but not all of the natural hormone's functions. It cannot be converted in the body to other hormones as needed, and it comes with a long list of unwanted side effects. (See Chapter 2.)

Diuretics, or water pills, are often recommended to relieve fluid retention in PMS sufferers.[3] However, these drugs work by forcing the kidneys to release body fluid, and along with the excess water go important minerals and chemicals, throwing off electrolyte and mineral balance. That's why most diuretics are prescription-only drugs. In fact, PMS is the *only* condition for which their over-the-counter use is approved, and that's only because the pills are intended for use only a few days each month.

Sarafem is a drug now being recommended for a PMS-related condition called PMDD—premenstrual dysphoric disorder. Sarafem is actually a renamed version of Prozac, a psychotropic antidepressant that affects the brain. It helps the depression associated with PMS by increasing serotonin levels, producing a drug-induced happy feeling. However, it comes with all the hazards of Prozac, a drug most women would be leary of taking if they knew what it was. (For some details about Prozac, see "Depression" on page 95.) Critics call Sarafem a marketing ploy. The patent on Prozac expired in the summer of 2001. Renaming it as a new drug generated new sales. Whether PMDD even exists has been questioned; if it does, only 5 percent of women may experience it. Yet Serafem's manufacturer spent $17 million promoting Serafem to the whole female population in the five months after the FDA approved it for sale.[4] As with Valium and amphetamines for weight loss, the result is liable to be a large class of women unwittingly and unnecessarily addicted to a psychotropic drug.

NATURAL REMEDIES

Natural Hormones

Although synthetic progesterone has not tested well for treating PMS, *natural* progesterone has. Significant improvements in PMS symptoms have been reported in only one controlled progesterone trial, and it used natural progesterone in oral micronized form.[5] Many doctors claim a high rate of success with the natural hormone, either in micronized pill form or as a transdermal cream derived from a type of Mexican yam. Dr. Ray Peat, who pioneered the transdermal form of natural progesterone, stated that in the approximately 400 women he observed, nearly all found the appropriate amount to control their PMS symptoms.[6] Transdermal natural progesterone has the advantage over the pill form that much lower amounts are required to get an effect. ProGest by Transitions for Health is a particularly effective brand. A full two-ounce jar of the cream is recommended per month to start, or about ½ teaspoon per day; requirements are very individual, however. The progesterone should be begun on day ten or twelve of the menstrual cycle (counting the first day of menstruation as day one), finishing on day twenty-five or twenty-six.[7]

Chinese and Western Herbal and Homeopathic Remedies

The approach of Chinese and homeopathic doctors is to aid the body in producing and balancing its own hormones.

Relaxed Wanderer, the brand name for a Chinese patent formula called *Hsiao Yao Wan* (or *Xiao Yao Wan*), is an excellent remedy not only for menopausal complaints but also for PMS. The remedy works particularly well for women with a tendency to be cold (for example, to have cold hands and feet). For women who are approaching menopause and tend to be hot, the Chinese remedy Bupleurum and Peony Formula is likely to be more effective. These Chinese patent remedies are made by different companies; follow directions on the label or take as directed by your practitioner. The European and native American Indian herbal traditions also include excellent botanicals for premenstrual and menopausal complaints. One is an American-made red raspberry leaf combination formula by Zand. It should be taken beginning a week before menstruation.

Homeopathic remedies are another effective alternative for treating PMS. For cramps, Cyclease by Boiron is good. For moodiness, bloating, and discomfort, try Natural Phases by Boiron. Contessa, a homeopathic remedy by Marco Pharma International, helps balance female hormones and relieve irritability. Follow label directions. Hormone Balance by Deseret is another excellent option. Take five to ten drops one to three times daily.

Nutritional Solutions

The high levels of estrogen on which PMS has been blamed may be the result of nutritional imbalances. One way to keep estrogen levels from going too high is by increasing your intake of dietary fiber. Fiber binds with the deactivated estrogen and moves it through the intestines. Studies show that women on high-fiber, low-fat diets have less PMS, less breast cancer, less premenstrual breast pain, and less trouble with their menstrual periods.[8]

Calcium can also help relieve PMS symptoms. In a Columbia University study reported in 1998, 466 women between the ages of 18 and 45 were randomly assigned to receive either 1,200 milligrams of elemental calcium daily in the form of calcium carbonate or a placebo for three menstrual cycles. Calcium supplementation resulted in a 48 percent reduction in PMS symptoms by the third menstrual cycle, compared to a 30 percent reduction with the placebo.[9]

For a calcium source, Bone-Up by Jarrow is particularly good. Take two capsules two to three times daily.

Other nutritional supplements shown to relieve PMS symptoms include vitamin B_6, vitamin E, essential fatty acids, evening primrose oil, black currant oil, and borage oil. Many brands are available. Follow label directions. Avoidance of caffeine and allergenic foods may also help.[10]

Multiple vitamin products are also available that are specifically prepared for PMS sufferers. Ask for recommendations at your local health food store.

PROLAPSE

See UTERINE PROLAPSE.

PSORIASIS

See SKIN PROBLEMS.

RASH

See SKIN PROBLEMS.

RHEUMATOID ARTHRITIS

See ARTHRITIS.

ROSACEA

See ACNE ROSACEA.

SCARS

See SKIN PROBLEMS.

SCIATICA

See BACK PAIN AND SCIATICA.

SEXUAL DYSFUNCTION

Sexual dysfunction can have organic causes, but it is much more likely to be due to stress, drugs, or hormone imbalance. About 15 percent of all couples are infertile (defined as unable to conceive after a year's effort), but in only 1 or 2 percent is conception physically ruled out.[1] In the rest, the problem is rooted in emotional or lifestyle factors. A lack of sexual desire is typically linked to emotional stress or hormonal changes. Many drugs can also cause or contribute to sexual dysfunction, including amphetamines, antihistamines, barbiturates, beta-blockers and other blood pressure medications, cimetidine (Tagamet), ketoconazole, sedatives, tricyclic antidepressants, cocaine, alcohol, marijuana, methadone, and Prozac. Prozac is so effective at numbing sexual feeling and drive, in fact, that it is sometimes prescribed as a remedy for men troubled with premature ejaculation.

CONVENTIONAL TREATMENT

For decreased libido in premenopausal women, pharmaceutical estrogen or low doses of testosterone are conventionally prescribed. The treatment generally works but can have side effects. For infertility, ovulation may be induced with hormones or fertility drugs. However, the drugs increase the chance of multiple births and can have other unwanted side effects, including hot flashes, breast tenderness, mood swings, visual problems, and an increased risk of ovarian cancer.

BODY-BALANCING REMEDIES ENCOURAGE PREGNANCY

Anna, age 42, had been incapacitated in her early childbearing years with chronic fatigue syndrome, but she had gotten better over time and had met the love of her life. She had gotten married and wanted to get pregnant but feared she wouldn't be able to, having failed when she had tried ten years earlier. Dr. Walker gave Anna a homeopathic remedy appropriate for her constitutional type, and gave her husband homeopathic *Aralia Q* 3X (homeopathic ginseng), a remedy that can help increase sperm count. The dosage was three to five pills one to three times daily. Within two months, to her delight, Anna was pregnant.

JOYS OF SEX REKINDLED

At age 44, Betsy had lost interest in sex, a distressing development that was jeopardizing her marriage. Her doctor had given her pharmaceutical testosterone, but it caused her to have an offensive body odor and made her facial hair thicken. When he insisted the amount was too low to cause side effects and proceeded to increase the dose, Betsy sought alternative relief from Dr. Walker. She went home with Jasmine and took it faithfully, ten drops three times daily. Two weeks later, she returned to report that she and her husband were having the best sexual relationship of their marriage. Her drive was up, her sleep was better, and she felt less stressed.

Kathleen was also age 44 when, after eight years of a very active sex life with her husband, she suddenly found she had no sex drive. After four months in this state, she wondered if her interest in sex would ever return. She was using natural progesterone cream, but it didn't seem to be enough. She began taking homeopathic Testosterone drops, ten drops three times daily. After a week, she reported that her sex drive was not only back but was also higher than it had been in years. Her husband was delighted, but it was actually more libido than she wanted. She was advised to decrease the dose to once a day, then decrease it further to ten drops two to three times per week. This seemed to be the right balance for her body.

NATURAL REMEDIES FOR INFERTILITY

While an inability to get pregnant may be organic, it is more likely to be due to simple imbalance. Women who think they can't get pregnant often achieve that result unexpectedly after using natural remedies, because the nature of natural medicine is to balance the body. When everything is working right, pregnancy is more likely.

Chinese doctors believe that the yin must be nourished for conception to occur. Many women are so yang at their jobs—they have to be so aggressive and assertive—that their yin gets out of balance. As a result, the womb can't support a baby. Chinese remedies called Infertility Pills help rebalance the hormones. Chinese midwives also recommend spending some time at home. Become soft and feminine, bake cookies, and avoid violent movies that stir up the adrenaline. Acupuncture rings can also help stimulate fertility. They are rubbed up and down on the finger, activating meridians attached to appropriate acupuncture points.

Liver congestion can be another cause of infertility. The Liver Cleanse Diet is recommended for this problem. For directions, see Chapter 4.

NATURAL REMEDIES FOR BOOSTING SEXUAL INTEREST

To stimulate sexual interest in women, several effective herbal and homeopathic remedies are available.

Natural progesterone cream (ProGest) is absorbed topically and increases the body's natural hormone levels. Progesterone is the hormone that kicks in during puberty in young girls and makes women feel younger, sexier, and more interested in having sex. The protocol varies depending on hormonal status. If you are still menstruating, rub ⅛ to ¼ teaspoon of the cream on the abdominal area each night for the fourteen days before your period, stopping the day or so before your period starts. For postmenopausal women, use this amount for twenty-five days out of the month.

For menopausal and postmenopausal women, OstaDerm by Bezwecken is a natural estrogen cream derived from plants that can offer the benefits of pharmaceutical estrogen without its side effects. Appropriate dosages vary from ⅛ to ½ teaspoon one to two times daily. OstaDerm V by Bezwecken is a natural estrogen cream intended for vaginal application, which is particularly good for vaginal dryness. Dosages vary from ⅛ to ½ teaspoon three times weekly.

In the homeopathic line, Sexual Stimulation Drops by PHP can effectively increase interest in sex. Another product reported to work is homeopathic Testosterone. It contains no actual testosterone but stimulates the body to produce its own.

Jasmine by Botanical Alchemy is an herbal and gem elixir formula that heals and increases sexual feelings toward a partner.

SKIN CANCER AND SUNBURN

Skin cancer is by far the most common cancer in the world. Despite the increasing use of sunblock, one out of six Americans can now expect to contract it. Fortunately, most cases are easily curable—so easily that at one time these conditions weren't classified as cancers for statistical purposes. (Skeptical statisticians have suggested that the classification was changed to improve the cancer "cure rate" from conventional treatment.)

The dangerous skin cancers are the 10 percent that are malignant melanomas. They progress much faster than other skin cancers, can spread beyond the skin, and are life-threatening. They are easily recognizable and are curable too, but they need to be detected early. Malignant melanoma is usually signaled by a change in the size, shape, or color of an existing mole, or as a new growth on normal skin. Factors to watch include asymmetry (a growth with unmatched halves); border irregularity (ragged or blurred edges); color (a mottled appearance, with shades of tan, brown, and black, sometimes mixed with red, white, or blue); and diameter (a growth more than 6 millimeters across—about the size of a pencil eraser—or any unusual increase in size).[1] *Warning: Suspicious growths should be examined by a dermatologist.*

CONVENTIONAL PREVENTION AND TREATMENT

Dermatologists remove skin tumors with electric current, freeze them with liquid nitrogen, kill them with low-dose radiation, treat them with chemotherapeutic agents, or remove them surgically.

For prevention, some dermatologists have gone so far as to recommend lathering up with sunscreen every morning, no matter what the weather, just to make sure the skin is protected from any sunshine that might chance to befall it. But other experts maintain there is insufficient scientific data to support the belief that sunscreens prevent skin cancer, and the products come with their own hazards. They interfere with the synthesis of vitamin D, which is essential for strong bones; they contain toxic chemicals such as titanium; and they give a false sense of security and encourage long periods in the sun. In a study reported in the *Journal of the National Cancer Institute* in 1998, the use of sunscreens was actually linked to an *increased* risk of melanoma, probably for the latter reason.[2] Most sunscreens, regardless of advertising claims, block out only UVB wavelengths, not the deeper-penetrating UVA wavelengths. The fact that the skin's surface doesn't burn doesn't mean it's not being exposed to harmful rays. The melanin produced on the skin by unblocked sunshine (the suntan) is actually what protects the tissues beneath.[3] Other studies have

SAFE SUNBATHING

The prudent approach to sunbathing is to build up exposure gradually—just to the point of a slight pinkish capillary dilation. This allows tolerance and still affords protection from vitamin D deficiency, which research has shown that even minimal exposure to blue sky is sufficient to prevent. If longer sun exposure can't be avoided, protect your skin with lightweight, light-colored, long-sleeved clothing and brimmed hats. If sunscreens need to be used, natural sunscreens without harmful chemical additives and preservatives are available at health food stores. Those containing PABA should be avoided. A recent FDA report concluded that fourteen out of seventeen suntan lotions containing PABA could be carcinogenic.[9]

found that sunbathing that does not involve blistering is actually protective against melanoma. Moderation and gradual adaptation to the sun appear to be the keys to safe sun exposure.[4]

NATURAL REMEDIES

Zane Kime, M.D., in the groundbreaking book *Sunlight,* demonstrates that the sun creates free-radical damage only in the absence of protective antioxidants and the presence of harmful fats. The antioxidants he discussed were vitamins A, C, and E and the trace mineral selenium, but there are many others. Harmful fats include hydrogenated oils, refined oils, and saturated fat; that is, the fats in the standard American (high-fat) diet.[5]

That antioxidants help prevent non-melanoma skin cancers has been confirmed in several studies. In 1992, Berkeley researchers found that exposing rats to ultraviolet rays depleted their skin of vitamins C and E.[6] In another study, people who took 200 mcg of selenium daily were found to have a reduced incidence of skin cancer. Good food sources of selenium include garlic, grains, sunflower seeds, seafood, and Brazil nuts.

In the herbal line, milk thistle (silymarin) has also been shown to curb skin cancer. Applying it to the skin of mice exposed to UVB light caused a 75 percent reduction in the total number of resulting tumors.[7] Ginger is another herb that has dramatically reduced the incidence and size of tumors when applied to the skin of mice exposed to a cancer-causing chemical.[8]

SKIN-PIERCING COMPLICATIONS

See SKIN PROBLEMS.

SKIN PROBLEMS

Dermatitis, or skin inflammation, is a term that includes a range of skin conditions characterized by dry, red, itchy skin. Eczema is chronically itchy, inflamed skin that is variously linked to allergies, asthma, stress, and heredity. Psoriasis is a baffling skin disorder in which skin cells multiply much faster than normal, producing raised, white-scaled patches. Other common skin problems include dry and aging skin, scars, and stretch marks. Itching, rashes, and hives can accompany the hormonal changes of menopause. See also "Acne" on page 31, "Acne Rosacea" on page 34, "Fungal Infections" on page 116, and "Menopause and Perimenopause" on page 174.

CONVENTIONAL TREATMENT

For serious skin conditions such as psoriasis, corticosteroids are sometimes prescribed. These drugs, however, are not only counterproductive but may actually *cause* psoriasis. Serious cases of that skin disease have been traced to the suppression of a simple skin infection with cortisone, which suppresses the immune system so the body can no longer heal itself. In the typical case, hydrocortisone cream is applied to a minor rash on the skin, which turns out to be ringworm or some other infection. The cortisone suppresses the immune system at that spot, so the infection is allowed to grow. When the rash comes back, it covers a much larger area of skin because the infection has spread. If hydrocortisone cream is then used on this rash, worse problems can result.

For minor skin problems, many drugstore topical remedies are available. These too require caution, since many contain hazardous chemicals. We tend to think of drugs applied to the skin as being relatively harmless, since they're not taken into the body like those that are swallowed, but this is a misconception. Drugs taken by mouth go through the normal detoxification processes for which the stomach, kidneys, and liver were designed. Drugs applied to the skin, although less well absorbed, go directly into the bloodstream without metabolic intervention. In fact, topical painkillers have produced adverse reactions more frequently when applied to the skin than when swallowed. People who are allergic to foods or other substances should be especially careful with them.[1]

A currently popular treatment for the complexion called Botox involves injecting botulism toxin into the face. It stops wrinkles by paralyzing the muscles, but botulism is a nerve poison that homeopaths believe suppresses the immune system and can affect the entire body. There are much safer natural alternatives.

NATURAL REMEDIES

The best approach to chronic skin conditions is to search for and eliminate the underlying cause. Often, it turns out to be food allergies. Sensitivity to the nightshades—potatoes, peppers, eggplant, and tomatoes—is a common cause of skin rashes.

SKIN PROBLEMS CLEARED NATURALLY

Tania's belly button had gotten severely infected from piercing. Her doctor wanted her to let the ring hole heal over, but Tania was bent on keeping it. She had taken antibiotics for the infection, but the drugs hadn't helped much. Two days after she began taking homeopathic Gunpowder 6X, the redness was gone and the infection had cleared.

Mary still had scars on her nose and face from a dog bite she had gotten fifteen years earlier. She also had rosacea. She applied the Bioptron light to her face for four minutes per spot each day. In a few weeks, the scars had faded and her rosacea disappeared. At 60, Mary has skin that looks beautiful.

Nutrition is also important for preserving the skin. Essential fatty acids are in short supply in the normal American diet and typically need to be supplemented. Omega-3 fatty acids help build efficient cell membranes that can exclude allergy-provoking proteins. Antioxidants and calcium can also help prevent wrinkled, sagging skin. An excellent oral combination product called the Missing Link contains omega-3 and omega-6 essential fatty acids, lignans, plant nutrients, enzymes, antioxidants, vitamins, minerals, friendly bacteria, fiber, and protein. Use according to label directions.

Women also report dramatic results when taking evening primrose oil (2,600 mg at bedtime), which helps the skin, hair, and nails from the inside out. Within a week, they say their skin is noticeably improved.

Vitamin E (400–800 IU daily), flaxseed oil (1 to 4 tablespoons daily), and alpha lipoic acid (ALA) are other helpful nutritional supplements. Oral nutritional remedies are particularly effective because they address the underlying deficiencies leading to dry and aging skin.

Topical ointments are also available that are made from all-natural, nontoxic components. Squalene, made from shark liver oil, softens the skin and is very good for psoriasis. Kukui Nut Oil from Hawaii is another option. Apply topically as needed. Also good is ProGest cream, a natural progesterone that is absorbed through the skin and helps restore it over a period of time. However, no more than ¼ or ½ teaspoon should be used daily.

Green tea can be applied topically too. Green tea has been shown to prevent and even reverse damage to the skin from the sun and aging, fighting viral as well as bacterial infection.[2] Steep a tea bag in water and apply the cooled bag directly to the skin.

For scars, a remedy called ScarGo applied topically as needed has produced dramatic results. Another remarkable therapy for scars, stretch marks, rosacea, and other skin blemishes involves a Swiss-made handheld device called a Bioptron machine. It emits polarized light that intensively stimulates the skin. Researched for twenty years in Europe, the Bioptron has been found to be particularly effective on skin problems and for the healing of wounds.

For cracks and splits in the fingers during winter, try homeopathic *Petroleum* 6X. Take two pills two to three times daily.

For cracks in the heel, use *Lycopodium* 6X, two pills orally three times daily.

For infection resulting from ear and body piercing, wash with homeopathic *Calendula* mother tincture to clear up the infected area and promote healing. Infection can also be inhibited in its early stages with homeopathic Gunpowder 6X. Take three pills every two hours on the first day, then take three pills four times daily. The infection usually clears in two days.

For inflammation caused by an allergic reaction to the base metal in jewelry, try switching to gold or silver.

Dark circles under the eyes may be indicative of kidney problems. Toxins or allergy complexes may be blocking kidney functions. Eliminating the problem requires locating and eliminating allergens, drinking lots of water to flush the kidneys, and taking detox homeopathic remedies. Ex Chem by Apex, for chemical sensitivity or chemical overload, is good. Start slowly with one drop daily in half a glass of water and work up to ten drops three times daily. (See "Multiple Chemical Sensitivity" on page 185.) Avoid known allergens and take remedies specific for clearing them. If you know you're allergic to nightshade vegetables, dairy, or wheat, for example, stay away from the offenders and use remedies to detoxify from them. (See "Allergies" on page 37.)

SPASTIC COLITIS

See BOWEL DISORDERS.

STAGE FRIGHT

See NERVOUSNESS, STAGE FRIGHT, AND LACK OF SELF-CONFIDENCE.

STRESS

The multitasking expected of today's supermom/career woman can be responsible for the adrenal exhaustion that underlies a range of women's diseases. (See Chapter 1.) Added to that burden are physical stressors that contribute to the overload overwhelming our bodies, including drugs, insecticides, synthetic fabrics, chemicals on and in our bodies, imported foods carrying parasites, and electronic pollution (electric lines, computer screens, TVs, cellular phones, and hair dryers). Crowds, noise, traffic, pain, travel, a new job, moving, a new baby, overwork, lack of sleep, illness, alcohol, and worry further compound the problem.

A recent study showed that half the patients who visit general physicians have conditions triggered or aggravated by stressful situations. The body responds with a number of physiological changes. All body functions and organs are now known to react to stress. Blood pressure, heart rate, and muscle tension increase. Digestion slows. Cholesterol levels rise to meet an increased need for cortisone. A rise in cortisol levels suppresses the immune system and inhibits the ability of white blood cells to help fight disease, and the cortisol is produced at the expense of the female hormones. Stress also increases the formation of free radicals, which damage and age the body.

CONVENTIONAL DRUG TREATMENT

The approach of conventional medicine is to suppress the symptoms of stress with drugs. Anxiety is suppressed with sedatives and tranquilizers, elevated blood pressure with antihypertensive medication, elevated cholesterol with cholesterol-lowering drugs, a racing or erratic heartbeat with antiarrhythmia drugs, and an upset stomach with antacids or H2-blockers. Besides side effects, the problem with the drug approach is that the remedies merely suppress symptoms without reaching the cause and without building up the defenses the body needs to deal with stress.

NATURAL REMEDIES

Nutritional and herbal remedies can boost the immune system and ease tension without side effects. Thymactive by NF Formulas and Immune Support by Deseret are effective homeopathic options. Colostrum (the first milk of mammals) is a nutrient that is useful for building immunity, now available in capsule form. A dosage of 1,000 mg may be taken two to four times daily.

Homeopathic remedies can address the underlying cause of stress. To be effective, however, the right remedy must be selected based on circumstances and personality traits. Below are some possibilities for different types of stress. The dosage for each is three pellets three times daily.

Adrenalinum 4X is for the person who "keeps on going" through a crisis, no matter how tired she is and no matter what else comes up. A few weeks after the crisis is over, she comes in seeking help. "I'm so tired," she says, "and I'm not sure why. I was fine during the crisis. Why should I be so tired now when it's all over?" The reason, of course, is that she has "burned out her adrenals." The Chinese say she has used up her excess *qi* (energy). For this personality type, a combination of homeopathic remedies containing *Adrenalinum in low potencies* is quite effective. Try *Adrenalinum* 4X by Dolisos.

Magnesia phosphorica 30C is for the person who is depressed, drowsy, dull, unable to study or think clearly, on edge, irritable, and overly sensitive.

Calcarea phosphorica 30C is for the person with a more serious depression (for example, after the death of a loved one). The person is slow to comprehend, disappointed, moaning, irritable, hard to please, peevish, discontented, complaining, never satisfied, and easily bored.

Phosphoricum acidum 30C is for the person so overwhelmed with grief or physical illness that she is emotionally drained. She seems fatigued, slow to answer, flat, indifferent, and even lifeless.

Cocculus 30C is for the stress of nursing a sick loved one, the ill effects of grief or anger, exhaustion from stress and anxiety over a loved one, sadness, grief, ailments from loss of sleep; the person who is sensitive to fear, anger, grief, noise, or touch; one who is easily startled.

Kali phosphoricum 30C is for the person at the breaking point, the worn-out business or professional woman, one very despondent about business, one for whom the slightest labor seems a heavy task; for weakened mental and physical states resulting from stress; for anxiety with nervous dread; and for lassitude and depression.

Nux vomica 30C is for the person who has stressed her body by overeating or with too much alcohol; for the person who loves to party.

Ignatia 30C is a remedy for grief and emotional upset, especially good for "disappointed love."

Lifestyle Modification

Stressed people tend to eat poorly. They say they don't have time. But proper nutrition and essential fatty acids are necessary to aid resistance to stress, and nutrients can detoxify and rebuild an overwhelmed system. Relaxation, sleep, and exercise are also important for reducing stress. Meditation can help as well. You may not be able to control the crises in your life, but you can control how you deal with them. Stress is a state of mind. Some people thrive on it.

STRESS CYCLE BROKEN

A few days after Debbie broke up with her boyfriend of three years—the man she thought she was going to marry—he was dating her best friend. Debbie was devastated. She couldn't sleep. She couldn't eat. She cried so much that she was sent home from work. She stayed in bed. She didn't shower or even get dressed. She dragged herself around without putting on makeup or fixing her hair. She kept repeating, "How could he do this to me?" That statement was the key to choosing the right homeopathic remedy for her—*Ignatia*. Three days after Debbie began taking it, she was a different woman. She was dressed to the teeth, her hair and nails were done, her makeup was perfect, and she was smiling. She joked and laughed. Asked if she had gotten back with her boyfriend, she said she hadn't. She had simply come to realize that she had made a bad choice. This man was not for her. Their breakup still hurt, but she was moving on.

STRETCH MARKS

See SKIN PROBLEMS.

STROKE

See HEART DISEASE.

SUNBURN

See SKIN CANCER AND SUNBURN.

SURGICAL TRAUMA

Surgeries are becoming increasingly popular not only in life-threatening situations but for merely cosmetic purposes. More than a million cosmetic surgical procedures are performed annually in the United States, including face-lifts, liposuctions, collagen treatments, chemical peels, and eyelid lifts. Procedural innovations, including the use of lasers and endoscopy, have made cosmetic surgeries cheaper, easier, and less traumatic. But surgery still represents a major stress to the body, and anesthetics and painkillers impose a sluggish drain on nerve and circulatory energy.

CONVENTIONAL POSTSURGICAL TREATMENT

For postsurgical trauma, narcotic analgesics are conventionally prescribed. They work by drugging the nerves. Morphine, codeine, and opium are narcotics that are natural plant derivatives. Synthetic or semi-synthetic narcotics include propoxyphene (Darvon), meperidine (Demerol), pentazocine (Talwin), oxycodone (contained in Percodan with aspirin and in Percocet with acetaminophen), and codeine (also used in cough medicines and for diarrhea). All narcotics can be addicting, and a virtually universal side effect is constipation. A less well-known side effect is a weakening of the body's immune defenses. In research reported in 1997, mice regularly receiving morphine died from bacterial infections that would not have been lethal to normal mice. The researcher conducting the study warned that patients receiving morphine for postsurgical pain may face an increased risk of sepsis, a massive, often fatal bacterial infection.[1]

NATURAL REMEDIES

Aiding Recovery with Homeopathic Remedies

Homeopathic remedies can cut the amount of narcotic analgesics needed after surgery. Plastic surgery is particularly appropriate for homeopathic treatment, since it's an elective surgery for which people have time to prepare in advance. Women have been impressed by how fast they healed, how little their surgery and recovery hurt, how little pain medication they required, how little bruising they experienced, and how quickly they were able to return to work as a result of using these simple remedies.

The best time to begin taking homeopathic remedies for surgical trauma is when you are being wheeled into the operating room. Since they are taken sublingually, they won't create nausea or vomiting as food will if taken immediately before anesthesia. The remedies may all be mixed and taken at once. Because they are vibrational remedies essentially consisting of nothing but water, they will not interfere in any way with the surgery.

MENOPAUSE PRECIPITATED BY SURGICAL SHOCK

A case illustrating the physical effects of shock involved a woman who had had a hysterectomy. Her doctor had assured her that her menstrual periods would not be affected by the surgery, since he wasn't removing the ovaries. However, her ovaries had quit working anyway. The shock of the surgery had evidently shut them down. Eight months later, her periods still had not returned. Contessa, a combination homeopathic remedy by Marco Pharma, brought her periods back. If she had taken *Aconitum* before and after her surgery, she may have been able to avoid this problem.

Choosing and Taking Homeopathic Remedies

Homeopathic remedies recommended in conjunction with surgery include the following:

1. *Arnica* stops the body from overreacting to trauma. *Arnica* at a potency of 200C should be taken immediately before surgery and every hour for the first four hours afterward. Then, *Arnica* 30C should be taken three times daily for two to three days. For cosmetic surgery, most of the doses need to be given right at the time of the surgical trauma, decreasing as time goes on. Ideally, have a friend come with you and give you a couple of pellets when you're being wheeled in, then immediately or soon after the trauma to your face, then every fifteen minutes for an hour or so, then every hour for the rest of the day. The following day, take the remedy in divided doses five times a day. Then, reduce to three

times a day. After the *Arnica* has done its job—once you're out of pain—you don't need it anymore.

2. *Ledum* helps in the treatment of injuries that result in bruising and puffy skin, as first aid, to prevent infection, and for eye injuries. After facial surgery, it's particularly useful for helping relieve black eyes. It should be taken in the same way as homeopathic *Arnica,* but after the second or third day, it can usually be discontinued.

3. *Bellis* is used to relieve blunt pain or trauma (the feeling of being hit in the face or of breaking the nose), to speed recovery after surgery, to help prevent infection, to treat abscesses, and to reduce swelling. Take three pills before and three pills after surgery.

4. *Calendula* is recommended for wounds that are slow to heal. Take three pills before and three pills after surgery.

5. *Hypericum* is used as a tonic for the nervous system and kidneys, and to treat puncture wounds and pain after dental work. For surgery, it's particularly useful for treating pain caused by injury to the nerve endings. Take three pills before and three pills after surgery.

SURGICAL SCARS DISSOLVED

When a woman took off her shirt for acupuncture, huge angry purplish-red scars were evident on her chest. She revealed that she had had a breast reduction a year and a half earlier. Dr. Walker treated the scars with ScarGo and the Bioptron light machine, and they completely faded after a month of treatment.

---

6. *Phosphorus* is used to treat anxiety, nervous and digestive ills, respiratory problems, and circulatory problems. In conjunction with surgical procedures, *Phosphorus* 6 or 30 helps relieve bleeding, nausea, and the lingering effects of anesthetics. Take three pills before and three pills after surgery.

7. *Staphysagria* aids in relieving the pain of incision. *Staphysagria* 30 may be taken four times a day following surgery until pain-free.

8. *Cantharis* is most often used for bladder and reproductive problems, particularly when there is inflammation in those regions; it is also useful in conjunction with surgery, for reducing the redness and swelling of burns. It should not be taken before a laser or face peel, however, since it neutralizes burns so well that it can nullify the surgery's effects. A face peel involves burning the skin in a way that removes wrinkles. These authors don't recommend it, because it leaves the skin plastic-looking and represents an unnatural stress to the skin; if homeopathic remedies are being used with a peel, however, they should be used only after the procedure has been performed, to speed healing. For other surgeries, take three pills before and three pills after surgery.

SAILING THROUGH COSMETIC SURGERY

A prominent woman in Sun Valley who was preparing to have extensive facial surgery and liposuction was quite skeptical of the homeopathic approach, but she was willing to try it because her sister, who had had the same surgery, had had a very difficult time with it. Her sister had suffered substantial pain, bruising, and swelling. She couldn't go out in public but had to stay "undercover" for a long time. The Sun Valley woman used the homeopathic remedies and was thrilled with the results. *She took no pain medications at all,* something her doctor said he had never seen. His patients typically required pain medication for two or three days after plastic surgery, which involves a great deal of trauma to the body. The woman experienced much less bruising, redness, and trauma to her face than in the usual case; her body healed very nicely; and she was quite comfortable through it all, although she had had liposuction at the same time.

The remarkable effectiveness of *Cantharis,* the homeopathic remedy for speeding recovery from burns, was demonstrated when a laser surgeon came to Sun Valley in 1997. He scheduled about ten patients for laser peels on the same day. Four of the women were Dr. Walker's patients and had been instructed to take *Cantharis* after the surgery. The day after the surgeries, the women all lined up for their rechecks. Comparing stories in the waiting room, those who had taken the *Cantharis* found they had slept better the night after the surgery, had had substantially less discomfort, and were noticeably more healed the following day.

PREPARING FOR SURGERY: NUTRITIONAL AND PSYCHOLOGICAL SUPPORT

Besides homeopathic treatment, the body's efforts to heal itself should be supported with nutritional and herbal supplements, proper diet, and toning exercises. Additional vitamin C, vitamin B$_6$, and magnesium are particularly important to counteract the stress of surgery on the body. Take according to product labels.

A week before surgery, avoid taking anything that encourages bleeding, including aspirin, vitamin E, evening primrose oil, some Chinese herbs (for example, *Hsiao Yao Wan* or *Xiao Yao Wan*), and certain prescription medications. Consult your doctor concerning specific products.

You should also try to enter surgery in a relaxed state of mind. Stress can exhaust nutritional stores and weaken the body's ability to recover. Use any technique at your disposal to maintain a positive and relaxed state of mind prior to your surgery: meditation, prayer, guided imagery, biofeedback, and so on.

RECOVERING FROM SURGERY

A fundamental principle of Chinese medicine is that the body is crisscrossed with "meridians," or lines of energy, which provide the vitality necessary not only for healing but for maintaining the workings of the body. Surgery inevitably cuts through these meridians, blocking both healing and bodily function. To reconnect them, Chinese doctors use acupuncture, a technique involving stimulating particular points on the body with very fine needles. Acupuncture treatments are helpful not only after surgery but before it, to increase energy flow and ensure that it's moving properly.

For patients who say they have never been well since their surgeries, homeopathic *Phosphorus* can help eliminate the effects of the anesthetics. Homeopathic remedies give the best results for patients who are armed with them in the operating room, but they can also aid recovery after surgery or from the drugs used with it. If your system can't eliminate the

RECOVERY ONLY AFTER REACHING THE CAUSE

A 35-year-old woman had serious pain in her gallbladder. Her doctor, finding that her gallbladder had shriveled to the size of a walnut, had surgically removed it. The woman thought the surgery would eliminate her problem, but she had the same pain after the operation as when she went in and now she couldn't get her vitality back. Homeopathic *Phosphorus* brought back her energy, but she continued to suffer from the pain. Further testing indicated that she was heavily infested with parasites. In fact, this was likely to have been the reason she had the gallbladder problem to begin with. She improved only after correcting this underlying problem.

anesthetics, you will continue to feel tired and sluggish. If you think this could be your problem, see a homeopath for recommendations and dosages.

Complete recovery, however, requires resolving the patient's underlying physical problems. Surgeries attack symptoms, but they often fail to address the real cause of disease. A practitioner can test for underlying problems and treat them homeopathically.

ALLEVIATING THE PHYSICAL EFFECTS OF SURGICAL SHOCK

Surgical shock can be responsible for unanticipated side effects. In one double-blind randomized trial involving fifty children undergoing surgery, a significant reduction in postoperative pain and agitation was experienced by those given homeopathic *Aconitum*.[2] *Aconitum* is a common remedy for ailments involving sudden and violent onset of shock or trauma and for fear and anxiety, such as before surgery. Three pellets of *Aconitum* 6 or 30 should be taken the night before the operation and again in the morning before the operation on awakening. If anxiety continues after surgery, take one to three more doses.

RECOVERY FROM SURGICAL SCARS

For speeding the healing of surgical scars, a cream called ScarGo, containing olive oil, peanut oil, lanolin, camphor, and yellow beeswax, does a remarkable job. Follow label directions. Also quite effective for reducing redness and swelling (resulting from burns after laser surgery, for example) is the Bioptron light machine. (See "Skin Problems" on page 222.)

SYPHILIS

Syphilis is among the most serious of sexually transmitted diseases, affecting over 100,000 Americans annually. Women contract syphilis only half as often as men, since gay men drive the male numbers up. However, the disease still afflicts more than 30,000 women per year. A painless sore on the genitals may signal the condition, but carriers may have no symptoms at all. Untreated syphilis can cause serious heart problems, blindness, paralysis, mental disorders, or death. It can be passed from mother to child, causing stillbirth, active infection, or birth defects.

Condoms can protect against the disease but are not foolproof, particularly if open sores are present in the carrier. Your best defenses remain abstention or careful choosing of partners and regular checkups.

CONVENTIONAL TREATMENT

People who contract syphilis are required by law to see a doctor. The doctor then must report the case to the health department. Patients who are diagnosed with the disease are treated with antibiotics. The syphilis bacteria is one that hasn't yet developed resistance to antibiotics, so the disease usually responds to penicillin. Drug treatment is often accompanied by fever, chills, headaches, worsening of lesions, and a general feeling of ill health. This complication, however, does not seem to be an allergic response to the drug. Rather, it's the result of the rapid release of antigens from the suddenly killed syphilis bacteria.[1]

NATURAL REMEDIES

As a complement to antibiotic treatment, homeopaths maintain that homeopathic treatment should also be sought from a qualified practitioner, to resolve not just the infection but any "miasms" (inherited tendencies) contributing to it. Children of a syphilitic parent may have psychotic tendencies. Homeopathic remedies clear the miasms along with the disease. After taking a detailed patient history, a homeopath can determine the appropriate remedies to resolve not just the syphilis but its inherited miasms.

SYSTEMIC LUPUS ERYTHEMATOSUS (SLE)

See LUPUS.

TOXIC SHOCK SYNDROME

Toxic shock syndrome is a sudden, potentially fatal shock response to the release of toxins by an overgrowth of a staphylococcus bacteria commonly found in women. An estimated 5,000 to 10,000 cases of staphylococcal toxic shock syndrome occur in the United States each year, and about half involve tampons or menstruation. Incidence of the condition declined in the 1980s, when certain highly absorbent tampons were taken off the market after a rash of cases was linked to them. But there has now been a sudden increase in the more dangerous streptococcal toxic shock, which has a death rate of up to 50 percent. Other precipitating causes of the syndrome besides tampons and menstruation include the use of contraceptive sponges, cervical caps, or diaphragms; childbirth; surgery; wounds; and influenza. Symptoms of toxic shock include sudden high fever, vomiting, diarrhea, a sunburnlike rash, low blood pressure, and shock.[1]

CONVENTIONAL TREATMENT

Conventional treatment is with antibiotics specific to staph infection, along with blood transfusions and other emergency treatment. The critical factor, however, is prompt diagnosis. Though potentially fatal, the disease is rare, so doctors may not recognize it.

Family members need to be alert to the possibility of toxic shock and to seek immediate treatment.

NATURAL REMEDIES

Effective homeopathic remedies are available for toxic shock syndrome from Staufen, Deseret, and CompliMed, but consultation with a homeopath is necessary. In this case, it's best simply to seek prompt conventional treatment.

To avoid acquiring toxic shock syndrome, avoid turning the vaginal area into a breeding medium for bacteria by closing it off for long periods with tampons, diaphragms, cervical caps, or sponges.

TRICHOMONIASIS

See VAGINITIS AND VAGINAL INFECTIONS.

URINARY TRACT INFECTION

See BLADDER INFECTION, IRRITATION, AND INFLAMMATION (CYSTITIS).

UTERINE CANCER

See CANCERS, HORMONAL.

UTERINE FIBROID TUMORS

Fibroid tumors are masses of connective tissue that tend to grow on the wall of the uterus before menopause, when estrogen secretion dominates. Symptoms suggesting fibroids include abdominal swelling, pelvic or back pain, heavy or irregular bleeding, painful periods, constipation, pressure on the bladder, and frequent urination. More than 40 percent of women over age 50 have benign fibroid tumors, the most common tumors of the female pelvic organs. Although rarely malignant, these tumors can still precipitate a hysterectomy by causing excessive menstrual bleeding and pelvic pain. They are, in fact, the most common reason given for this surgery. Researchers in one study concluded that more than a quarter of a million uteri were removed annually to excise fibroid tumors.[1]

CONVENTIONAL TREATMENT

Medical wisdom says that fibroids cannot be dissolved. Small ones may disappear by themselves after menopause, but the conventional treatment for eliminating large or painful fibroids remains surgical removal by hysterectomy.[2] For downsides, see "Hysterectomy" on page 153.

SURGICAL ALTERNATIVES

Even if surgery is required, there may be alternatives to removing the female organs. Vicki Hufnagel, M.D., author of *No More Hysterectomies,* favors a modified surgery that can eliminate fibroids while preserving the uterus and ovaries. Called "female reconstructive surgery," the procedure involves a surgical resectioning of the organ. The abdomen is opened with a bikini-type incision and the uterus is lifted out for complete inspection. The tissue connected to the uterus is clamped off with a special clamp and a drug is injected to stop the flow of blood, to allow maximum surgical time without bleeding. Fibroid tumors are then removed. In the case of prolapse, the ligaments and organs are also restructured and resuspended.

NATURAL REMEDIES

Nonsurgical Alternatives: Natural Progesterone

Hormone researcher John Lee, M.D., maintains that uterine fibroids can be prevented and treated without surgery by using natural progesterone cream—not the synthetic form of the hormone, but a plant derivative of a type of yam. Estrogen stimulates the growth of fibroids, which are common in the estrogen-dominant phase of perimenopause (early-stage menopause, before menses have ceased). If estrogen levels are allowed to drop off naturally after menopause, existing uterine tumors will typically atrophy by themselves. Problems arise when estrogen is artificially supplied, stimulating fibroid tumors to grow. These fibroids usually remain nonmalignant, but they can cause excessive menstrual bleeding and pelvic pain, precipitating a hysterectomy.

Supplementing before menopause with natural progesterone, estrogen's antagonist, not only may help prevent fibroids from developing but also can help shrink them once they have developed.[3] ProGest by Transitions for Health is a particularly effective over-the-counter natural progesterone cream. Dosages vary depending on hormonal status; see Chapter 2. *Note: Synthetic progestin (as opposed to natural progesterone) is contraindicated for fibroids; it tends to make them grow.*[4]

SURGERY AVOIDED WITH SIMPLE CREAM

Dr. Lee cites the case of a former patient who telephoned to say she had developed a large fibroid tumor. Her gynecologist, concerned that its rapid growth suggested cancer, recommended immediate removal of her uterus and ovaries. Dr. Lee suggested that she try natural progesterone cream instead, and she agreed. When the woman returned to her gynecologist a month later, the tumor was about 10 percent smaller. After three months, it was 25 percent reduced; six months later (or ten months from when she began using natural progesterone), it was gone.[5]

Both authors of this book have had similar experiences. Both were diagnosed with large fibroid tumors and were told surgical removal was required. In both cases, before menopause, the tumors shrank on their own and hysterectomy was avoided, with the aid of natural remedies including natural progesterone cream, acupuncture, homeopathy, and herbs.

Other Natural Remedies for Shrinking Fibroids

Eastern herbs can also help shrink tumors, but professional help should be sought in choosing a remedy and determining dosages. Among other possibilities, the following are some Chinese herbal products by Seven Forests useful for shrinking unwanted growths:

◆ Laminaria 4—for fatty type swellings.

◆ Zedoria tablets—for hard masses.

◆ Chih-ko and Curcuma—for phlegm or blood stagnation, considered in Chinese medicine to be the cause of many fibroids.

Even malignant tumors have responded to Chinese herbs. In a recent study, proteins extracted from Chinese medicinal herbs were shown to selectively injure tumor cell lines while preserving normal cell lines. Conventional cytotoxic ("cell-killing") chemotherapy, by contrast, kills normal cells along with aberrant cells.[6]

Natural Remedies to Counteract Bleeding and Balance Hormones

Dr. Ray Peat, developer of natural progesterone in topical cream form, observes that the heavy and irregular menstrual bleeding accompanying a uterine tumor can be a symptom of an underactive thyroid gland. He suggests that before the uterus is removed for excessive bleeding, thyroid therapy should be tried.[7] For remedies, see Hypothyroidism on page 150.

Other natural remedies can also help stop the heavy bleeding that often accompanies a fibroid. Natural progesterone cream is one option. ProGest by Transitions for Health is a particularly good product. If you are still menstruating, rub ⅛ to ¼ teaspoon of the cream on your abdominal area each night for the fourteen days before your period, stopping the day or so before your period starts. For postmenopausal women, use this amount for twenty-five days out of the month.

Another option is the herb chasteberry, which stimulates progesterone synthesis and secretion. It not only can help regulate periods involving too frequent or too much bleeding but also is a good treatment for fibroids and for inflammation of the lining of the uterus. Follow label directions. *Note: Chasteberry should not be used during pregnancy, since it is a strong uterine stimulant.*[8]

Other natural remedies for heavy bleeding include the following:

◆ Homeopathic Mother Tincture of *Thlaspi bursa pastoris* (shepherd's purse)—take ten drops in water every hour until bleeding slows.

◆ Bleeding (a combination homeopathic remedy by BHI)—take one pill every fifteen minutes as needed until bleeding slows, then four times daily until it stops.

◆ Luvos Earth (a powdered clay) and Trillium (an herbal liquid)—take twenty drops of Trillium in water three times daily, or in cases of acute bleeding, use fifty drops in half a glass of water followed by twenty drops every hour.

◆ *Yunnan Pai Yao*—take two capsules every hour until bleeding stops. This Chinese formula is highly effective both topically and orally to stop bleeding on which nothing else seems to work. It was used by Vietnamese soldiers, who put it on their wounds to avoid leaving a bloody trail when they got shot.

Once bleeding is stopped, steps should be taken to build up the blood and balance the body to avoid repeating the problem each month. (See "Anemia" on page 44.) Useful remedies for toning and balancing when fibroid tumors are present include the following:

◆ Female Tonic by MPI—take one tablespoonful twice daily.

◆ Fibrozolve by Apex—take ten drops three to four times daily.

◆ Female Balance—take ten drops three times daily.

◆ Vita Gyn by Eclectic Institute—take four pills twice daily for five days after the period.

◆ Grapeseed extract—take 1 mg per pound of body weight daily.

◆ Cat's claw—take two capsules three times daily.

Caution: Although fewer than 0.2 percent of fibroid tumors are found to be malignant, malignancy remains a possibility.[9] *If you have symptoms suggesting fibroids, see a gynecologist. While the natural remedies discussed here are safe, you should not attempt self-treatment. If you are interested in exploring natural remedies, see an Eastern medical, homeopathic, or naturopathic physician.*

UTERINE PROLAPSE

Uterine prolapse is a condition in which the uterus descends into the lower part of the vagina or, in some cases, actually outside the vaginal opening. Childbirth is considered the most common precipitating cause, since it substantially stretches the muscles of the uterus. Age-related loss of the collagen that keeps the muscles elastic can also precipitate pelvic-floor disorders. Heavy lifting and other exercise that causes the abdominal wall muscles to contract are other possible precipitating causes.[1]

CONVENTIONAL TREATMENT

No known drug will reverse a prolapsed uterus. The conventional treatment is hysterectomy—surgical removal of the uterus. A less drastic option that preserves the female organs is a surgical resectioning of the uterus called "female reconstructive surgery." Both are discussed under "Hysterectomy" on page 153. A mechanical stopgap measure for prolapse is the pessary, a device placed within the vagina to support the bladder, vagina, and rectum. Kegel exercises, involving contracting and relaxing the uterine muscles, are also recommended for uterine prolapse. They may forestall the condition but won't reverse it.

UTERINE PROLAPSE REVERSED

Ellen, a coauthor of this book, was scheduled at the age of 50 for female reconstructive surgery to repair a prolapsed uterus and remove a large fibroid tumor. The surgery had been recommended several years earlier, but she ignored the advice until her symptoms got so pronounced that she had to quit going for walks because they resulted in a quite uncomfortable drop in the subject organ. She canceled the operation, however, after both the prolapse and the fibroid disappeared of their own volition. She attributed this rather remarkable result primarily to the use of natural progesterone cream (ProGest) along with several courses of live cell therapy, a treatment developed in Germany consisting of injections of fetal cells of animal organs. This therapy has evidently been kept off the U.S. market by the high cost of FDA approval but is available in Central America (where she lived at the time) and is offered in many Tijuana alternative clinics. The ProGest link has been confirmed by an experiment she has tried on numerous occasions over a period of several years, always with the same result. Whenever she allows several days to pass without rubbing ¼ to ½ teaspoon of this cream on her abdominal area at night, her uterus invariably drops uncomfortably. She has tried switching brands and has found that ProGest is the only over-the-counter formulation that keeps her uterus in suspension, although she can't explain why. Another product that has this effect but is available only by prescription is a 6 percent natural progesterone cream made by Women's International Pharmacy in Madison, Wisconsin. Ellen also uses a number of other natural hormone boosters, including the precursor hormones DHEA and pregnenolone and a natural estrogen cream derived from plants (OstaDerm). She abandoned the use of contraceptive creams after learning that they could be contributing to the problem. She has delivered two large babies, but so have many other women who managed to avoid uterine prolapse.

NATURAL REMEDIES

Natural progesterone cream (ProGest) can help reverse or forestall uterine prolapse. If you are still menstruating, rub ⅛ to ¼ teaspoon of the cream on your abdominal area each night for the fourteen days before your period, stopping the day or so before your period starts. For postmenopausal women, use this amount for twenty-five days out of the month.

Sepia is a homeopathic remedy that helps counteract a loss of energy that leaves the body with insufficient resources to hold the organs in place or the blood in the blood vessels. Women of the *Sepia* constitutional type are tired, tend to bruise easily, and have hemorrhoids, varicose veins, and prolapse. Appropriate strengths can range from 200 to 1M; see a homeopath for recommendations in your own case.

In China, a form of the herb black cohosh called *Sheng Ma* is traditionally used for uterine and bladder prolapse—as well as for measles, toothache, and canker sores. Black cohosh (*Cimicifuga racemosa*) is also native to North America, where it was first used by Native Americans to ease the pain of menstruation and childbirth and to antidote rattlesnake bites. Black cohosh is an estrogenic herb that has a regulating and normalizing effect on hormone production and is contained in many formulas for balancing women's hormones. A powerful uterine tonic, it is useful for bladder and uterine prolapse and vaginal atrophy. *Caution: Black cohosh should not be used during abnormally heavy menstrual periods.*[2]

Other Chinese herbal formulas recommended for uterine prolapse include Ginseng and Astragalus and Tang Kuei Formula, both by Zand. Follow label directions.

Contraceptive creams containing monoxynol have been linked to uterine prolapse and should be discontinued. Nonoxynol-9 breaks down into nonylphenol when it comes in contact with the body. Nonylphenols are estrogen-mimicking chemicals that are toxic to the body and can disrupt its hormone balance even in very low concentrations. They are absorbed not only from contraceptive creams but also from ubiquitous sources including plastic products, polystyrene food containers, detergents, personal-care products, and the polyvinyl chloride tubing through which water passes.[3]

VAGINAL DISCHARGE

See VAGINITIS AND VAGINAL INFECTIONS.

VAGINAL DRYNESS

Lack of vaginal lubrication during intercourse means hormone levels are dropping. It can be one of the first symptoms of menopause. Classic symptoms of vaginal atrophy are dryness, irritation, burning, and a feeling of pressure. There may also be a yellowish discharge. The vagina gets progressively shorter and narrower, its skin tissue thins, and its muscular layer is replaced with fibrous tissue. The vagina shrivels and shrinks and loses its flexibility, while the labia become small, colorless, and flat.[1] The vagina also becomes susceptible to infection. This is because its thin walls lack the normal secretions that cleanse the vaginal tissues. Vaginal pH rises (meaning it becomes more alkaline instead of the normal acid), allowing undesirable bacteria to replace the friendly bacterial flora. The result can be urinary tract infections. (See "Vaginitis and Vaginal Infections" on page 240 and "Bladder Infection, Irritation, and Inflammation [Cystitis]" on page 63.)

CONVENTIONAL TREATMENT

Antibiotics are usually prescribed for vaginal infections; however, because the problem in this case is the alkalinity of the vagina, the infections tend to recur, leading to long-term drug use that can be dangerous and expensive.[2] Many physicians resort to chronic suppressive therapy with sulfonamides, but these drugs can also be dangerous, with complications that are sometimes life-threatening.[3]

For vaginal dryness, lubricants and moisturizers are available. A vaginal suppository called Replens is effective but expensive. Cheaper options are K-Y jelly and Mennen's Baby Magic. A drawback of these drugstore products is that they contain mineral oil, which blocks pores and congests tissue. Mineral oil is difficult for the body to dispose of and tends to be allergenic.

For menopausal vaginal infections, hormone treatment is an effective alternative to antibiotics. In a University of Florida Medical School study, when postmenopausal women with a history of recurrent infection and antibiotics were treated with pharmaceutical estrogen, vaginitis was cured and urinary tract infections went away for good. The estrogen worked by restoring the normal vaginal flora and pH.[4] At first, the women took estrogen by mouth, but they were already past menopause and were upset by the return of their periods, painful enlargement of their breasts, and nausea. Some of the women were, therefore, switched to a vaginal estrogen cream taken twice weekly. The cream, which avoided passage through the digestive tract, proved to be just as effective as the pills without their unpleasant side effects.

LUBRICATION AND SEX DRIVE RETURN WITH NATURAL REMEDY

Peggy, age 62, was married but hadn't had sex for years, due to bladder problems and vaginal dryness. After taking Hormone Combination for just a few weeks, to her husband's delight, her sex drive returned. Sex no longer hurt, and she found that she liked it after all!

European research shows that hormone therapy can help in cases not only of vaginal infection but also of vaginal dryness and atrophy. In a 1991 study, twenty postmenopausal women (average age 73) were treated with oral pharmaceutical estrogen in the form of estriol. When their flora and epithelial cells were compared to those of twenty untreated women of similar age and twenty healthy younger women (average age 28), they more nearly resembled those of the younger women than of the untreated postmenopausal women.[5] A Norwegian review concluded that estriol is a safe, inexpensive, and effective therapy for the symptoms of estrogen deficiency after menopause, including atrophy of the vagina, urethra, and bladder, urinary tract infections, and abnormal function of the lower urinary tract. The researchers found that estriol had no metabolic effects or serious side effects at recommended doses and was safe for long-term use.[6]

NATURAL REMEDIES

The estrogen in these studies was in drug form, but natural options are also available. Estriol is the major estrogen component in "OstaDerm V," a natural estrogen/progesterone cream derived from plants that is designed for vaginal use. David Shefrin, N.D., uses this cream for cases of severe atrophic vaginitis. He observes, "It has always amazed me how easily the vaginal problems can be reversed. Women whose vaginas bled just with the introduction of a small speculum or from taking a Pap smear return literally after six weeks with a moist, pink, youthful vagina. Not all cases can be completely reversed in just six weeks, however. In those women with profound atrophy, the process may take a few months. Prognosis then depends on how great the loss of estrogen was and for how long. So it's very important to educate these women early on."[7] Recommended dosage of OstaDerm V is 1/8 to 1/2 teaspoon as needed three times weekly.

The natural way to maintain vaginal lubrication is to remain sexually active, but lack of vaginal lubrication can keep you from that therapy. Natural estrogen cream (OstaDerm V) or progesterone cream (ProGest) can be used vaginally for lubrication. A product that is petroleum-free is Lubricating Gel by Women's Health Institute.

Vitamin E has also been shown to be effective in relieving atrophic vaginitis. You can insert the capsules vaginally, take them by mouth, or open them up and apply the oil directly to the vaginal tissues. The dosage by mouth is 400–800 IU daily. Evening primrose oil can be used in the same way. The dosage by mouth is 500–2,600 mg daily.

Hormone Combination by Deseret is an excellent homeopathic product that helps to balance the hormones in the brain and stimulates the body to increase hormone production. It works not only for perimenopausal, menopausal, and postmenopausal women but also for men. Both men and women with low sex drive often report increased interest in sex and increased sexual function after using this remedy for just a few weeks. Take five to ten drops one to three times daily.

VAGINAL WARTS

See GENITAL WARTS.

VAGINITIS AND VAGINAL INFECTIONS

Vaginal inflammation (vaginitis) and vaginal infection are the most common gynecological disorders, prompting more than 10 million doctor visits annually. Vaginal infections include the following:

◆ Candidiasis (yeast infection): a fungal infection caused by an overgrowth of yeast cells (*Candida*). Symptoms include itching, burning, and a white discharge resembling cottage cheese.

◆ Bacterial vaginosis: vaginitis caused by bacteria. Bacteria are found naturally in the vagina, but this disorder results from a change in the balance of vaginal bacteria, as from antibiotics. The condition is characterized by a milky discharge with a fishy odor. It can precipitate pelvic infection leading to infertility or complications of pregnancy.[1]

◆ Trichomoniasis ("trich"): a sexually transmitted disease caused by a parasite. Affecting about 2.5 million women yearly, it may have no symptoms or may involve vaginal itching, burning, and a yellow or creamy white vaginal discharge with a strong odor. A mother affected with this infection during pregnancy may pass it on to her female baby at delivery.

See also "Fungal Infections" on page 116 and "Vaginal Dryness" on page 238.

Conventional Treatment

Antifungal creams such as clotrimazole and miconazole were once available only by prescription, but they can now be purchased over the counter for vaginal infections. The National Vaginitis Association warns, however, that unless the sufferer has had yeast infections before and is sure of the symptoms, treatment should not be attempted without getting a diagnosis first, since antifungals won't cure the bacterial and parasitic infections that have similar symptoms but more hazardous outcomes. For these, prescription medications are recommended. Recurrent yeast infections can also be an indication of something more serious, like diabetes or the HIV virus. Other downsides of the popular nonprescription antifungals are that they can have side effects and don't deal with the underlying cause, so the infection is liable to recur.

The usual treatment for trichomoniasis is with the antiparasitic drug metronidazole (Flagyl), but again the infection is liable to recur, and the drug can have substantial side effects. (See "Parasitic Infection" on page 212.) *Caution: Metronidazole is carcinogenic to rodents and should not be taken by pregnant women. Metronidazole taken with alcohol can result in nausea, vomiting, flushing, and difficulty breathing.*

VAGINAL *"CANDIDA"* ELIMINATED WITH CONSTITUTIONAL HOMEOPATHIC REMEDY

Linda complained of a *Candida* infection, but she had no yeasty discharge or specific pain or itch. She was just uncomfortable in the vaginal area. She was also quite unhappy. Questioning revealed underlying emotional trauma. The key to her case seemed to be an incident when she was 8 years old, when a man grabbed her as she was riding her bicycle and pulled off her underwear. She was terrified by this incident and had never really gotten over it. Her fear of men had caused her to make some bad choices in relationships, and she was generally unsettled and disturbed.

Dr. Walker gave Linda a constitutional remedy specific to her case, *Staphysagria* 1M, for women who were abused or mistreated as children and grew up to accept abuse in their relationships with men or to be attracted to abusive men. The remedy changed her life. She broke off her current unsatisfactory relationship and soon met a man everyone said was perfect for her, although she conceded she would not previously have been attracted to his type. She had tried before to get pregnant and had been unable to, but now she got pregnant without trying. Her boyfriend was delighted and said he wanted to marry her. She is happy for the first time in years and feels her successful relationship was the result of changes in her that allowed her to attract this sort of mate. Meanwhile, she no longer complains of her *Candida,* which has been forgotten. She probably never had it. What she had was a nonspecific awareness of something wrong in the vaginal area, a traumatic childhood imprint that constitutional remedies relieved.

NATURAL REMEDIES

To discourage overgrowths of yeast and other invaders, a proper acid-alkaline balance needs to be restored and maintained within the vagina. Yeast can't live in an acid environment. To acidify the vaginal area, a douche can be made of acidophilus. Mix liquid acidophilus or a teaspoon of acidophilus powder into an ounce of water or milk. Another option is apple cider vinegar (four tablespoons to one cup of water). Yogurt that contains active *Lactobacillus acidophilus* culture may also be included in the diet.

Another alternative is boric acid capsules, which increase vaginal acidity. Boric acid has been found to reverse yeast infections in 98 percent of women for whom other treatments were unsuccessful. Recommended dosage is one capsule inserted vaginally every night at bedtime for a week, then two or three times a week for three more weeks. (You can use an "O"-sized gelatin capsule filled with powdered boric acid, which is about 600 mg.) *Caution: Professional advice should be sought before undertaking boric acid treatment, since sensitive women occasionally experience some burning or watery discharge. Keep boric acid out of the reach of children, for whom it can be fatal at doses of as little as 5 grams.* [2]

An herbal douche containing forty drops of echinacea, forty drops of goldenseal, forty drops of calendula, and two tablespoons of aloe vera in a pint of water can also relieve symptoms. A sitz bath containing calendula and goldenseal can soothe burning and itching. For other herbal remedies for yeast infection, see "Fungal Infections" on page 116.

To discourage vaginal yeast, it's best to omit foods from the diet on which yeast thrive. These include foods containing sugar, molds, or yeasts, and aged or fermented foods, including breads made with yeast, aged cheeses, vinegar, and beer. No anti-*Candida* diet will effect a permanent cure, however, unless the underlying problem is also corrected.

Homeopathic options for vaginitis include *Kreosotum, Cantharis,* and *Sulfur.* A good combination remedy is Vaginitis by Hyland's. Follow label directions.

For trichomoniasis, Staufen makes a safe, effective, nontoxic homeopathic series therapy called Trichomonas Vaginitis. Comparable series therapy is available in the

United States from Deseret Biologicals. Directions are on the box. The remedy should be used even if conventional treatment is used, to prevent future recurrences.

In some cases, the underlying problem is emotional rather than physical. A homeopath may be able to correct the problem in those cases with an appropriate constitutional remedy.

VARICOSE VEINS

Varicose veins are prominent dark-blue blood vessels running just beneath the surface of the skin, usually in the legs and feet. Between 20 and 25 percent of women suffer from them, nearly twice the male percentages. Sufferers may experience aching, fatigue, or heat that is relieved by elevation or wearing compressive hosiery. Risk factors associated with developing varicose veins include obesity, high systolic blood pressure, cigarette smoking, low levels of physical activity, pregnancy, abdominal or pelvic masses, and occupations that require prolonged standing.[1]

Chinese doctors say varicose veins result when the vital life force is weak as a result of physical or adrenal stress. (See "Adrenal Stress" on page 36.) The body becomes too weak to hold the organs in place. The blood falls out of the veins and they "varicose," or pool rather than flow, on the model of a hose that is shut off at one end while the water is still running. Women often get varicose veins during childbirth. Chinese medical theory attributes this phenomenon not only to the weight of the fetus pressing on the mother's leg veins but also to the fact that her body is under stress and her baby uses much of her vital life force.

CONVENTIONAL TREATMENT

Standard treatment for varicose veins is mechanical compression, sclerotherapy (injection of a substance that causes the veins to shrink), or surgery. Compression therapy is done with lightweight hosiery for small varicose veins. Advanced cases require a heavier elastic support stocking.

Many physicians consider the first line of therapy to be a high-fiber diet with commercial fiber supplements and enough oral fluids to produce soft but well-formed and regular bowel movements. A low-fiber diet can result in small, hard stools that can cause straining during bowel movements. This strain increases pressure on the veins of the lower legs and the hemorrhoidal cushions, deteriorating the veins over time. A high-fiber diet is important for the prevention and treatment of both hemorrhoids and varicose veins. (See "Hemorrhoids" on page 139.) Activities that require strain should also be avoided.

NATURAL REMEDIES

Homeopathic remedies can help relieve varicose veins. *Sepia* 30 is one that helps counteract a loss of energy that leaves the body with insufficient resources to hold the organs in place or the blood in the blood vessels. Women of the *Sepia* constitutional type are tired, tend to bruise easily, and have hemorrhoids, varicose veins, and organ prolapse. Other

BUSY PRACTITIONER'S VARICOSE VEINS RELIEVED

Susan, a chiropractor, began developing varicose veins that were painful when she slept. Her stress came from a busy practice where she stood on her feet all day and worked very hard, causing her veins to varicose. She began taking Dolisos European Horse Chestnut along with *Sepia*, a homeopathic remedy that was appropriate for her constitutional type and supported her overall body energy. Her veins stopped hurting at night almost immediately, and in the succeeding months, they got progressively smaller and less purple.

possibilities include *Lachesis* 200, *Calc fluor* 30, and *Lycopodium* 200. See a homeopath for recommendations and dosage for your own case.

European Horse Chestnut, a gemmotherapy by Dolisos, can help support the veins. Take fifty drops in water every morning.

WATER RETENTION

See BLOATING, GAS, AND EDEMA.

WEIGHT LOSS

See OVERWEIGHT.

WEIGHT, LOW

Inability to put on weight is a far less common problem than inability to take it off, but some women are afflicted with it. Women who have lost weight from illness or toxic drug therapies are particularly affected.

CONVENTIONAL TREATMENT

The usual recommendation is a weight supplement, such as Ensure, drunk four times a day between meals. The problem is that a woman already suffering from lack of appetite is then liable to be too full to eat properly during meals.

NATURAL REMEDIES

Alfalfa can help by cleansing the liver and stimulating the appetite. (Overweight women should avoid using this supplement.)

Other recommendations are to eat regular meals and to reduce stress. For the latter, Skullcap Oats can help (one to two droppersful three times daily).

CANCER PATIENT GAINS WEIGHT WITH NATURAL REMEDY

Bea was painfully thin after receiving chemotherapy and radiation treatments for cancer. She began taking alfalfa supplements (one capsule three times daily) and was pleased to report that she had gained forty pounds a month and a half later, putting her at a weight she felt was healthy for her.

Low thyroid hormone levels can be a cause of underweight. If these are found by a practitioner, homeopathic remedies can help. To balance an overactive thyroid, take Pituitary 9C by Dolisos (three pills once or twice daily). For other options, see "Hyperthyroidism" on page 148.

YEAST INFECTIONS

See FUNGAL INFECTIONS.

NOTES

PART ONE

Chapter 1. What Makes Women Different: Understanding Hormones

1 R. Peat, *Nutrition for Women* (Eugene, Oreg.: Kenogen, 1981), pages 11–22; J. Prior, "Progesterone as a Bone-tropic Hormone," *Endocrine Reviews* 11(2):386–98 (1990); J. Lee, M.D., "Significance of Molecular Configuration Specificity: The Case of Progesterone and Osteoporosis," *Townsend Letter for Doctors* 119:558–62 (1993).

2 L. Swartzman, et al., "Impact of Stress on Objectively Recorded Menopausal Hot Flushes and on Flush Report Bias," *Health Psychology* 9(5):529–45 (1990).

3 R. Peat, *op. cit.*, pages 17–18.

4 J. Lee, M.D., "Slowing the Aging Process with Natural Progesterone" (Sebastopol, Calif.; unpublished research paper).

5 H. Lewis, et al., *Psychosomatics* (New York: Pinnacle Books, 1975).

6 H. Aldercreutz, et al., "Dietary Estrogens and the Menopause in Japan," *The Lancet* 339:1233 (1992).

7 Y. Beyenne, "Cultural Significance and Physiological Manifestations of Menopause: A Biocultural Analysis," *Culture, Med. Psychiatry* 10:58 (1986).

8 See E. Brown, L. Walker, *Menopause and Estrogen* (Berkeley, Calif.: Frog Ltd., 1996), chapter 14.

9 S. Sellman, "The Physiology of Hormones," *Health and Natural Journal* (October 2000).

10 *Ibid.*

Chapter 2. Hormone Replacement Therapy: Pros, Cons, and Alternatives

1 J. Healey, "The Cancer Weapon America Needs Most," *Reader's Digest* (June 1992), pages 69–72.

2 L. Huppert, "Hormonal Replacement Therapy: Benefits, Risks, Doses," *Medical Clinics of North America* 71(1):23–39 (1987).

3 M. Whitehead, et al., "The Role and Use of Progestogens," *Obstetrics and Gynecology* 75(4):59S–76S (1990).

4 "The Top Ten Drugs—1997," www.chiroweb.com (2002).

5 Writing Group for the Women's Health Initiative, "Risks and Benefits of Estrogen Plus Progestin in Healthy Postmenopausal Women," *JAMA* 288(3):321–33 (July 17, 2002); "Menopausal Hormone Therapy and the Risk of Ovarian Cancer," *Ibid.*, 334–41, 368–69.

6 A. Skolnick, "At Third Meeting, Menopause Experts Make the Most of Insufficient Data," *JAMA* 268(18):2483–85 (1992).

7 R. Peat, "Origins of Progesterone Therapy," *Townsend Letter for Doctors* (November 1992), pages 1016–17; R. Sitruk-Ware, et al., "Oral Micronized Progesterone," *Contraception* 36(4):373–402 (1987); S. Whitcroft, et al., "Hormone Replacement Therapy: Risks and Benefits," *Clinical Endocrinology* 36:15–20 (1992); N. Lauersen, M.D., *PMS: Premenstrual Syndrome and You* (New York: Simon & Schuster, 1983).

8 M. Whitehead, *op. cit.*

9 P. Stumpf, "Pharmacokinetics of Estrogen," *Obstetrics and Gynecology* 75:9S–14S (1990).

10 J. Mercola, "Dangers of Estrogen," www.mercola.com (October 4, 1998), citing *The Lancet* 350:1041–44, 1047–59 (October 11, 1997).

11 The increased risk was 41 percent for women on HRT vs. 32 percent for women on estrogen alone. G. Colditz, et al., "The Use of Estrogens and Progestins and the Risk of Breast Cancer in Postmenopausal Women," *New England Journal of Medicine* 332:1589–93 (June 15, 1995).

12 C. Schairer, et al., "Menopausal Estrogen and Estrogen-progestin Replacement Therapy and Breast Cancer Risk," *JAMA* 283:485–91 (2000), discussed in "Studies Link Combination HRT to Breast Cancer," *Clinician Reviews* (April 2000).

13 R. Ross, et al., "Effect of Hormone Replacement Therapy on Breast Cancer Risk: Estrogen Versus Estrogen Plus Progestin," *Journal of the National Cancer Institute* 92:328–32 (2000).

14 W. Willett, et al., "Postmenopausal Estrogens—Opposed, Unopposed, or None of the Above [Editorial]," *JAMA* 283:534–35 (2000).

15 S. Okie, "Hormones Don't Protect Women from Heart Disease, Study Says," *Washington Post* (July 23, 2001); *Circulation* 104:499–503 (July 24, 2001).

16 "Study Says Estrogen No Help to Women with Alzheimer's," *Dallas Morning News* (February 23, 2000).

17 "Meta-analysis of Randomized Trials," *JAMA* 285(22):2891–97 (June 13, 2001).

18 "Prevalence and Predictive Factors for Regional Osteopenia in Women with Anorexia Nervosa," *Annals of Internal Medicine* 133(10):790–94 (November 21, 2000).

19 J. Lee, "The Case of Estrogen and Osteoporosis," *Townsend Letter for Doctors* 119:558–62 (1993).

20 R. Peat, *op. cit.*; J. Lee, "Osteoporosis Reversal: The Role of Progesterone," *International Clinical Nutrition Review* 10(3):384–91 (1990); J. Lee, "Significance of Molecular Configuration Specificity," *op. cit.*; "The Case of Progesterone and Osteoporosis," *op. cit.*; L. Huppert, *op. cit.*; S. Roan, "Study Urges Use of 2nd Hormone in Estrogen Therapy," *Los Angeles Times*, Home Edition, Part A, page 1 (February 7, 1996).

21 See E. Brown, L. Walker, *Menopause and Estrogen* (Berkeley, Calif.: Frog Ltd., 1996).

22 M. Key, "Data on Estrogens in Soybeans May Make ERT More Acceptable," *Cancer Biotechnology Weekly* (October 23, 1995), page 10; E. Braverman, et al., "Natural Estrogen and Progesterone: Research Indicates Health Benefits of Natural vs. Synthetic Hormones," *Total Health* (October 1991), page 55.

23 T. Hudson, "Current Natural Hormone Replacement Therapy Prescription Options," *Townsend Letter for Doctors and Patients* (May 2001); M. Napoli, "Plant-derived Estrogens: Safer Than Premarin?" *HealthFacts* (September 1999).

Chapter 3. Going Natural: Remedies That Correct Underlying Imbalances

1 J. Lazarou, et al., "Incidence of Adverse Drug Reactions in Hospitalized Patients," *JAMA* 279:1, 200–205 (1998).

2 D. Klinghardt. "Neural Therapy" [seminar] (1994–95); see www.neuraltherapy.com.

3 *Ibid.*

4 J. Diamond, M.D. *Life Energy* (St. Paul, Minn.: Paragon House, 1990).

5 J. Duke, "Death by Pharmaceuticals?" *Better Nutrition* (June 2001).

6 See M. Castleman, *Nature's Cures* (Emmaus, Penn.: Rodale Press, 1996).

7 I. Kirsch, et al., "Listening to Prozac but Hearing Placebo: A Meta-analysis of Antidepressant Medication," *Prevention & Treatment* (June 26, 1998) (American Psychological Association, www. journals.apa.org.)

Chapter 4. Nutritional Balance: Supplementing Nutrient Needs and Clearing Metabolic Wastes

1 U.S. Senate Document No. 264, 74th Congress, 2nd Session, 1936.

2 The Burton Goldberg Group, *Alternative Medicine: The Definitive Guide* (Puyallup, Wash.: Future Medicine Publishing, 1994), pages 215–23; M. Murray, *Arthritis* (Rocklin, Calif.: Prima Publishing, 1994), pages 59–66; J. Theodosakis, *Maximizing the Arthritis Cure* (New York: St. Martin's Press, 1998), pages 206–15.

3 T. Baroody, *Alkalize or Die* (Waynesville, N.C.: Holographic Health, 1991; telephone [800] 566-1522).

4 F. Batmanghelidj, M.D., *Your Body's Many Cries for Water* (Falls Church, Va.: Global Health Solutions, 1995).

5 D. Dupler, "Detoxification," *Gale Encyclopedia of Alternative Medicine*, www.gale.com (2001).

6 B. Jensen, D. C., *Dr. Jensen's Guide to Better Bowel Care* (New York: Avery, 1998), page 132.

7 P. Airola, N.D., *Are You Confused?* (Phoenix, Ariz.: Health Plus Publishers, 1971), pages 112–13, 137.

8 P. Serure, *Three Days to Vitality* (New York: HarperCollins, 1997).

9 B. Jensen, *op. cit.*

Chapter 5. Deloxifying from Chemical and Heavy Metal Buildup

1 D. Williams, "Cleaning House," *Alternatives* 4(12):97–100 (July 1992), citing *Environmental Pollution* 10(3):183–200 (1976); *Canadian Journal of Physiology* 52:1080–94 (1974).

2 See E. Brown, R. Hansen, *The Key to Ultimate Health* (La Mirada, Calif.: Advanced Health Research Publishing, 1998); E. Brown, L. Walker, *The Informed Consumer's Pharmacy* (New York: Carroll & Graf, 1990).

3 D. Dupler, *op. cit.*

4 D. Ullman, *The Consumer's Guide to Homeopathy* (New York: Dorling Kindersley, 1995), page 56.

5 J. Kotter, "Chemical Contamination and Human Detoxification," *Townsend Letter for Doctors and Patients* (January 2001), page 15.

6 D. Schnare, et al., "Evaluation of a Detoxification Regimen for Fat Stored Xenobiotics," *Medical Hypotheses* 9(3):265–82 (1982). For a detailed protocol, see Ellen Brown, *Healing Joint Pain Naturally* (New York: Broadway Books, 2001), chapter 9.

7 See N. Clarke, et al., "Treatment of Occlusive Vascular Disease with Disodium Ethylene Diamine Tetra-acetic Acid (EDTA)," *American Journal of Medical Science* 239:732 (1960); N. Clarke, et al., "Treatment of Angina Pectoris with Disodium Ethylene Diamine Tetra-acetic Acid," *ibid.* 232:645 (1956); C. Lamar, "Chelation Therapy of Occlusive Arteriosclerosis in Diabetic Patients," *Angiology* 15:379 (1964).

8 R. Evers, M.D., "A Successful Therapy for the Relief of Chronic Degenerative Diseases" (200 Beta St., Belle Chasse, Louisiana 70037; undated).

9 See T. Warren, *Beating Alzheimer's* (Garden City Park, N.Y.: Avery Publishing Group, 1991).

10 Y. Omura, et al., *Acupuncture Electrotherapy Research* 21(2):133–60 (1996).

11 G. Bushkin, et al., "ALA Fights Free Radical Damage," *Nutrition Science News* 2(11):572 (November 1997).

PART TWO

Acne

1 S. Bharija, M. Belhaj, "Acetylsalicylic Acid May Induce a Lichenoid Eruption," *Dermatologica* 177:19 (1988).

2 S. Roan, "Sufferers of Acne, Beware: Pimples May Be Winning," *Los Angeles Times* (May 8, 1996).

3 T. Halvorson, "Warning Issued for Painkiller," *Gannet News Service* (March 7, 1995); "Acne Drugs Cause Serious Side Effects: M.D.s Prescribe Anyway," www.chiropage.com (April 1997).

4 "Gray Hair and Acne," *University of California, Berkeley Wellness Letter* 4(8):7 (1988); J. Trowbridge, M. Walker, *The Yeast Syndrome* (New York: Bantam Books, 1986).

5 "Acne Drugs Cause Serious Side Effects," *ibid.*

6 "What's the Connection between Hormones and Skin?" *Pharmacy Times* (May 1989), pages 49–51.

7 P. Boyer, et al., "Can Hormone Therapy Save Your Skin?" *Prevention* (January 1, 1997).

8 J. Sheppard, "Acne Anguish," www.healthychild.com.

9 S. Vedantam, "Plane Crash Reinforces That Accutane Can Cause Suicide," www.mercola.com (2002).

10 A. Shalita, et al., "Isotretinoin Revisited," *Cutis* 42:1–19 (1988).

11 J. Trowbridge, et al., *op cit.*, pages 301–20.

12 See D. Gates, et al., *The Body Ecology Diet* (Atlanta, Ga.: B.E.D. Publications, 1993).

13 J. Sheppard, *op. cit.*

14 For other home cosmetic ideas, see T. Jeffries, "Healthy Hints for Looking Good . . . Naturally," *Health Quest* (February 28, 1995); and T. Moore, *Kitchen Cosmetics,* reviewed in *Health Quest* (March 31, 1994).

Acne Rosacea

1 American Academy of Dermatology, "Acne Rosacea," www.aad.org (1999).

2 A. Salomon, "Acne Drug Can Kill, British Doctors Warn," *Reuters* (January 18, 1996).

3 T. Halvorson, *op. cit.*

4 "Gray Hair and Acne," *op. cit.;* J. Trowbridge, et al., *op. cit.*

5 *Drug Facts and Comparisons* (St. Louis: Facts and Comparisons, 1998).

Allergies

1 S. Squires, "Allergy Season Returns," *Washington Post Health* (April 18, 1989), pages 6–7.

2 L. Aesoph, *How to Eat Away Arthritis* (Englewood Cliffs, N.J.: Prentice Hall, 1996), pages 51–56.

3 N. Freundlich, "Health: Fight Sneezing—Without Snoozing," *Business Week* (April 7, 1997); D. Levy, "Allergy-relief Alternatives to Seldane," *USA Today* (January 14, 1997); "Slow, and Then Too Slow: FDA Falls Short in Dealing with an Already Approved Drug," *Los Angeles Times* (Home Edition) (January 15, 1997); *Drug Facts and Comparisons, op. cit.,* page 1229.

4 S. Stolberg, "Inhalers Linked to Cataracts," *Los Angeles Daily News* (July 2, 1997).

5 N. Freundlich, *op. cit.;* K. Painter, "Allergy Shots Give Little Help in Asthma Battle," *USA Today* (January 30, 1997).

6 The Burton Goldberg Group, *Alternative Medicine: The Definitive Guide* (Puyallup, Wash.: Future Medicine Publishing, 1994), pages 215–23; M. Murray, *Arthritis* (Rocklin, Calif.: Prima Publishing, 1994), pages 59–66; J. Theodosakis, *Maximizing the Arthritis Cure* (New York: St. Martin's Press, 1998), pages 206–15.

7 See R. Mendelsohn, M.D., *How to Raise a Healthy Child in Spite of Your Doctor* (Chicago: Contemporary Books, 1984), pages 205–206; L. Moll, "The Link Between Food and Mood," *Vegetarian Times* (August 1986), pages 28–30; R. Wunderlich, M.D., et al., "Nourishing Your Hyperactive Child to Health," *Good Health* 2(5):16–19 (1984).

8 F. Batmanghelidj, M.D., *Your Body's Many Cries for Water* (Falls Church, Va.: Global Health Solutions, 1995).

Alzheimer's Disease

1 T. Friend, "Alzheimer's Deaths 'Underestimated,'" *USA Today* (March 4, 1996); M. Aronson, "Alzheimer's Disease," *Colliers Encyclopedia CD-ROM* (February 28, 1996); D. Chopra, M.D., *Ageless Body, Timeless Mind* (New York: Harmony Books, 1993), page 242.

2 "Study Says Estrogen No Help to Women with Alzheimer's," *Dallas Morning News* (February 23, 2000).

3 University of California, Irvine, "New Evidence Links Herpes and Alzheimer's," *UCI News* (May 24, 2000); "Herpes Could Cause Alzheimer's," *Reuters* (January 23, 1997).

4 J. Talan, "Alzheimer's Drug Gets Mixed Results," *Newsday* (April 6, 1994).

5 M. Werbach, *op. cit.*

6 Dr. H. R. Casdorph, Dr. M. Walker, *Toxic Metal Syndrome* (Garden City Park, N.Y.: Avery Publishing Group, 1995).

7 D. Crapper, et al., "Brain Aluminum Distribution in Alzheimer's Disease and Experimental Neurofibrillary Degeneration," *Science* 180:511–13 (1973); D. Crapper, et al., "Aluminum, Neurofibrillary Degeneration and Alzheimer's Disease," *Brain* 99:67–80 (1976); D. Perl, A. Brody, "Alzheimer's Disease: X-ray Spectrometric Evidence of Aluminum Accumulation in Neurofibrillary Tangle-bearing Neurons," *Science* 208:297–99 (1980); J. Candy, et al., "New Observations on the Nature of Senile Plaque Cores," in E. Vizi, et al., eds., *Regulation of Transmitter Function: Basic and Clinical Aspects* (Amsterdam: Elsevier Press, 1984), pages 301–304; O. Bugiani, B. Ghetti, "Progressing Encephalomyelopathy with Muscular Atrophy, Induced by Aluminum Powder," *Neurobiol. Aging* 3:209–22 (1982). See P. Altmann, et al., "Serum Aluminum Levels and Erythrocyte Dihydropteridine Reductase Activity in Patients on Hemodialysis," *New England Journal of Medicine* 317(2):80–84 (1987).

8 C. Starr, "Aluminum and Alzheimer's," *Drug Topics* (April 17, 1989), page 30, citing *The Lancet* 1:59 (1989).

9 M. Werbach, M.D., "Does Aluminum Exposure Promote Alzheimer's?" *Nutrition Science News* (January 1998), page 16.

10 H. Casdorph, et al., *op. cit.*, page 156, citing D. Wenstrup, et al., "Trace Element Imbalances in Isolated Subcellular Fractions of Alzheimer's Disease Brains," *Brain Research* 553:125–31 (1990).

11 H. Casdorph, et al., *op. cit.*, pages 140, 162.

12 J. Pleva, "Mercury Poisoning from Dental Amalgam," *Journal of Orthomolecular Psychiatry* 12:184–93 (1983); M. Vimy, et al., "Serial Measurements of Intra-oral Air Mercury: Estimation of Daily Dose from Dental Amalgams," *Journal of Dental Research* 64(8):1072–75 (1985); R. Siblerud, "The Relationship between Mercury from Dental Amalgam and the Cardiovascular System," *Science of the Total Environment* 99:23–35 (1990).

13 D. Eggleston, et al., "Correlation of Dental Amalgam with Mercury in Brain Tissue," *Journal of Prosthetic Dentistry* 58:704–707 (1987); M. Nylander, et al., "Mercury Concentrations in the Human Brain and Kidneys in Relation to Exposure from Dental Amalgam Fillings," *Swedish Dental Journal* 11:179–87 (1987).

14 K. Sehnert, M.D., et al., "Is Mercury Toxicity an Autoimmune Disorder?" *Townsend Letter for Doctors and Patients* (October 1995), pages 134–37.

15 See E. Brown, R. Hansen, *The Key to Ultimate Health* (La Mirada, Calif.: Advanced Health Research Publishing, 1998).

16 D. Williams, "Alzheimer's Remedy Found in the Remote Mountain Villages of China," *Alternatives* 5(9):70 (March 1994).

17 M. Zucker, "The Miracle of E," *Let's Live* (November 1997), citing the April 24, 1997, *New England Journal of Medicine*.

18 T. Warren, *Beating Alzheimer's* (Garden City Park, N.Y.: Avery Publishing Group, 1991); T. Warren, "Reversing Alzheimer's Disease," www.halcyon.com/alzh9.

19 J. Birkmayer, et al., "Coenzyme Nicotinamide Adenine Dinucleotide: New Therapeutic Approach for Improving Dementia of the Alzheimer's Type," *Annals of Clinical and Laboratory Science* 26(1):1–9 (1996).

20 *Ibid.*

21 M. Castleman, *Nature's Cures* (Emmaus, Penn.: Rodale Press, 1996), page 421.

22 C. Johnston, et al., "Holotranscobalamin Levels in Plasma Are Related to Dementia in Older People," *Journal of the American Geriatric Society* 45:779–80 (June 1997).

23 D. Williams, "More Suggestions for Alzheimer's Victims," *Alternatives* 4(22):175 (April 1993).

Anemia

1 S. Sellman, "The Physiology of Hormones," *Healthy and Natural Journal* (October 2000); N. Shaw, et al., "A Vegetarian Diet Rich in Soybean Products Compromises Iron Status in Young Students," *Journal of Nutrition* 125:212–19 (1995).

Anorexia Nervosa and Bulimia

1 P. Rowan, "A Brief Introduction to Bulimia Nervosa," www.priory-hospital.co.uk.

Anxiety and Panic Disorders

1 D. Cross, M.D., "Anxiety Disorders in Women," *Psychiatry & Women* (December 1997).

2 C. Kilham, "Kava for Anxiety and Insomnia," *Nutrition Science News* 2(5):232–34 (May 1997).

3 D. Cross, *op. cit.*

4 "Top 200 drugs of 1988," *Pharmacy Times* (April 1989), page 40.

5 W. Leary, "F.D.A. Asks Stronger Label on Sleeping Pill under Scrutiny," *New York Times* (September 23, 1989), page 6.

6 R. Greene, "The Mellow Market," *Forbes* (October 31, 1988), page 106.

7 D. Greenblatt, et al., "Effect of Gradual Withdrawal on the Rebound Sleep Disorder after Discontinuation of Triazolam," *New England Journal of Medicine* 317(12):722–28 (1987); P. Roy-Byrne, et al., "Relapse and Rebound Following Discontinuation of Benzodiazepine Treatment of Panic Attacks: Alprazolam Versus Diazepam," *American Journal of Psychiatry* 146(7):860–65 (1989).

8 C. Kilham, *op. cit.*

9 D. Cross, *op. cit.*

10 D. Manders, "The Curious Continuing Ban of L-tryptophan: The Serotonin Connection," *Townsend Letter for Doctors* (October 1992), pages 880–81; Citizens for Health, "Prepare for the Worst: FDA Propaganda Ready to Barrage Media," *Townsend Letter for Doctors* (August/September 1993), pages 860–61.

11 "PMS? Let 'Em Eat Carbs," *Vegetarian Times* (March 1990), page 7.

12 M. Shangold, "Exercise in the Menopausal Woman," *Obstetrics and Gynecology* 75:53S–58S (1990).

13 R. Peat, *Nutrition for Women* (Eugene, Oreg.: Kenogen, 1981), page 92.

14 G. Lewis, "An Alternative Approach to Premedication: Comparing Diazepam with Auriculotherapy and a Relaxation Method," *American Journal of Acupuncture* 15(3):205–13 (1987); B. Brown, *Stress and the Art of Biofeedback* (New York: Harper & Row Publishers, 1977).

Arthritis

1 Arthritis Foundation, "Women and Arthritis," www.intelihealth.com (April 22, 1998). For a fuller discussion of arthritis and its treatment, see E. Brown, *Healing Joint Pain Naturally* (New York: Broadway Books, 2001).

2 R. Steyer, "For Arthritis Sufferers, Fighting the Pain Becomes a Way of Life: A New Drug from Monsanto's Searle Shows Promise," *St. Louis Post-Dispatch* (February 14, 1999), page A10; J. Cashman, et al., "Nonsteroidal Anti-inflammatory Drugs in Perisurgical Pain Management," *Practical Therapeutics* 49(1):51–70 (1995).

3 J. Foreman, "Arthritis Drugs Kill Pain Without Irritating Stomach," *Minneapolis Star Tribune* (October 11, 1998), page 05E.

4 P. Galewitz, "New Drug to Battle Arthritis Causes Stir," *The Washington Times* (February 16, 1999), page B7; "FDA Approves New Arthritis Painkiller But Won't Say It's Easier on Stomachs," *The Dallas Morning News* (January 1, 1999), page 9A.

5 J. Mercola, "FDA Panel Votes to Approve New Celebrex Alternative," *Townsend Letter for Doctors and Patients* (July 1999), pages 27–28.

6 J. Foreman, *op. cit.*

7 J. Mercola, *op. cit.*

8 "Questions & Answers: Painful Dilemma," *Newsweek* (May 25, 2001).

9 S. Washington, "Drug Company Lies About Celebrex in *JAMA*," *Washington Post* (August 5, 2001), page A11.

10 S. Rashad, et al., "Effect of Non-steroidal Anti-inflammatory Drugs on the Course of Osteoarthritis," *The Lancet* (September 2, 1989), pages 519–21; J. DeCava, "Osteoarthritis," *Nutrition News and Views* 1(4):1–8 (July/August 1997).

11 L. Coles, et al., "From Experiment to Experience: Side Effects of Nonsteroidal Anti-inflammatory Drugs," *American Journal of Medicine* 74:820–28 (1983).

12 P. Brooks, et al., "Effects of NSAID on PG Metabolism," *Journal of Rheumatology* 9:1 (1982).

13 B. Absher, O.D., *New Discovery Proves That Arthritis Can Be Stopped and Joints Repaired in Three Months* (Marina del Rey, Calif.: Health Quest Publications, 1998), page 17.

14 S. Jacob, M.D., et al., *The Miracle of MSM: The Natural Solution for Pain* (New York: G. P. Putnam's Sons, 1999).

15 "Glucosamine," *The Natural Pharmacist*, www.tnp.com (1999–2000).

16 Julian Whitaker, M.D., "A Safe, Simple Treatment for Arthritis," *Human Events* (April 7, 1995).

17 L. Aesoph, *How to Eat Away Arthritis* (Englewood Cliffs, N.J.: Prentice Hall, 1996), page 237.

18 M. Murray, *Arthritis* (Rocklin, Calif.: Prima Publishing, 1994), pages 19–21, 83–92, citing studies.

19 B. Goldberg, *Alternative Medicine*, (Puyallup, Wash.: Future Medicine Publishing, 1994), page 532; L. Power, "Exploring the Link Between Diet, Arthritis," *Los Angeles Times* (May 6, 1986), page 3; L. Aesoph, *op. cit.*

20 B. Goldberg, *op. cit.*, pages 215–23; M. Murray, *op. cit.*, pages 59–66; J. Theodosakis, *Maximizing the Arthritis Cure* (New York: St. Martin's Press, 1998), pages 206–15.

21 R. Evers, M.D., *op. cit.*

22 See K. Sehnert, M.D., et al., "Is Mercury Toxicity an Autoimmune Disorder?" *Townsend Letter for Doctors and Patients* (October 1995), pages 134–37.

23 W. Price, D.D.S., *Dental Infections—Oral and Systemic* [vol. 1] and *Dental Infections and the Degenerative Diseases* [vol. 2] (Cleveland, Ohio: Penton Publishing Co., 1923). See E. Brown, R. Hansen, *The Key to Ultimate Health, op. cit.*

24 A. Hoffer, M.D., "Arthritis," *Townsend Letter for Doctors* (December 1997), page 104.

25 C. Keough, et al., *Natural Relief for Arthritis* (Emmaus, Penn.: Rodale Press, 1983), pages 167–68, citing P. Sechzer, M.D., et al., *Bulletin of the New York Academy of Medicine.*

26 Zane Kime, M.D., *Sunlight* (Penryn, Calif.: World Health Publications, 1980), pages 229–31.

27 Research summarized in J. Heimlich, *What Your Doctor Won't Tell You* (New York: HarperCollins, 1990), page 156.

Aspartame, Adverse Reactions To

1 See M. Stoddard, *The Deadly Deception* (Dallas, Tex.: Aspartame Consumer Safety Network, 1996); H. Roberts, "Reactions Attributed to Aspartame-containing Products: 551 Cases," *Journal of Applied Nutrition* 40:85–94 (1988); H. Roberts, *Sweet'ner Dearest: Bittersweet Vignettes About Aspartame (NutraSweet)* (West Palm Beach, Fla.: Sunshine Sentinel Press, 1989).

2 M. Gold, "The Bitter Truth About Artificial Sweeteners," extracted from *Nexus Magazine* 2(28) (October/November 1995) and 3(1)(December 1995–January 1996), www.nexusmagazine.com.

3 See D. Richard, *Stevia: Nature's Sweet Secret* (Bloomingdale, Ill.: Blue Heron Press, 1996).

Asthma

1 A. Marcus, "Asthma Hits Women Harder Than Men," www.drkoop.com (January 24, 2001).

2 P. Harrison, "Obesity Linked to Asthma in Women But Not Men," www.nycallergist.com (June 20, 2001).

3 A. Buist, "Asthma Mortality: What Have We Learned?" *Journal of Allergy and Clinical Immunology;* B. Lanier, "Who Is Dying of Asthma and Why?" *Journal of Pediatrics* 115:838–40 (1989).

4 American Lung Association, "About Asthma Medicines," www.lungusa.org (2002).

5 S. Stolberg, "Inhalers Linked to Cataracts," *Daily News* (Los Angeles), July 2, 1997.

6 "Are Asthma Drugs Harmful to Young Women?" *Tufts e-news,* www.tufts.edu (October 2001).

7 L. Thompson, "The Asthma Dilemma: With Better Treatment Available, Why Are More Patients Dying?" *Washington Post Health* (August 25, 1987), pages 12–14; R. Henig, "The Big Sneeze," *Washington Post Health* (May 31, 1988), pages 12–15; D. DeSilver, "Powerful Drugs, Disturbing Effects," *Vegetarian Times* (August 1989), page 24.

8 "Keep Your Asthma at Bay with Magnesium," www.hom.net, citing Dr. Julian Whitaker's *Health and Healing* newsletter (July 1994).

9 *Ibid.*

10 S. Lingling, et al., "Effect of Needling Sensation Reaching the Site of Disease on the Results of Acupuncture Treatment of Bronchial Asthma," *Journal of Traditional Chinese Medicine* 9(2):140–43 (1989).

11 See R. Roberts, et al., *Asthma: An Alternative Approach* (New Canaan, Conn.: Keats Publishing, 1997).

12 B. Brown, *Stress and the Art of Biofeedback* (New York: Harper & Row Publishers, 1977); "Asthma and Biofeedback," www.channel4000.com (2002).

13 See G. Maleskey, "Stuffed Up? Try These Natural Remedies," *Prevention* (September 1984), pages 63–66.

14 F. Batmanghelidj, M.D., *Your Body's Many Cries for Water* (Falls Church, Va.: Global Health Solutions, 1995).

Back Pain and Sciatica

1 Burton Goldberg Group, *Alternative Medicine, op. cit.,* page 546.
2 BackCare, National Organization for Healthy Backs, "Women and Back Pain—Some Facts and Figures," www.backpain.org.
3 "Back Pain: Conventional Treatment," www.holistic-online.com (January 20, 2002).
4 *Ibid.*
5 P. Manga, et al., "A Study to Examine the Effectiveness and Cost-Effectiveness of Chiropractic Management of Low-Back Pain," www.chiropage.com/research (August 1993).
6 A good resource is *The Healthy Back Book* by Elizabeth Sharp (New York: HarperCollins, 1994).

Bladder Infection, Irritation, and Inflammation (Cystitis)

1 L. Goldstein, "Home Remedies," *Prevention* (July 2001).
2 C. Houck, "The Infection that Drives Women Absolutely Crazy," *Redbook* (May 1, 1996).
3 D. Vergano, "The Trouble with Condoms," *Science News* 150(11):165 (1996).
4 C. Houck, *op. cit.*
5 S. Weeks, "Cystitis and Antibiotics," *Quackbusters Chronicles,* www.quackbusters.com (2001).
6 R. Morrison, *Desktop Guide* (Albany, Calif.: Hahnemann Clinic Publishing, 1993), page 338.

Bloating, Gas, and Edema

1 J. Lee, M.D., "Slowing the Aging Process with Natural Progesterone" (Sebastopol, Calif.; unpublished research paper).
2 D. Hoffman, "Dandelion," *Herbal Material Medica,* www.healthy.net.
3 T. Gossel, "Antiflatulence Agents," *U.S. Pharmacist* (August 1989), pages 18ff.

Bowel Disorders

1 Crohn's & Colitis Foundation of America, "Common Gastrointestinal & Medical Problems in Women: Irritable Bowel Syndrome," www.ccfa.org (1996–2001).
2 S. Kane, M.D., "Women's Issues in Inflammatory Bowel Disease," *Foundation Focus* (summer 1999).
3 *Ibid.*

Breast Pain and Tenderness, Breast Lumps, and Fibrocystic Breasts

1 J. Lee, "Slowing the Aging Process with Natural Progesterone," *op. cit.* See J. Lee, et al., *What Your Doctor May Not Tell You About Menopause* (New York: Warner Books, 1996).
2 V. Hufnagel, M.D., *No More Hysterectomies* (New York: Penguin Books, 1989), page 108.

Cancer, Cervical

1 T. Canavan, et al., "Cervical Cancer," *American Family Physician* 60:1369–76 (2000).
2 L. Harris, "Postmenopausal Women May Not Need Annual Pap Smear, UCSF Study Finds," www.UCSF/edu/daybreak (December 20, 2000).
3 J. Mercola, "CDC Says Annual Pap Smears May Do More Harm Than Good," www.mercola.com (December 3, 2000).

4 J. Mercola, ibid., citing the CDC's "Morbidity and Mortality Weekly Report," 49:1001–1003 (2000).

5 See E. Robin, *op. cit.*

6 J. McCormick, "Cervical Smears: A Questionable Practice?" *The Lancet* (July 22, 1989), pages 207–209.

7 M. Kelley, "Hypercholesterolemia: The Cost of Treatment in Perspective," *Southern Medical Journal* 83:1421–25 (1990).

8 J. Littell, M.D., "Further Discussion on the Role of Pap Smear Screening," *American Family Physician* (November 15, 2000).

9 L. Harris, *op. cit.*

Cancers, Hormonal

1 R. Walters, *Options: The Alternative Cancer Therapy Book* (Garden City Park, N.Y.: Avery Publishing Group, 1993).

2 "Author of Canadian Breast Cancer Study Retracts Warnings," *Journal of the National Cancer Institute* 84(11):832–34 (June 3, 1992).

3 A. Miller, et al., "Canadian National Breast Screening Study: 1. Breast Cancer Detection and Death Rates among Women Aged 40 to 49 Years," *Canadian Medical Association Journal* 147(10):1459–76 (1992).

4 M. Napoli (October 2000), "An Equally Effective and Safer Alternative to Mammography Screening," *HealthFacts* (October 2000).

5 K. Kerlikowske, et al., "Continuing Screening Mammography in Women Aged 70 to 79 Years," *JAMA* 282:2156–63 (1999).

6 M. Napoli, "Mammography: No Major Drop in Breast Cancer Deaths," *HealthFacts* (March 1999), citing the Swedish medical journal *Laekaren Tidningen* (February 1999).

7 P. Gotzsche, *op. cit.*

8 "New Cancer Statistics Show Losses, Gains," *Journal of the National Cancer Institute* 82(15):1238 (1990), quoting Brenda Edwards, Ph.D., acting associate director of NCI's Surveillance Program.

9 See G. Cowley, et al., "In Pursuit of a Terrible Killer," *Newsweek* (December 10, 1990), pages 66–68.

10 J. Gofman, M.D., *Radiation from Medical Procedures in the Pathogenesis of Cancer and Ischemic Heart Disease: Dose-Response Studies with Physicians Per 100,000 Population* (San Francisco: Committee for Nuclear Responsibility, 1999).

11 D. Josefson, "Mammography Is No Better Than Physical Examination, Study Shows," *British Medical Journal* (September 30, 2000).

12 A. Miller, *op. cit.* (emphasis added).

13 A. Lang, "Cancer Patients Organized Against FDA Violations," *Townsend Letter for Doctors* (May 1988), pages 178–80.

14 J. Bailar, et al., "Cancer Undefeated," *New England Journal of Medicine* 336(22):1569–74 (May 29, 1997).

15 See R. Moss, *Questioning Chemotherapy* (New York: Equinox Press, 1995); J. Cairns, "The Treatment of Diseases and the War Against Cancer," *Scientific American* 253(5):51 (1985).

16 Dr. Moss cited the research of German biostatician Dr. Ulrich Abel, who observed that reduction of tumor mass doesn't necessarily prolong survival. In fact, it can cause the cancer to return more aggressively, since killing off most of the cancer mass allows drug-resistant cell lines to grow. Dr. Abel observed that for breast cancer, there is no direct evidence that chemotherapy prolongs survival, making its use "ethically questionable." His work was reviewed in the popular German magazine *Der Spiegel* in 1990.

17 R. Moss, "The War on Cancer," *Townsend Letter for Doctors and Patients* (January 2001), page 136.

18   See R. Houston, "Misinformation from OTA," *Townsend Letter for Doctors* (August/September 1990), page 600; J. Weese, et al., "Do Operations Facilitate Tumor Growth?" *Surgery* 100(2):273–77 (1986) (surgery and anesthesia enhance the implanting of tumors and facilitate metastasis); J. Stjernsward, "Decreased Survival Related to Irradiation Postoperatively in Early Operable Breast Cancer," *The Lancet* (November 30, 1974), pages 1285–86; R. Moss, *The Cancer Industry: Unravelling the Politics* (New York: Paragon House, 1989), *op. cit.*, pages 59–72.

19   See, e.g., J. Cuzick, et al., "Overview of Randomized Trials of Postoperative Adjuvant Radiotherapy in Breast Cancer," *Cancer Treatment Reports* 71(1):15–29 (1987), a review of eight trials from around the world finding that the risk of death after ten years for women who had not gotten radiation after their breast surgeries was 26 percent *lower* than for women who had gotten it. See also J. Cairns, *op. cit.*, observing that the majority of cancers cannot be cured by radiation because the dose of X rays required to kill all the cancer cells would also kill the patient; and that chemotherapy prevents death in only 2 to 5 percent of cancer cases. See also R. Walters, *op. cit.*, page 13, observing that, as early as 1953, Benedict Fitzgerald, special counsel for the Department of Justice, presented studies to Congress showing that patients who received no radiation lived longer than those who were irradiated.

20   See "A Questionable Cure," *Jim Lehrer NewsHour*, www.pbc.com (May 13, 1999).

21   S. Boodman, "Marrow Transplants No Better Than Regular Treatment: Studies," *The Toronto Star* (April 30, 1999).

22   R. O'Regan, et al., "Selective Estrogen-receptor Modulators in 2001," *Oncology*, 1177–85, 1189–90 (September 2001); F. Jelovsek, M.D., "Designer Estrogens—Are They for Me?" *Woman's Diagnostic Cyber*, www.wdxcyber.com (October 31, 2000).

23   M. Paulsen, "The Cancer Business," *Mother Jones* (May/June 1994).

24   "What's Hot: #1 Breast Cancer Tamoxifen Drug Increases Risk of Uterine Cancer, Hot Flashes and Blood Clots," www.alternativemedicine.com (June 11, 1999).

25   "What's Hot," *ibid.*; J. Lee, et al., *What Your Doctor May Not Tell You About Menopause* (New York: Warner Books, 1996).

26   G. Griffin, *World Without Cancer* (Westlake Village, Calif.: American Media, 1974), pages 79–82.

27   As early as 1902, John Beard, a professor of embryology at the University of Edinburgh in Scotland, showed in the British medical journal *The Lancet* that there was no detectable difference between highly malignant cancer cells and certain pre-embryonic cells (trophoblasts) that are normal to the early stages of pregnancy. Work on the trophoblast-cancer link was continued by Dr. Ernest T. Krebs, Jr., until his death in 1996 and has formed the basis of other recent cancer theories in the United States and abroad. See R. Moss, "HCG vs. Kaposi's Sarcoma: NCI Scientist Claims Priority in Pregnancy Hormone Study," *The Cancer Chronicles* (September 1995).

28   See R. Peat, *Nutrition for Women, op. cit.*, pages 11 and 22.

29   "Medicine Mum on Mammography: Do the Math—Think Thermography," www.AlternativeMedicine.com (October 23, 2000).

30   See, e.g., *Alternative Medicine Definitive Guide to Cancer* (Tiburon, Calif.: Future Medicine Publishing, 1997), by W. John Diamond, M.D., W. Lee Cowden, M.D. (in collaboration with Burton Goldberg and a long list of M.D. contributors); Dr. Ralph W. Moss's *Cancer Therapy: The Independent Consumer's Guide* (New York: Equinox Press, 1992); and R. Walters' *Options: The Alternative Cancer Therapy Book* (New York: Avery Publishing Group, 1993), among other resources.

31   Ellen Brown, *Forbidden Medicine* (Hurricane, W.Va.: Third Millennium Press, 1998; telephone [800] 891-0390).

32   C. Pert, "Your Body Is Your Subconscious Mind" [audiotape] (Boulder, Colo.: Sounds True, 2000) (text condensed).

33   M. Paulsen, "The Cancer Business," *Mother Jones* (May/June 1994).

34   P. Gotzsche, et al., "Is Screening for Breast Cancer with Mammography Justifiable?" *The Lancet* 355(9198):129–34 (January 8, 2000); M. Napoli, *op. cit.*, citing *Journal of the National Cancer Institute* (September 20, 2000). See also M. Napoli, "Mammography Screening Does Not Save Lives," *HealthFacts* (February 2000).

35   C. Pert, *op. cit.*

Carpal Tunnel Syndrome

1   T. Hayes, "Local Physician Cuts Carpal Tunnel Surgery Time," *Indianapolis Business Journal* 16:34 (1995).

Chlamydia

1   N. Hicks, "Chlamydia Infection in General Practice," *British Medical Journal* (March 20, 1999).

2   See "Sexually Transmitted Diseases," *National Women's Health Report* (March 1, 1993); E. Brown, L. Walker, *The Informed Consumer's Pharmacy* (New York: Carroll & Graf, 1990).

3   D. Vergano, "The Trouble with Condoms," *Science News* 150(11):165 (1996).

Cholesterol, High

1   P. Krisetnerton, "Over-the-counter Statin Medications: Emerging Opportunities for MDs," *American Dietetic Association* (October 2000).

2   G. Cowley, "What's High Cholesterol?" *Newsweek* (November 14, 1994), page 63.

3   J. Golier, et al., "Low Serum Cholesterol Level and Attempted Suicide," *American Journal of Psychiatry* 152:419–23 (1995), discussed by Alan Gaby, M.D., in *Townsend Letter for Doctors* (December 1995), page 21.

4   M. Mercola, *op. cit.*

5   C. Blum, R. Levy, "Current Therapy for Hypercholesterolemia," *JAMA* 261(24):3582–87 (1989).

6   R. Safeer, "Choosing Drug Therapy for Patients with Hyperlipidemia," *American Family Physician* (June 1, 2000).

7   M. Mercola, "Half of Population Will Be Taking Statins," *Optimal Wellness Health News* (July 9, 2000).

8   M. Pignone, "Use of Lipid Lowering Drugs for Primary Prevention of Coronary Heart Disease: Meta-analysis of Randomised Trials," www.bmj.com (October 21, 2000).

9   M. Mercola, *op. cit.*, citing *JAMA* 275: 55–60 (1996).

10   "Bayer Voluntarily Withdraws Baycol," *FDA News Page*, www.fda.gov (August 8, 2001).

11   See "Lower Your Cholesterol Naturally," *The Neighborhood Doctor*, www.yourneighborhooddoctor.com.

12   J. Mercola, "Red Rice Yeast Extract Taken Off Market by FDA as It Violates Merck Patent?" www.mercola.com (June 29, 1998), citing *Family Practice News* (June 15, 1998), page 20.

13   P. Canner, et al., "Fifteen Year Mortality in Coronary Drug Project Patients: Long-term Benefit with Niacin," *American Journal of Cardiology* 8:1245–55 (1986).

14   D. Schnare, et al., "Evaluation of a Detoxification Regimen for Fat Stored Xenobiotics," *Medical Hypotheses* 9(3):265–82 (1982). For a more detailed protocol, see E. Brown, *Healing Joint Pain Naturally* (New York: Broadway Books, 2001).

15   S. Squires, "Heart Researchers Find Diet Alone Can Help," *Washington Post Health* (November 15, 1988); "It's True, You Can Reverse Heart Disease through Vegetarianism," *Vegetarian Times* (February 1990), page 18.

16 S. Pratt, "Body and Soy: New Study Indicates Soy-rich Diet Can Lower Cholesterol," *Chicago Tribune* (August 22, 1995).

17 M. Anderson, M.D., "Soy Protein and Risk for Coronary Heart Disease," paper presented at American Dietetic Association 80th Annual Meeting in Boston, Massachusetts, October 27–30, 1997, www.soyfoods.com.

18 S. Sellman, "The Physiology of Hormones," *Healthy and Natural Journal* (October, 2000); N. Shaw, et al., "A Vegetarian Diet Rich in Soybean Products Compromises Iron Status in Young Students," *Journal of Nutrition* 125:212–19 (1995).

19 L. Nicholson, "Focus on Fiber," *Center Post* 10(9):1 (1989).

20 "Psyllium and Cholesterol," *Harvard Medical School Health Letter* 13(8):1 (1988), citing *Archives of Internal Medicine* (February 1988), pages 292–96.

21 "Mystery of High-fiber Diet Unraveled," *Washington Post* (October 26, 1987), page A7; S. Siwolop, "Curbing Killer Choleserol," *BusinessWeek* (October 26, 1987), pages 122–23.

Chronic Fatigue Syndrome

1 S. Wessely, "The Epidemiology of Chronic Fatigue Syndrome," *Epidemiological Reviews* 17:1–13 (1995); D. Buchwald, et al., "Chronic Fatigue and the Chronic Fatigue Syndrome in a Pacific Northwest Health Care System," *Annals of Internal Medicine* 123(2):81(8) (1995).

2 M. Ali, M.D., *The Canary and Chronic Fatigue* (Denville, N.J.: Life Span Press, 1994), pages 325–27, quoting *American Journal of Medicine* 90:730 (1991).

3 D. Nambudripad, *Say Goodbye to Illness* (Buena Park, Calif.: Delta Publishing Co., 1993), page 287; L. Casura, "Sick of Being Patient, Part 1," *Townsend Letter for Doctors* (June 1996), pages 36–41.

4 L. Casura, "Sick of Being Patient, Part 2," *Townsend Letter for Doctors* (June 1996), pages 54–63.

5 Dr. H. R. Casdorph, Dr. M. Walker, *Toxic Metal Syndrome* (Garden City Park, N.Y.: Avery Publishing Group, 1995), pages 151–52.

6 S. Rogers, M.D., *Wellness Against All Odds* (Syracuse, N.Y.: Prestige Publishing, 1994), page 240.

7 E. Brown, R. Hansen, D.M.D., *The Key to Ultimate Health* (La Mirada, Calif.: Advanced Health Research Publishing, 1998).

Cold Sores and Canker Sores

1 McKinley Health Center, University of Illinois, "Herpes Simplex (Cold Sores)," www.mckinley.uiuc.edu (1999).

2 A. Orfuss, "Cold Sore," *Colliers Encyclopedia CD-ROM* (February 28, 1996).

Constipation

1 "Constipation," *Colliers Encyclopedia CD-ROM* (February 28, 1996).

2 J. Whitaker, "The Natural Cure for Constipation," *Human Events* (August 12, 1994).

3 C. Inlander, "Is It Time to Get Off the Bran Wagon?" *People's Medical Society Newsletter* (February 1, 1995).

4 J. Whitaker, *op. cit.*

5 S. Gilbert, "Eight Drugstore Remedies That Can Make You Sick," *Redbook* (February 1, 1996).

6 B. Hunter, "Beneficial Bacteria (Bifidobacteria)," *Consumers' Research Magazine* (January 1, 1996).

Depression

1   S. Nolen-Hoeksema, et al., "Why Women Experience Depression More Than Men Do," *Self Help Magazine* (October 19, 1999).

2   S. Satel, et al., "Stimulants in the Treatment of Depression: A Critical Overview," *Journal of Clinical Psychiatry* 50(7):241–49 (1989); "Advances in the Diagnosis and Management of Depression (II)," *American Pharmacy* (February 1988), pages 33–37.

3   C. Starr, "Introducing Wellbutrin, a One-of-a-kind Antidepressant," *Drug Topics* (August 7, 1989); "Advances in the Diagnosis and Management of Depression (II)," *American Pharmacy* (February 1988), pages 33–37; G. Cowley, et al., "The Promise of Prozac," *Newsweek* (March 26, 1990), pages 38–41.

4   J. Whitaker, M.D., "Depression: Drug Company Found 80% Guilty of Murder," www. DrWhitaker.com (August 12, 2001).

5   A. Tracy, *Prozac: Panacea or Pandora?* (Salt Lake City: Cassia Publications, 1994).

6   S. Roan, "Dangerous Combinations," *Newsday* (January 14, 1997).

7   G. Greenberg, "Do Antidepressants Permanently Rewire the Human Brain?" *Discover* (July 2001).

8   A. Tracy, *op. cit.*

9   S. Roan, *op. cit.*; G. Cowley, et al., "The Promise of Prozac," *Newsweek* (March 26, 1990), pages 38–41; G. Null, "Prozac, Eli Lilly and the FDA," *Townsend Letter for Doctors* (March 1993), pages 1ff.; "A Prozac Backlash," *Newsweek* (April 1, 1991), pages 64–67.

10   J. Whitaker, "Depression," *op. cit.*

11   "Lawsuit Alleges Paxil an Addictive Drug," *Baton Rouge Sunday Advocate* (August 26, 2001), page 2A.

12   D. Manders, "The Curious Continuing Ban of L-tryptophan: The Serotonin Connection," *Townsend Letter for Doctors* (October 1992), pages 880–81; Citizens for Health, "Prepare for the Worst: FDA Propaganda Ready to Barrage Media," *Townsend Letter for Doctors* (August/September 1993), pages 860–61.

13   "PMS? Let 'Em Eat Carbs," *Vegetarian Times* (March 1990), page 7.

14   M. Shangold, "Exercise in the Menopausal Woman," *Obstetrics and Gynecology* 75:53S–58S (1990).

15   R. Peat, *Nutrition for Women* (Eugene, Oreg.: Kenogen, 1981), page 92.

16   S. Miller, "A Natural Mood Booster," *Newsweek* (May 5, 1997), page 74; C. Jones, "St.-John's-Wort Gets New Attention," *Nutrition Science News* (September 1997), page 436.

17   R. Podell, "Inositol Found Effective for Depression and Panic-Anxiety," *NFM's Nutrition Science News* (October 1996), page 18; W. Poldinger, et al., "A Functional-dimensional Approach to Depression," *Psychopathology* 24:53–81 (1991).

18   A. Stoll, "Choline in the Treatment of Rapid-cycling Bipolar Disorder," *Biological Psychiatry* 40:382–88 (1996).

Diabetes

1   G. Johnson, et al., *Harvard Medical School Health Letter Book* (Cambridge, Mass.: Harvard University Press, 1981); T. Pollare, et al., "A Comparison of the Effects of Hydrochlorothiazide and Captopril on Glucose and Lipid Metabolism in Patients with Hypertension," *New England Journal of Medicine* 321:868–73 (1989).

2   See R. Campbell, "Clinical Use of Insulin: Side Effects & Dosing Factors," *Pharmacy Times* (November 1988), pages 154–63.

3   Centers for Disease Control and Prevention, "Fact Sheet: Diabetes and Women's Health Across the Life Stages," www.cdc.gov/od/oc/media (April 30, 2001).

4   See J. Lauerman, "Diabetes: How Scary Is It?" *Cosmopolitan* (May 1, 1994).

5 See M. Billingham, et al., "Lipoprotein Subfraction Composition in Non-insulin-dependent Diabetes Treated by Diet, Sylphonylurea, and Insulin," *Metabolism* 38(9):850–57 (1989).

6 A. Thorburn, et al., "Slowly Digested and Absorbed Carbohydrate in Traditional Bushfoods: A Protective Factor Against Diabetes?" *American Journal of Clinical Nutrition* 45:98–106 (1987); B. Karlstrom, et al., "Effect of Leguminous Seeds in a Mixed Diet in Non-insulin-dependent Diabetic Patients," *Diabetes Research* 5:199–205 (1987).

7 T. Byfield, "Developing Diabetes," *Body Bulletin* (August 1, 1996).

8 J. Anderson, K. Ward, "High-Carbohydrate, High-fiber Diets for Insulin-treated Men with Diabetes Mellitus," *American Journal of Clinical Nutrition* 32:2312–21 (1979).

9 L. Nicholson, "Focus on Fiber," *Center Post* 10(9):1, 7 (1989). See E. Brown, *With the Grain* (New York: Carroll & Graf, 1990).

10 R. Rizek, E. Jackson, "Current Food Consumption Practices and Nutrient Sources in the American Diet," in *Animal Products in Human Nutrition* (New York: Academic Press, 1982), pages 150–51; C. Adams, *Nutritive Value of American Foods in Common Units* (Washington D.C.: Agricultural Research Service, USDA, 1975); J. Gear, et al., "Biochemical and Haematological Variables in Vegetarians," *British Medical Journal* 1:1415 (1980); K. West, *Epidemiology of Diabetes and Its Vascular Lesions* (New York: Elsevier North-Holland, 1978); D. Snowdon, "Animal Product Consumption and Mortality Because of All Causes Combined, Coronary Heart Disease, Stroke, Diabetes, and Cancer in Seventh-day Adventists," *American Journal of Clinical Nutrition* 48:739–48 (1988).

11 T. Friend, "Chromium Test on Diabetics 'Spectacular,'" *USA Today* (June 10, 1996); J. Carper, "Chromium, the Forgotten Fuel," *USA Weekend* (January 12, 1997) .

12 "Alpha Lipoic Acid Lowers Diabetes Risk," *Let's Live* (November 1997), page 4, citing *Metabolism* 46:763–68 (1997).

13 "Natural Approaches to Diabetes," *American Journal of Natural Medicine* 5:8–12 (January/February 1998).

14 "Silymarin May Help in Diabetes," *Let's Live Nutrition Insights* (November 1997), page 9.

15 D. Richard, *Stevia: Nature's Sweet Secret* (Bloomingdale, Ill.: Blue Heron Press, 1996).

16 Zane Kime, M.D., *Sunlight* (Penryn, Calif.: World Health Publications, 1980), pages 39–41, 58–62.

Digestive Problems

1 "What Causes Heartburn? What Can I Do about It?" *University of California Berkeley Wellness Letter* 3(9):8 (1987); L. Altman, M.D., "Scientists Track Clues Linking Bacterium to Stomach Disorders," *New York Times* (January 3, 1989), page C3.

2 See J. Williams, et al., "Biliary Excretion of Aluminum in Aluminum Osteodystrophy with Liver Disease," *Annals of Internal Medicine* 104:782–85 (1986), reviewed in "Toxicologic Consequences of Oral Aluminum," *Nutrition Reviews* 45(3):72–74 (1987); H. Casdorph, M. Walker, *Toxic Metal Syndrome* (Garden City Park, N.Y.: Avery Publishing Group, 1995).

3 See "Nutritional Consequences of Antacids for Hyperacidity," *Nutrition & the M.D.* (November 1986), page 1.

4 A. Wade, ed., *Martindale: The Extra Pharmacopoeia*, 29th ed. (London: Pharmaceutical Press, 1989), pages 891, 1547.

5 *O'Malia v. Oakes*, Docket No. 360174, Superior Court, Alameda County, Cal. 1971.

6 D. Zimmerman, *Essential Guide to Nonprescription Drugs* (New York: Harper & Row Publishers, 1983).

7 "Aluminum and Orange Juice," *U.S. Pharmacist* (April 1989), page 30, citing *The Lancet* 2:849 (1988); A. Bakir, et al., "Hyperaluminemia in Renal Failure: The Influence of Age and Citrate Intake," *Clinical Nephrology* 31(1):40–44 (1989).

8 M. Sax, "Clinically Important Adverse Effects and Drug Interactions with H2-receptor Antagonists," *Pharmacotherapy* 7 (6, pt. 2):110–15S (1987); J. Aymard, et al., "Haematological Adverse Effects of Histamine H2-receptor Antagonists," *Medical Toxicology* 3:430–48 (1988).

9 M. Driks, et al., "Nosocomial Pneumonia in Intubated Patients Given Sucralfate as Compared with Antacids or Histamine Type 2 Blockers: The Role of Gastric Colonization," *New England Journal of Medicine* 317(22):1376–82 (1987).

10 T. Baroody, *Alkalize or Die* (Holographic Health, 1991; telephone [800] 566–1522).

Endometriosis

1 The Endometriosis Association, Milwaukee, "Facts and Figures on Endometriosis," *U.S. Pharmacist* (February 1993), page 42.

2 *Drug Facts and Comparisons*, 1993 edition (St. Louis: Facts and Comparisons), pages 2549–52.

3 *Planta Medica* (August 1993).

4 "Natural Tampons: An Alternative to Dioxin-Bleached Products," *Health Foods Business* (June 1997), page 22.

Fibromyalgia

1 L. Casura, "'(Don't) Touch Me in the Morning': Fibromyalgia Sufferers Want Natural Relief," *Townsend Letter for Doctors and Patients* (January 2000), page 70.

2 D. Clauw, "The Pathogenesis of Chronic Pain and Fatigue Syndromes with Special Reference to Fibromyalgia," *Medical Hypotheses* 44(5):369–78 (May 1995); M. Yunus, et al., "Primary Fibromyalgia," *American Family Physician* 25:115–21 (1982).

3 P. Davidson, M.D., *Are You Sure It's Arthritis?* (New York: Macmillan Publishing Co., 1985), page 164.

4 B. Berman, et al., "Is Acupuncture Effective in the Treatment of Fibromyalgia?" *Journal of Family Practice* 48(3):213–18 (1999).

5 P. Davidson, *op. cit.*

6 "Researchers Present Latest Findings on Pycnogenol," *Nutrition Science News* (July 1997), page 308.

7 A. Tavoni, et al., "SAMe in Primary Fibromyalgia," *American Journal of Medicine* 83(5A):107–10 (1987).

Fungal Infections

1 P. Phillips, "New Drugs for the Nail Fungus Prevalent in Elderly," *JAMA* 276(1):12–13 (July 3, 1996).

2 S. Sellman, "The Physiology of Hormones," *Health and Natural Journal* (October 2000).

3 P. Phillips, *op. cit.*

4 *Drug Facts and Comparisons* (St. Louis: Facts and Comparisons, 1998); C. Foster, M.D., "Medication Dangers," www.startthehealing.com (2000); "FDA Says Nail-Fungus Drugs Need Stronger Warnings of Liver, Heart Damage," www.webmd.com (2001).

5 R. Blake, "When a Toenail Turns Yellow," www.webmd.com (2000).

6 See W. Crook, M.D., *The Yeast Connection* (Jackson, Tenn.: Professional Books, 1985), pages 291–92.

7 "Quelling Candida," *Nutrition Science News* 2(5):236 (May 1997).

8 R. Blake, *op. cit.*

9 R. Shelley, et al., *The pH Miracle* (New York: Warner Books, 2002).

Gallbladder Disease and Gallstones

1 T. Cornforth, "Gallstones: Symptoms, Treatments, Prevention," www.womenshealth.about.com (2001).

2 B. Apgar, M.D., "Gallbladder Disease in Women Receiving ERT," *American Family Physician*, www.aafp.org (November 1, 2000).

3 J. Emes, et al., *Introduction to Pathophysiology* (Baltimore: University Park Press, 1983), pages 264–65; Royal College of Physicians of London, *Medical Aspects of Dietary Fibre* (London: Pitman Medical, 1980), pages 95–98.

4 A. Levin, "The New Gallbladder Surgery: Too Much, Too Soon," *HealthFacts* (March 1, 1993).

5 See F. Fessenden, "A Closer Look: The Rewards and Hidden Risks of Laparoscopy," *Newsday* (November 3, 1996).

6 See A. Levin, *op. cit.*

7 C. SerVaas, "Dr. Denis Burkitt: A Passion for Preventing Disease," *Saturday Evening Post* (March 1, 1995).

8 J. Carper, *The Food Pharmacy* (New York: Bantam Trade Paperback Books, 1989), page 275.

9 P. Pitchford, *Healing with Whole Foods* (Berkeley, Calif.: North Atlantic Books, 1993), page 283.

10 "Vitamin C May Help Prevent Gallbladder Disease in Women, Study Shows," www.CNN.com/2000/HEALTH/women (April 9, 2000).

11 M. Murray, et al., *Encyclopedia of Natural Healing* (Rocklin, Calif.: Prima Publishing, 1991), page 325.

12 P. Pitchford, *op. cit.*; B. Jensen, D.C., *Tissue Cleansing Through Bowel Management* (Escondido, Calif.: Bernard Jensen, D.C., 1981).

Genital Warts

1 University of Illinois, McKinley Health Center, "Genital Warts and Human Papillomavirus (HPV)," www.mckinley.uiuc.edu/health-info (2002).

2 "Sexually Transmitted Diseases," *National Women's Health Report* (March 1, 1993); "Cosmo's Guide to Sexual Wellness," *Cosmopolitan* (September 1, 1994); "Interferon for Treatment of Genital Warts," *Medical Letter* 30(770):70–92 (1988).

Gonorrhea

1 Centers for Disease Control, "Gonorrhea," *STD Prevention*, www.cdc.gov (May 2001).

2 "Gonorrhea Increasingly Resistant to Antibiotics," www.CNN.com (September 22, 2000).

Hair Loss

1 M. Howe, "Hair Loss," *Country Living* (July 1, 1995); J. Balch, M.D., et al., *Prescription for Nutritional Healing* (Garden City Park, N.Y.: Avery Publishing Group, 1990).

2 "Myth: There's a Cure for Male Pattern Baldness," *University of California Berkeley Wellness Letter* 5(2):8 (1988); "Minoxidil: A Few of the Questions You're Likely to Hear," *American Pharmacy* NS28(11):47–50 (1988).

Headaches

1 R. Ochs, "Headaches: The Causes of and Cures for a Painful Malady That Afflicts Millions," *Newsday* (September 29, 1996).

2 American Council for Headache Education, "Women and Headaches," www.achenet.org (2000).

3 *Ibid.*

4 *Ibid.*

5 N. Regush, et al., "Migraine Killer," *Mother Jones* (September 19, 1995).

6 "Doctor Discovers Aspirin-free Headache Cure," *Vegetarian Times* (April 1987), page 10.

7 J. Carper, "Can Herbs Heal You?" *USA Weekend* (July 13, 1997).

8 "The Natural Way to Get Relief," *Redbook* (February 1, 1996).

9 "Magnesium Boosts Energy, Helps Migraines," *Let's Live Nutrition Insights* (November 1977), page 6.

10 "Feverfew," *Vegetarian Times* (November 1988), page 15; J. Carper, *op. cit.*

11 "Herbal Aspirin Relieves Pain," *Catalist* (July/August 1994).

12 B. Brown, *Stress and the Art of Biofeedback* (New York: Harper & Row Publishers, 1977).

13 R. Ochs, *op. cit.*

14 See E. Brown, R. Hansen, *The Key to Ultimate Health* (La Mirada, Calif.: Advanced Health Research Publishing, 1998).

Heart Disease

1 S. Okie, "Hormones Don't Protect Women from Heart Disease, Study Says," *Washington Post* (July 23, 2001); *Circulation* 104:499–503 (July 24, 2001).

2 J. Sullivan, "Iron and the Sex Difference in Heart Disease Risk," *The Lancet* (June 13, 1981), pages 1293–95.

3 T. Gordon, et al., "Premature Mortality from Coronary Heart Disease. The Framingham Study," *JAMA* 215:1617–25 (1971).

4 See R. Frentzel-Beyme, et al., "Mortality among German Vegetarians: First Results after Five Years of Follow-up," *Nutrition and Cancer* 11:117–26 (1988); H. Kahn, et al., "Association between Reported Diet and All-cause Mortality," *American Journal of Epidiology* 119:775–87 (1984); D. Snowdon, "Animal Product Consumption and Mortality Because of All Causes Combined, Coronary Heart Disease, Stroke, Diabetes and Cancer in Seventh-day Adventists," *American Journal of Clinical Nutrition* 48:739–48 (1988); and other studies cited in E. Brown, *With the Grain* (New York: Carroll & Graf, 1990).

5 See also E. Brown, L. Walker, *The Informed Consumer's Pharmacy, op. cit.*

6 W. Martin, "Reducing Deaths from Heart Attacks and Cancer," *Townsend Letter for Doctors* (January 1998), page 72.

7 *Ibid.*

8 "Aspirin after Myocardial Infarction," *The Lancet* i:1172–73 (1980); W. Fields, et al., "Controlled Trial of Aspirin in Cerebral Ischaemia," *Stroke* 8:310–16 (1977); Canadian Cooperative Study Group, "A Randomised Trial of Aspirin and Sulfinpyrazone in Threatened Stroke," *New England Journal of Medicine* 299:53–59 (1978); A. Leaf, P. Weber, "Cardiovascular Effects of N-3 Fatty Acids," *New England Journal of Medicine* 318(9):549–57 (1988); "Fish Oil Pills: Jumping the Gun," *University of California Berkeley Wellness Letter* 3(5):1 (1987).

9 Julian Whitaker, *Health & Healing* (newsletter) (April 1995).

10 D. Chopra, M.D., *Perfect Health: The Complete Mind/Body Guide* (New York: Harmony Books, 1990), pages 8–9.

11 S. Squires, "Heart Researchers Find Diet Alone Can Help," *Washington Post Health* (November 15, 1988); "It's True, You Can Reverse Heart Disease through Vegetarianism," *Vegetarian Times* (February 1990), page 18.

12 S. Squires, *op. cit.*

13 S. Fallon, et al., "Diet and Heart Disease: Not What You Think," *Consumers' Research Magazine* (July 1, 1996).

14 L. McKeown, "Vitamin E May Cut Heart Risk," *Medical Tribune* (November 26, 1992), page 1.

15 See Life Extension Foundation, "The Vitamin C Controversy," www.lef.org (May 5, 2000).

16 G. Bushkin, et al., "ALA Fights Free Radical Damage," *Nutrition Science News* (November 1997), page 572.

17 "Crataegus—More than the Heart?" *MediHerb Professional Newsletter,* nos. 28–29, citing J. Graham, *BMJ* (November 1939), page 951; E. Frank, et al., *Arztl Forsch* 10:3 (1956); J. Kandziora, *MMW* 111:295 (1969); M. Iwamoto, et al., *Planta Med* 42:1 (1981).

18 *Thorne Research Abstracts* (March 10, 1995), citing *Fortschr Med* 111:352–54 (1993) and 110:290–92 (1992).

19 C. Morisco, et al., "Effect of Coenzyme Q10 Therapy in Patients with Congestive Heart Failure: A Long-term Multicenter Randomized Study," *Clinical Investigation* 71:S134–36 (1993).

20 C. Jiang, et al., "Progesterone Induces Endothelium-independent Relaxation of Rabbit Coronary Artery in Vitro," *Europe Journal of Pharmacology* 211:163–67 (1992).

21 K. Miyagawa, et al., "Medroxyprogesterone Interferes with Ovarian Steroid Protection Against Coronary Vasospasm," *Nature Med* 3:324–27 (1997).

22 O. Fonorow, "Counterattack," *Townsend Letter for Doctors* (April 1997), page 98.

23 A. Wolf, et al., "Dietary L-arginine Supplementation Normalizes Platelet Aggregation in Hypercholesterolemic Humans," *Journal of the American College of Cardiology* 29:479–85 (1997).

24 T. Gower, "The New Villain in Your Veins," *Esquire* (March 1997), page 110.

25 "Raynaud's Sufferers Warm to Acupuncture," *Nutrition Science News* (November 1997), page 539.

Hemorrhoids

1 A. Levin, "A Primer on Hemorrhoids," *HealthFacts* (June 1, 1993).

2 See J. Kaufman, et al., *Over the Counter Pills That Don't Work* (New York: Pantheon Books, 1983), page 144; Consumers Union, *The Medicine Show* (New York: Pantheon Books, 1980), pages 136–39.

3 A. Fisher, *Contact Dermatitis* (Philadelphia: Lea & Febiger, 1973), pages 42, 312, and 313; North American Contact Dermatitis Group, "Epidemiology of Contact Dermatitis in North America," *Archive of Dermatology* 108:537–40 (1973).

4 Consumers Union, *op. cit.:* Kaufman, et al., *op. cit.*

5 A. Levin, "A Primer on Hemorrhoids," *op. cit.*

Herpes, Genital

1 Centers for Disease Control, "Preventing Neonatal Herpes," *STD Prevention,* www.cdc.gov (December 8, 2001).

2 See E. Brown, L. Walker, *The Informed Consumer's Pharmacy* (New York: Carroll & Graf, 1990).

3 "Worried Sick: Hassles and Herpes," *Science News* (December 5, 1987), page 360; H. Nelson, "Sensitive Armor," *Los Angeles Times* (September 19, 1988), page II:3.

High Blood Pressure (Hypertension)

1 E. Reynolds, et al., "Hypertension in Women and the Elderly," *Postgraduate Medicine* (October 1996).

2 *Ibid.*

3 "High Blood Pressure Drugs: Making Patients Sick and Tired," *Alternative Medicine* (November 15, 1999).

4 See O. Andersson, "Survival in Treated Hypertension: Follow Up Study after Two Decades," *British Medical Journal* (July 18, 1998).

5 S. Guttmacher, et al., "Ethics and Preventive Medicine: The Case of Borderline Hypertension," *Hastings Center Report* 11:12–20 (1981); N. Kaplan, "Non-drug Treatment of Hypertension," *Annals of Internal Medicine* 102:359–73 (1985).

6 E. Reynolds, *op. cit.*

7 Hypertension Detection and Follow-up Program Cooperative Group, "Five-year Findings of the Hypertension Detection and Follow-up Program I &II," *JAMA* 242(23):2562–71, 2572–77 (1979); The Women's Caucus, Working Group on Women's Health of the Society of General Internal Medicine, "Hypertension in Women: What is Really Known?" *Annals of Internal Medicine* 115(4):287–93 (1991).

8 Australian National Blood Pressure Management Committee, "The Australian Therapeutic Trial in Mild Hypertension," *The Lancet* 1(8181):1261–67 (1980).

9 Medical Research Council Working Party, "MRC Trial of Treatment of Mild Hypertension: Principal Results," *British Medical Journal* (Clin Res Ed) 291(6488):97–104 (1985).

10 A. Breckenridge, "Treating Mild Hypertension" (editorial), *British Medical Journal* (Clin Res Ed) 291(6488):89–90 (1985).

11 M. Weinberger, "Diuretics and Their Side Effects," *Hypertension* 11 (Supp. II):II-16—II-20 (1988), citing W. Kannel, et al., "Hypertension, Antihypertensive Treatment and Sudden Death," *CVD Epidemiol. Newsletter* 37:34 (1985), and T. Morgan, et al., "Failure of Therapy to Improve Prognosis in Elderly Males with Hypertension," *Medical Journal of Australia* 2:27–32 (1980).

12 M. Weinberger, *op. cit.*

13 T. Pollare, H. Lithell, et al., "A Comparison of the Effects of Hydrochlorothiazide and Captopril on Glucose and Lipid Metabolism in Patients with Hypertension," *New England Journal of Medicine* 321:868–73 (1989).

14 "Magnesium in Human Nutrition," *Nutrition & the M.D.* 14(11):1–3 (1988).

15 M. Weinberger, *op. cit.*

16 P. Peck, "Blood Pressure Drug May Increase Risk of Death," my.webmd.com (2000).

17 R. Ochs, "A High-Tension Drug Study," *Newsday* (October 22, 1996); R. Ochs, "Hypertension Drug Fuels Debate," *Newsday* (September 11, 1996).

18 E. Reynolds, *op. cit.*, citing J. Insua, et al., "Drug Treatment of Hypertension in the Elderly: A Meta-analysis," *Annals of Internal Medicine* 121(5):355–62 (1994); C. Mulrow, et al., "Hypertension in the Elderly," *JAMA* 272(24):1932–38 (1994).

19 Z. Shah, "Management of Hypertension," *Drugstore News* (January 12, 1998).

20 "High Blood Pressure Drugs: Making Patients Sick and Tired," *Alternative Medicine* (November 15, 1999).

21 D. Hoffman, "Dandelion," *Herbal Material Medica,* www.healthy.net.

22 S. Briggs, "Magnesium—A Forgotten Mineral," *Nutrition Science News* (September 1997), page 430.

23 T. Maugh II, "Diet Alone Found to Lower Blood Pressure," *Los Angeles Times* (April 17, 1997).

24 O. Lindahl, et al., "A Vegan Regimen with Reduced Medication in the Treatment of Hypertension," *British Journal of Nutrition* 52:11–20 (1984).

25 F. Batmanghelidj, M.D., *Your Body's Many Cries for Water* (Falls Church, Va.: Global Health Solutions, 1995).

26 B. Hunter, "Should Everyone Cut Back on Sodium?" *Consumers' Research Magazine* (February 1, 1995).

27 R. Siblerud, "The Relationship Between Mercury from Dental Amalgam and the Cardiovascular System," *Science of the Total Environment* 99:22–35 (1990); See E. Brown, R. Hansen, *The Key to Ultimate Health* (La Mirada, Calif.: Advanced Health Research Publishing, 1998).

28 See C. Patel, et al., "Relaxation and Biofeedback Techniques in the Management of Hypertension," *Angiology* 27(2):106–13 (1976).

29 *Ibid.*; K. Datey, et al., "'Shavasan'—a Yogic Exercise in the Management of Hypertension," *Angiology* 20:325–33 (1969); N. Kaplan, "Non-drug Treatment of Hypertension," *Annals of Internal Medicine* 102:359–73 (1985). Simple relaxation also works, but not as well. See, e.g., R. Jacob, et al., "Relaxation Therapy for Hypertension: Comparison of Effects with Concomitant Placebo, Diuretic, and Beta-blocker," *Archives of Internal Medicine* 146:2335–40 (1986).

30 See N. Kaplan, *op. cit.*

31 G. Mancia, et al., "Effects of Blood Pressure Measurement by the Doctor on Patient's Blood Pressure and Heart Rate," *The Lancet* 2:695–98 (1983).

Hyperthyroidism

1 B. Eskin, et al., "The Disease in Disguise," *Good Housekeeping* (April 1, 1995); J. Lippert, "The Disease Doctors Ignore," *Redbook* (August 1, 1994).

Hypothyroidism

1 M. Mercola, "Thyroid Disease Far More Widespread Than Originally Thought, 13 Million May Be at Risk," www.mercola.com (March 5, 2000), citing *Archives of Internal Medicine* 160:526–34 (2000).

2 S. Sellman, "The Physiology of Hormones," *Healthy and Natural Journal* (October 2000).

3 *Ibid.*

4 J. Lee, "Osteoporosis Reversal: The Role of Progesterone," *International Clinical Nutrition Review* 10(3):384–91 (1990). Compare J. Franklyn, et al., "Long-term Thyroxine Treatment and Bone Mineral Density," *The Lancet* 340:9–13 (1992), finding no significant difference in bone mineral density between patients on thyroid treatment and controls. Evidently, thyroid supplementation itself is not detrimental; it is excess thyroid that does harm.

5 S. Sellman, *op. cit.*

Hysterectomy

1 L. Zussman, et al., "Sexual Response after Hysterectomy-oophorectomy: Recent Studies and Reconsideration of Psychogenesis," *American Journal of Obstetrics and Gynecology* 140(7):725–29 (1981).

2 V. Hufnagel, M.D., *No More Hysterectomies* (New York: Penguin Books, 1989), pages 4–5, 59–64, 114.

3 *Ibid.*, page 108; L. Nachtigall, M.D., et al., *Estrogen* (New York: HarperCollins, 1991), page 192.

4 G. Colditz, et al., "Menopause and the Risk of Coronary Heart Disease in Women," *New England Journal of Medicine* 316(18):1105–10 (1987).

5 V. Hufnagel, *op.cit.*, citing *Arch. Gynaekol* 35:1 (1989).

6 See, e.g., M. Kobayashi, et al., "Immunohistochemical Localization of Pituitary Gonadotrophins and Estrogen in Human Postmenopausal Ovaries," *Acta Obstetrica et Gynecologica Scandinavica* 72:76–80 (1993).

7 L. Zussman, et al., *op. cit.*

8 A. Kinsey, *Sexual Behavior in the Human Female* (Philadelphia: W. B. Saunders Co., 1953).

9 V. Hufnagel, *op. cit.*, pages 4–5, 59–64, 114, 124.

10 J. Lee, M.D., "Osteoporosis Reversal," *op. cit.* See J. Lee, et al., *What Your Doctor May Not Tell You About Menopause* (New York: Warner Books, 1996).

11 V. Hufnagel, *op. cit.*, pages 108, 117; S. Lark, M.D., *Menopause Self Help Book* (Berkeley, Calif.: Celestial Arts, 1990, 1992), pages 220–21.

12 R. Peat, *Nutrition for Women* (Eugene, Oreg.: Kenogen, 1981).

13 J. Lee, M.D., "Slowing the Aging Process with Natural Progesterone" (Sebastopol, Calif.; unpublished research paper).

14 V. Hufnagel, *op. cit.*, page 108.

15 See Directory of Alternative Medicine, "Live Cell Therapy," www.healthplusweb.com (1998), page 38.

16 See J. McDougall, M.D., "Balancing the Estrogen Issue," *Vegetarian Times* (August 1986), page 44.

17 Directory of Alternative Medicine, *op. cit.*

18 See "Dr. John Lee Speaking on Natural Progesterone, 1992," audiotape (Sebastopol, Calif.); R. Peat, *op. cit.*, pages 11, 21; N. Lauersen, M.D., *PMS: Premenstrual Syndrome and You* (New York: Simon & Schuster, 1983); Lita Lee, "Estrogen, Progesterone and Female Problems," *Earthletter* 1(2):1–4 (1991); V. Hufnagel, *op. cit.*

Incontinence

1 "Incontinence in Women," www.the dailyapple.com (2000).

2 *Ibid.*

Infections, Bacterial and Viral

1 R. Weiss, "Common Staph Bacteria Found Resisting Powerful Antibiotic," *Washington Post* (August 22, 1997), page A02.

2 W. Crook, M.D., *The Yeast Connection* (Jackson, Tenn.: Professional Books 1985).

3 J. Whitaker, M.D., "Getting the Jump on Colds and Flu," *Human Events* (December 16, 1996).

4 "Cold and Flus," *The Natural Pharmacist*, www.tnp.com.

5 "Vitamin C Overdose," *Santa Clara University Wellness Newsletter*, www.scu.edu/wellness/newsletter (1999).

6 S. Eauclaire, "Preventing Colds and Flu," *Vegetarian Times* (December 1996).

7 De Flora, et al., "Attenuation of Influenza-like Symptomatology and Improvement of Cell-mediated Immunity with Long-term N-acetylcysteine Treatment," *European Respiratory Journal* 1:1535–41 (1997), reported in *Life Extension* (January 1998), page 25.

8 S. Fishkoff, "A Berry Good Idea to Cure the Flu," *Jerusalem Post* (January 19, 1996).

9 M. Walker, "Olive Leaf Extract," *Nutrition Science News* (January 1998), page 18.

10 J. Ferley, et al., "A Controlled Evaluation of a Homoeopathic Preparation in the Treatment of Influenza-like Syndromes," *British Journal of Clinical Pharmacology* 27:329–35 (1989).

11 J. Orient, "Risk vs. Benefits of Vaccinations," *Congressional Testimony* (August 3, 1999); H. Buttram, M.D., "Measles-mumps-rubella (MMR) Vaccine as a Potential Cause of Encephalitis (Brain Inflammation) in Children," *Townsend Letter for Doctors* (December 1997), page 100; "Plagued by Cures," *The Economist* (November 22, 1997), page 95. See L. Smith, L. Walker, E. Brown, *Nature's Pharmacy for Children* (New York: Three Rivers Press, 2002).

12 N. Regush, "Will the Vaccine Work?" www.ABCNEWS.com (October 8, 2001).

13 W. Jonas, M.D., "Do Homeopathic Nosodes Protect Against Infection? An Experimental Test," *Alternative Therapies in Health and Medicine* 5(5):32–34 (September 1999). For a detailed discussion, see E. Brown, *Homeopathy and the Bioterrorist Challenge* (Hurricane, W.Va.: Third Millennium Press, 2001; telephone [800] 891-0390).

Insomnia

1 "Women and Sleep Poll," *PR Newswire* (October 22, 1998).
2 D. McCree, "The Appropriate Use of Sedatives and Hypnotics in Geriatric Insomnia," *American Pharmacy* NS29(5):49–53 (1989).
3 P. Sanberg, et al., *Over-the-counter Drugs: Harmless or Hazardous?* (New York: Chelsea House, 1986), pages 76–83; J. Kaufman, et al., *Over the Counter Pills That Don't Work* (New York: Pantheon Books, 1983), pages 159–61.
4 G. Cowley, "Melatonin Mania," *Newsweek* (November 6, 1995), pages 60–63.

Irregular Heartbeat

1 The Cardiac Arrhythmia Suppression Trial Investigators, "Preliminary Report: Encainide and Flecainide on Mortality in A Randomized Trial of Arrhythmia Suppression After Myocardial Infarction," *New England Journal of Medicine* 321(6):406–12 (1989).
2 S. Kopecky, et al., "The Natural History of Lone Atrial Fibrillation," *New England Journal of Medicine* 317(11):669–74 (1987).

Jet Lag and Jet Travel

1 "Frequent Fliers Saying Fresh Air Is Awfully Thin at 30,000 Feet," *New York Times* (June 6, 1993), section 1, page 1.
2 W. Leary, "F.D.A. Asks Stronger Label on Sleeping Pill under Scrutiny," *New York Times* (September 23, 1989), page 6.
3 R. Becker, M.D., *Cross Currents* (Los Angeles: Jeremy P. Tarcher, 1990), page 70.

Lupus

1 "Lupus Special Edition," *Townsend Letter for Doctors and Patients* (August 1999), www.tldp.com.
2 P. Glover, "Treating Systemic Lupus Erythematosus," *Minority Health Today* (July 2000).
3 E. Hess, "Drug-related Lupus," *New England Journal of Medicine* 318(22):1460–62 (1988).
4 A. Melville, C. Johnson, *Cured to Death* (New York: Stein & Day, 1982), pages 136–40.

Lyme Disease

1 D. Fletcher, et al., "Lyme Disease: The Unknown Epidemic," *Alternative Medicine* (May 2001).
2 *Ibid.*
3 *Ibid.*
4 See B. Arnot, "The Lowdown on Lyme Disease," *Good Housekeeping* (June 1, 1995).
5 D. Fletcher, *op. cit.*

Memory Loss

1 S. Starr, "Supplements for the Brain," *Health Foods Business* (May 1997), page 28.

Menopause and Perimenopause

1 H. Aldercreutz, et al., "Dietary Estrogens and the Menopause in Japan," *The Lancet* 339:1233 (1992); Y. Beyenne, "Cultural Significance and Physiological Manifestations of Menopause: A Biocultural Analysis," *Culture, Medicine and Psychiatry* 10:58 (1986).

2 G. Sheehy, *The Silent Passage: Menopause* (New York: Random House, 1991, 1992); S. Whitcroft, et al., "Hormone Replacement Therapy: Risks and Benefits," *Clinical Endocrinology* 36:15–20 (1992).

3 E. Darj, et al., "Clinical and Endometrial Effects of Gestradiol and Progesterone in Post-Menopausal Women," *Maturitas* 13:109–15 (1991); G. Lane, et al., "Dose Dependent Effects of Oral Progesterone on the Estrogenised Postmenopausal Endometrium," *British Medical Journal* 287:1241–45 (1983).

4 "Dr. John Lee Speaking on Natural Progesterone, 1992," audiotape (Sebastopol, Calif.).

5 M. Key, "Data on Estrogens in Soybeans May Make ERT More Acceptable," *Cancer Biotechnology Weekly* (October 23, 1995), page 10; E. Braverman, et al., "Natural Estrogen and Progesterone: Research Indicates Health Benefits of Natural vs. Synthetic Hormones," *Total Health* (October 1991), page 55.

6 B. Borho, "Therapy of the Menopausal Syndrome with Mulimen—Results of a Multicentre Post-marketing Survey," *Biological Therapy* 10(2):226–29 (1992).

7 L. Lee, "Estrogen, Progesterone and Female Problems," *Earthletter* 1(2):1–4 (June 1991).

8 J. Chen, "Pharmacologic Actions and Therapeutic Uses of Ginseng and Tang Kwei," *International Journal of Chinese Medicine* 1(3):23–27 (1984).

9 D. Bensky, et al., *Chinese Herbal Medicine: Materia Medica* (Seattle: Eastland Press, 1986), page 476.

10 E. Duker, et al., "Effects of Extracts from *Cimicifuga racemosa* on Gonadotropin Release in Menopausal Women and Ovariectomized Rats," *Planta Medica* 57:420–24 (1991).

11 P. Holmes, *The Energetics of Western Herbs* (Boulder, Colo.: Artemis, 1989), pages 471–73.

12 K. Keville, "A Total Approach to Fighting PMS," *Vegetarian Times* (August 1986), page 40ff.

13 L. Barbach, Ph.D., *The Pause* (New York: Penguin Books, 1993), page 174, citing S. Weed, *Menopausal Years.*

14 H. Aldercreutz, et al., *op. cit.*

15 G. Wilcox, et al., "Oestrogenic Effects of Plant Foods in Postmenopausal Women," *British Medical Journal* 301(6757):905–906 (1990).

16 See, e.g., A. Hain, et al., "The Control of Menopausal Flushes by Vitamin E," *British Medical Journal* 7:9 (1943).

17 G. Burton, et al, "Comparison of Free Alpha-tocopherol & Alpha-tocopheryl Acetate as Sources of Vitamin E in Rats and Humans," *Lipids* 23:834–40 (1988).

18 See L. Barbach, *op. cit.*; J. Balch, M.D., et al., *Prescription for Nutritional Healing* (Garden City Park, N.Y.: Avery Publishing Group, 1990), page 241.

19 L. Nachtigall, M.D., et al., *Estrogen* (New York: HarperCollins, 1991), page 75; J. Balch, M.D., *op. cit.*

Mononucleosis

1 Centers for Disease Control and Prevention, "Chronic Fatigue Syndrome," www.cdc.gov (September 7, 2000).

2 A. Rochell, "Chronic Fatigue Syndrome Is Still a Mystery," *The Atlanta Journal and Constitution* (March 27, 1996).

3 L. Vorhaus, "Infectious Mononucleosis," *Colliers Encyclopedia CD-ROM* (February 28, 1996).

Multiple Chemical Sensitivity

1 H. Cass, M.D., "Women's Depression: An Integrated Approach," in J. Strohecker, et al., eds., *Natural Healing for Depression* (New York: Penguin Putnam, 1999), pages 70–91.

2 R. Walker, "Fungus May Be Linked to Lung Disease," *Call and Post* (Cleveland) (January 19, 1995); "Health Problems Linked to Mold," *Detroit News* (March 30, 2000).

Multiple Sclerosis

1 W. Craelius, "Comparative Epidemiology of Multiple Sclerosis and Dental Caries," *Journal of Epidemiology and Community Health* 32:155–65 (1978); T. Ingalls, "Epidemiology, Etiology, and Prevention of Multiple Sclerosis," *American Journal for Medicine and Pathology* 4(1):55–61 (1983); R. Siblerud, "A Comparison of Mental Health of Multiple Sclerosis Patients with Silver/Mercury Dental Fillings and Those with Fillings Removed," *Psychological Reports* 70:1139–51 (1992); H. Casdorph, M. Walker, *Toxic Metal Syndrome* (Garden City Park, N.Y.: Avery Publishing Group, 1995), page 149; K. Sehnert, M.D., et al., "Is Mercury Toxicity an Autoimmune Disorder?" *Townsend Letter for Doctors and Patients* (October 1995), pages 134–37.

2 R. Siblerud, et al., "Evidence that Mercury from Silver Dental Fillings May Be an Etiological Factor in Multiple Sclerosis," *Science of the Total Environment* 142:191–205 (1994).

3 R. Siblerud, *op. cit.* A 1969 study comparing MS patients to patients with muscular dystrophy found that twice as many MS as muscular dystrophy patients suffered from depression, countering the argument that MS patients are depressed just because they have a crippling disease. See D. Surridge, "Investigation into Some Psychiatric Aspects of Multiple Sclerosis," *British Journal of Psychiatry* 115:749–64 (1969).

4 D. Swartzendruber, "The Possible Relationship Between Mercury from Dental Amalgam and Diseases I: Effects Within the Oral Cavity," *Medical Hypotheses* 41:31–34 (1993).

5 R. Evers, M.D., "A Successful Therapy for the Relief of Chronic Degenerative Diseases" (200 Beta St., Belle Chasse, Louisiana 70037; undated).

6 T. Levy, M.D., "Teeth—the Root of Most Disease?" *Extraordinary Science* (April/May/June 1994); D. Williams, "The Dangers of Root Canal Therapy," *Alternatives* 5(8):57–61 (February 1994).

7 M. Vimy, D.D.S., *Toxic Teeth* (University of Calgary, Alberta, Canada, 1993), pages 36–37.

Nausea and Vomiting

1 "Myth: Carbonated Beverages Relieve Nausea," *University of California Berkeley Wellness Letter* 3(4):8 (1987).

Osteoporosis

1 C. Danielson, et al., "Hip Fractures and Fluoridation in Utah's Elderly Population," *JAMA* 268(6):746–48 (August 12, 1992).

2 J. Reginster, et al., "Prevention of Postmenopausal Bone Loss by Tiludronate," *The Lancet* (December 23/30, 1989), pages 1469–71.

3 L. Huppert, "Hormonal Replacement Therapy," *Medical Clinics of North America* 71(1):23–39 (1987).

4 U. Barzel, "Estrogens in the Prevention and Treatment of Postmenopausal Osteoporosis: A Review," *American Journal of Medicine* 85:847–50 (1988).

5 R. O'Regan, et al., "Selective Estrogen-receptor Modulators in 2001," *Oncology* 1177–85, 1189–90 (September 2001); F. Jelovsek, M.D., "Designer Estrogens—Are They for Me?" *Woman's Diagnostic Cyber*, www.wdxcyber.com (October 31, 2000).

6 F. Cody, "Doctor Claims New Drug (Evista) Poses Risk of Ovarian Cancer," www.inmotionmagazine.com (undated).

7 A. Fontana, et al., "Clinical Use of Selective Estrogen Receptor Modulators," *Current Opinion Rheumatology* 13(4):333–39 (July 2001).

8 S. Godbey, et al., "Boning Up: Old-fashioned Calcium Helps Newfangled Drugs," *Prevention* (February 1, 1997).

9 J. Mercola, "Does Fosamax (Alendrouate) Prevent Bone Loss?" www.mercola.com (1998); M. Abramowicz, "New Drugs for Osteoporosis," *Medical Letter* (January 1, 1996), page 1; E. Tanouye, "Delicate Balance: Estrogen Study Shifts Ground for Women—and for Drug Firms," *Wall Street Journal* (June 15, 1995), pages A1 ff.; R. Ochs, "Promising Drugs for Osteoporosis," *Newsday* (September 30, 1995); W. Kuznar, "New Cautions for Osteoporosis Drug," *Modern Medicine* (June 1, 1996).

10 J. Lee, "Osteoporosis Reversal: The Role of Progesterone," *International Clinical Nutrition Review* 10(3):384–91 (1990); J. Lee, "Is Natural Progesterone the Missing Link in Osteoporosis Prevention and Treatment?" *Medical Hypotheses* 35:314–16 (1991).

11 J. Lee, "Is Natural Progesterone the Missing Link . . . ," *op. cit.*; J. Lee, "Osteoporosis Reversal," *op. cit.* Dr. Lee notes that while these other factors were necessary to prevent bone loss, they could not alone account for the impressive results of this study. See E. Brown, L. Walker, *Menopause and Estrogen* (Berkeley, Calif.: Frog Ltd., 1996).

12 Dr. Lee feels that the beneficial effects on bone attributed to estrogen in earlier studies may have been due largely to the progesterone that accompanied it. Studies before 1976 lacked adequate measurement of bone mineral density; and in those after 1976, estrogen was routinely accompanied by a progestin. J. Lee, "Successful Menopausal Osteoporosis Treatment: Restoring Osteoclast/osteoblast Equilibrium" [unpublished paper]; "Dr. John Lee Speaking on Natural Progesterone, 1992," audiotape (Sebastopol, Calif.).

13 B. Beeley, "Profile: Alan Gaby, M.D.," *Meno Times* (March 1, 1996).

14 *Ibid.*

15 See G. Anderson, et al., "Effect of Dietary Phosphorus on Calcium Metabolism . . . ," *Journal of Nutrition* 102:1123–32 (1972); J. Froom, "Selections from Current Literature: Hormone Therapy in Postmenopausal Women," *Family Practice* 8(3):288–92 (1991); E. Brown, L. Walker, *The Informed Consumer's Pharmacy* (New York: Carroll & Graf, 1990), pages 342–43.

16 N. Fuchs, "Calcium Controversy," *Townsend Letter for Doctors* (August/September 1993), pages 906–908; "Nutritional Consequences of Antacids for Hyperacidity," *Nutrition & the M.D.* (November 1986), page 1.

17 O. Epstein, et al., "Vitamin D, Hydroxyapatite, and Calcium Gluconate in Treatment of Cortical Bone Thinning in Postmenopausal Women with Primary Biliary Cirrhosis," *American Journal of Clinical Nutrition* 35:426–30 (1982); "Microcrystalline Hydroxyapatite Versus Calcium Gluconate," *Meta Update* 90(3):4 (March 1990); *Townsend Letter for Doctors* (December 1990), page 863.

18 J. Lieberman, O.D., Ph.D., *Light: Medicine of the Future* (Santa Fe, N.Mex.: Bear & Co. Publishing, 1991), page 70.

19 D. Lawson, et al., "Relative Contributions of Diet and Sunlight to Vitamin D State in the Elderly," *British Medical Journal* 2:303–305 (1979); M. Poskitt, et al., "Diet, Sunlight, and 25-hydroxy Vitamin D in Healthy Children and Adults," *British Medical Journal* 1:221–23 (1979).

20 M. Holick, "Photosynthesis of Vitamin D in the Skin: Effect of Environmental and Life-style Variables," *Federation Proceedings* 46:1876–82 (1987).

21 B. Beeley, *op. cit.*

22 N. Fuchs, *op. cit.*

23 S. Cummings, et al., "Epidemiology of Osteoporosis and Osteoporotic Fractures," *Epidemiologic Reviews* 7:178–208 (1985); J. Chalmers, et al., "Geographical Variations in Senile Osteoporosis," *Journal of Bone and Joint Surgery* 52-B:667–75 (1970); G. Lewinnek, et al., "The Significance and a Comparative Epidemiology of Hip Fractures," *Clinical Orthopaedics and Related Research* 152:35–43 (1980). See E. Brown, *With the Grain* (New York: Carroll & Graf, 1990).

24 R. Walker, et al., "Calcium Retention in the Adult Human Male as Affected by Protein Intake," *Journal of Nutrition* 102:1297–1302 (1972); M. Hegsted, et al., "Urinary Calcium and Cal-

cium Balance in Young Men as Affected by Level of Protein and Phosphorus Intake," *Journal of Nutrition* III:553–62 (1981).

25 R. Peat, *Nutrition for Women* (Eugene, Oreg.: Kenogen, 1981), page 23.

26 M. Shangold, "Exercise in the Menopausal Woman," *Obstetrics and Gynecology* 75:53S–58S (1990).

27 D. Swartzendruber, "The Possible Relationship Between Mercury from Dental Amalgam and Diseases I: Effects Within the Oral Cavity," *Medical Hypotheses* 41:31–34 (1993). See E. Brown, R. Hansen, D.M.D., *The Key to Ultimate Health* (La Mirada, Calif.: Advanced Health Research Publishing, 1998).

28 See E. Brown, R. Hansen, *ibid.*

29 W. Ray, et al.,"Psychotropic Drug Use and the Risk of Hip Fracture," *New England Journal of Medicine* 316:363–69 (1987).

30 J. Williams, et al., "Biliary Excretion of Aluminum in Aluminum Osteodystrophy with Liver Disease," *Annals of Internal Medicine* 104:782–85 (1986), reviewed in "Toxicologic Consequences of Oral Aluminum," *Nutrition Reviews* 45(3):72–74 (1987).

Ovarian Cysts

1 "Ovarian Cysts—Surgery Not Always Necessary," *Health Facts* (December 1, 1996), citing *British Medical Journal* (November 2, 1996).

Overweight

1 N. Hellmich, "Obesity Getting Worse, Especially in Kids," *USA Today* (March 7, 1997), page 1; L. Brody, "The Diet Years," *Los Angeles Times* (February 1, 1996).

2 SNB Publications, "Women and Weight Loss," www.weight-loss-for-women.net (2001).

3 R. Abcarian, "A Growing Body of Evidence," *Los Angeles Times* (July 16, 1997).

4 J. Talan, et al., "Popular Diet Pills Recalled," *Newsday* (September 16, 1997).

5 E. Bravo, "Phenylpropanolamine and Other Over-the-counter Vasoactive Compounds," *Hypertension* II (Supp. II):II-7—II-10 (1988); R. Glick, et al., "Phenylpropanolamine: An Over-the-counter Drug Causing Central Nervous System Vasculitis and Intracerebral Hemorrhage," *Neurosurgery* 20(6):969–74 (1987).

6 Associated Press, "Ephedrine Crackdown," www.hcrc.org/news (June 2, 1997).

7 J. Whitaker, "How to Win the Weight Loss Battle," *Human Events* (June 3, 1994).

8 "Sweetener, Brain Tumors Linked?" *The Atlanta Journal* (November 5, 1996); "Olestra: Just Say No," *University of California Berkeley Wellness Letter* 12(5):1–2 (February 1996).

9 SNB Publications, *op. cit.*

10 M. Rhodes, "America's Top 6 Fad Diets," *Good Housekeeping* (July 1, 1996).

11 B. Jensen, D.C., *Dr. Jensen's Guide to Better Bowel Care* (New York: Avery, 1999).

12 R. Moss, "Coffee: The Royal Flush," *The Cancer Chronicles* (autumn 1990), www.ralphmoss.com.

Pain and Inflammation

1 "Women and Pain Management," newschannel2000.com (August 31, 1999).

2 "Effects of Analgesics May Differ Between the Sexes," www.drugdigest.com (August 27, 1999).

3 S. Squires, "Happy 100th, Aspirin," *Los Angeles Times* (August 13, 1997).

4 "Toxicity of Nonsteroidal Anti-inflammatory Drugs," *Medical Letter* 25:15–16 (1983).

5 See R. Steyer, "For Arthritis Sufferers, Fighting the Pain Becomes a Way of Life," *St. Louis Post-Dispatch* (February 14, 1999), page A10.

6   E. Neus, "Got a Cold? Is There a Pill Safe to Take?" *Gannett News Service* (January 18, 1995).

7   "Elderly Users," *Vegetarian Times* (May 1989), page 13.

8   "Herbal Aspirin Relieves Pain," *Catalist* (July/August 1994).

9   "Magnesium Boosts Energy, Helps Migraines," *Let's Live Nutrition Insights* (November 1977), page 6.

10   J. Barilla, "Natural Remedies Show Effectiveness," *Health News & Review* (June 1, 1995).

11   See Consumers Union, *The Medicine Show* (New York: Pantheon Books, 1980), pages 25–26.

12   M. Kapp, "Placebo Therapy and the Law: Prescribe with Care," *American Journal of Law and Medicine* 8(4):371 (1982).

13   See P. Sanberg, R. Krenna, *Over-the-Counter Drugs: Harmless or Hazardous?* (New York: Chelsea House Publishers, 1986), pages 96–98.

Parasitic Infection

1   S. Rochlitz, "Breakthroughs for Chronic Fatigue/Fibromyalgia, Allergic Disorders, Candidiasis, Parasites and Permeability," *Townsend Letter for Doctors and Patients* (May 2001).

2   See D. Kotz, "How Safe Is Your Water?" *Good Housekeeping* (November 1, 1995); "Study Says 2 Million a Year Suffer Water-borne Illness," *All Things Considered* (NPR) (July 17, 1994).

3   A. Gittleman, *Guess What Came to Dinner: Parasites and Your Health* (Garden City Park, N.Y.: Avery Publishing Group, 1993).

4   K. Krzystyniak, et al., "Approaches to the Evaluation of Chemical-induced Immunotoxicity," *Environmental Health Perspectives* (December 1, 1995).

Premenstrual Syndrome (PMS)

1   D. Williams, "The Forgotten Hormone," *Alternatives for the Health Conscious Individual* 4(6):41–46 (December 1991).

2   G. Robinson, et al., "Problems in the Treatment of Premenstrual Syndrome," *Canadian Journal of Psychiatry* 35:199–206 (1990), citing studies.

3   J. Lee, M.D., "Slowing the Aging Process with Natural Progesterone" (Sebastopol, Calif.; unpublished research paper).

4   E. Silverman, "Prozac Profit Ploy—Rename and Sell Under," *New Jersey Star Ledger* (June 6, 2001).

5   L. Dennerstein, et al., "Progesterone and the Premenstrual Syndrome: A Double Blind Crossover Trial," *British Medical Journal* 290:1617–21 (1985).

6   See R. Peat, "Progesterone: Essential to Your Well-being," *Let's Live* (April 1982); "Dr. John Lee Speaking on Natural Progesterone, 1992," audiotape (Sebastopol, Calif.); L. Dusky, "Progesterone: Safe antidote for PMS," *McCall's* (October 1990), pages 152–56.

7   For more detailed information, see E. Brown, L. Walker, *Menopause and Estrogen* (Berkeley, Calif.: Frog Ltd., 1996).

8   B. Goldin, et al., "Estrogen Excretion Patterns and Plasma Levels in Vegetarian and Omnivorous Women," *New England Journal of Medicine* 307:1542–47 (1982); "Less Fat, More Grain Can Ease Breast Pain," *Vegetarian Times* (May 1989), page 11; "PMS? Let 'Em Eat Carbs," *Vegetarian Times* (March 1990), page 17.

Sexual Dysfunction

1   The Editors of Time-Life Books, *The Medical Advisor* (Alexandria, Va.: Time-Life Books, 1996), page 503.

Skin Cancer and Sunburn

1 American Society of Plastic Surgeons, "Skin Cancer," www.plasticsurgery.org (1996).

2 P. Autier, et al., "Sunscreen Use, Wearing Clothes, and Number of Nevi in 6- to 7-year-old European Children," *Journal of the National Cancer Institute* 90(24):1873–80 (1998).

3 "Is the Sunscreen Craze Actually Causing More Skin Cancer?" *Alternatives* (April 1993), page 2.

4 P. Wolf, et al., "Phenotypic Markers, Sunlight-related Factors and Sunscreen Use in Patients with Cutaneous Melanoma: An Austrian Case-control Study," *Melanoma Research* 8(4):370–78 (1998).

5 Zane Kime, M.D., *Sunlight* (Penryn, Calif.: World Health Publications, 1980).

6 D. Sullivan, "Better Diet, Healthier Skin," *Health* (November 1996), pages 44–46.

7 "Milk Thistle May Thwart Skin Cancer," *Nutrition Science News* (July 1997), page 317.

8 "Ginger May Curb Skin Cancer," *Let's Live Nutrition Insights* (November 1997), page 9.

9 J. Lieberman, *Light: Medicine of the Future* (Santa Fe, N.Mex.: Bear & Co. Publishing, 1991), pages 152–54, citing W. Allen, "Suspected Carcinogen Found in 14 of 17 Sunscreens," *St. Louis Post-Dispatch* (March 9, 1989).

Skin Problems

1 See D. Zimmerman, *Essential Guide to Nonprescription Drugs,* pages 449–71.

2 J. McEnaney, "Herbal Concentrates, Extracts Wave of the Future," *Filipino Reporter* (December 7, 1995).

Surgical Trauma

1 "Morphine's Actions Outside the Brain," *Science News* (May 24, 1997), page 322.

2 D. Ullman, *The Consumer's Guide to Homeopathy* (New York: Dorling Kindersley, 1995), page 344, note 1.

Syphilis

1 "Sexually Transmitted Diseases," *National Women's Health Report* (March 1, 1993); "Cosmo's Guide to Sexual Wellness," *Cosmopolitan* (September 1, 1994); E. Brown, L. Walker, *The Informed Consumer's Pharmacy* (New York: Carroll & Graf, 1990).

Toxic Shock Syndrome

1 "Toxic Shock Syndrome," *Iris: A Journal About Women* (December 1, 1994); C. Drinkall, "Toxic Shock Syndrome," *Colliers Encyclopedia CD-ROM* (February 28, 1996).

Uterine Fibroid Tumors

1 V. Hufnagel, M.D., *No More Hysterectomies* (New York: Penguin Books, 1989), page 108, 117; L. Nachtigall, M.D., et al., *Estrogen* (New York: HarperCollins, 1991), page 192.

2 V. Hufnagel, *op. cit.,* page 124.

3 J. Lee, M.D., "Slowing the Aging Process with Natural Progesterone," (Sebastopol, Calif.; unpublished research paper). See J. Lee, et al., *What Your Doctor May Not Tell You About Menopause* (New York: Warner Books, 1996).

4 See S. Lark, M.D., *Menopause Self Help Book* (Berkeley, Calif.: Celestial Arts, 1990, 1992), pages 220–21; V. Hufnagel, M.D., *op. cit.*; J. Lee, M.D., "Slowing the Aging Process with Natural Progesterone," *op. cit.*

5 J. Lee, *ibid.*

6 S. Tsao, et al., "Toxicities of Trichosanthin and Alpha-momorcharin, Abortifacient Proteins from Chinese Medicinal Plants, on Cultured Tumor Cell Lines," *Toxicon* 28(10):1183–92 (1990).

7 R. Peat, *Nutrition for Women* (Eugene, Oreg.: Kenogen, 1981), page 17.

8 P. Holmes, *The Energetics of Western Herbs* (Boulder, Colo.: Artemis, 1989), pages 471–73.

9 V. Hufnagel, *op. cit.*, page 108.

Uterine Prolapse

1 C. Harris, "Doctors Still Prescribe Drugs that Don't Mix," *Gannett News Service* (April 30, 1996).

2 "Herbal Wisdom," *Meno Times* (September 1, 1996).

3 T. Colburn, et al., *Our Stolen Future* (New York: Penguin Books, 1996).

Vaginal Dryness

1 M. Beard, "Atrophic Vaginitis: Can It Be Prevented As Well As Treated?" *Postgraduate Medicine* 91(6):257–60 (1992).

2 *Ibid.*; D. Shefrin, N.D., T. Hudson, N.D., "Menopause," audiotape (undated) (Naturopathic Educational Series; telephone [800] 743-2256).

3 M. Privette, et al., "Prevention of Recurrent Urinary Tract Infections in Postmenopausal Women," *Nephron* 50:24–27 (1988). See also J. Baldassarre, et al., "Special Problems of Urinary Tract Infection in the Elderly," *Medical Clinics of North America* 75(2):375–90 (1991).

4 M. Privette, *ibid.*

5 I. Milsom, et al., "Vaginal Immunoglobulin A (IgA) Levels in Post-menopausal Women: Influence of Oestriol Therapy," *Maturitas* 13(2):129–35 (1991).

6 B. Eriksen, et al., "Urogenital Estrogen Deficiency Syndrome: Investigation and Treatment with Special Reference to Hormone Substitution," *Tidsskrift for den Norske Laegeforening* 111(24):2949–51 (1991). See also U. Molander, et al., "Effect of Oral Oestriol on Vaginal Flora and Cytology and Urogenital Symptoms in the Post-menopause," *Maturitas* 12(2):113–20 (1990); D. Gerbaldo, et al., "Endometrial Morphology After 12 Months of Vaginal Oestriol Therapy in Post-menopausal Women," *Maturitas* 13(4):269–74 (1991).

7 D. Shefrin, et al., *op. cit.*

Vaginitis and Vaginal Infections

1 A. Hardie, "Women Seek Irritation Relief—Now," *The Atlanta Journal and Constitution* (April 24, 1997). For a free booklet, "Women's Guide to Vaginal Infections," write the National Vaginitis Association, 117 S. Cook St., Suite 315, Barrington, Illinois 60010.

Varicose Veins

1 D. Mackay, "Hemorrhoids and Varicose Veins: A Review of Treatment Options," *Alternative Medicine Review* (April 2001).

for menopause and perimenopause, 180
for overweight, 205–206
for pain and inflammation, 211
for parasitic infection, 214
for premenstrual syndrome, 217
for uterine fibroid tumors, 235
Herpes, 40
genital, 140–42
simplex virus, 90, 140
Hiatal hernia. *See* Digestive problems
High blood pressure (hypertension), 142–48
Hip fractures. *See* Osteoporosis
Hives. *See* Skin problems
Hoffer, Abram, Dr., 55
Homeopathic remedies, 14, 16–17
for acne, 33
for adrenal stress, 36–37
for allergies, 38–39
for anorexia, 46
for anxiety, 48–49
for arthritis, 55
for asthma, 59–60
for back pain/sciatica, 62
for bladder infection, 65
for bloating, gas, and edema, 67–68
for bone spurs, 69
for bowel disorders, 71
for carpal tunnel syndrome, 81
for cervical cancer, 75
for chlamydia, 82
for chronic fatigue syndrome, 87–88
for cold sores and canker sores, 90–91
for constipation, 93
for cytomegalovirus, 94
for depression, 98
for detox, 26
for diabetes, 102
for digestive problems, 106–107
dosages and scheduling, 18–19
for emotional trauma, 17
for empty nest syndrome, 109
for endometriosis, 111
for fibrocystic breasts, 73
for fibromyalgia, 114
for fungal infections, 118
for gallbladder disease and gallstones, 122
for genital herpes, 141
for genital warts, 125
for headaches, 130–33
for heart disease, 138
for hemorrhoids, 140
for high blood pressure (hypertension), 146
for hyperthyroidism, 149
for hypothyroidism, 152
for hysterectomy, 155
for infections, bacterial and viral, 160
for insomnia, 163
for irregular heartbeat, 165

for jet lag and jet travel, 167
for low weight, 244
for Lyme disease, 173
for menopause and perimenopause, 177
for menstrual problems, 184
for multiple chemical sensitivity, 186–88
for multiple sclerosis, 192
for muscle cramps and spasms, 193
for nail health, 193–94
for nausea and vomiting, 194–95
need for professional advice, 17–18
for nervousness, stage fright, and lack of self-confidence, 196–97
for ovarian cysts, 203–204
for overweight, 206
for pain and inflammation, 211
for parasitic infection, 214–15
for premenstrual syndrome, 217
rules for, 19
for skin problems, 224
for stress, 226
for surgical trauma, 228–31
for syphilis, 232
for toxic shock syndrome, 233
for uterine fibroid tumors, 235–36
for vaginal dryness, 239
for vaginitis and vaginal infections, 241–42
for varicose veins, 242–43
Homocysteine, 137
Honeymoon cystitis, 63
Hormone Balance (Deseret), 217
Hormone Combination (Deseret), 43, 177, 200, 239
Hormone creams, natural, 176
Hormone imbalance, 203–204, 216
Hormone replacement therapy (HRT), 8–9, 14, 134, 175
and breast cancer risk, 10–11
natural, 198–200, 217
plant hormone alternative, 12–13
Hormones, 3–4
Hot flashes. *See* Menopause and perimenopause
Household Chemicals (Molecular Biologics), 186
Hsiao Yao Wan, 183, 188, 217, 230
Hufnagel, Vicki, Dr., 153–54, 234
Human growth hormone (hGH), 176, 199–200
Human Herpes 6 Virus series, 125
Human papilloma virus (HPV), 74, 125
Huperzine A, 41
Hydrastis MT (mother tincture), 91
Hydrocortisone cream, 223
Hyperglycemia, 99
Hypericum, 133, 192, 211, 229
Hypertension. *See* High blood pressure
Hypertension Detection and Follow-Up Program, 143
Hyperthyroidism, 148–50
Hypoglycemia, 149